CARDIAC PACEMAKERS – BIOLOGICAL ASPECTS, CLINICAL APPLICATIONS AND POSSIBLE COMPLICATIONS

Edited by **Mart Min**

Cardiac Pacemakers – Biological Aspects, Clinical Applications and Possible Complications
Edited by Mart Min

Published by InTech
Janeza Trdine 9, 51000 Rijeka, Croatia

Publishing Process Manager Dragana Manestar

Technical Editor Teodora Smiljanic

Cover Designer InTech Design Team

Additional hard copies can be obtained from orders@intechopen.com

Cardiac Pacemakers – Biological Aspects, Clinical Applications and Possible Complications,
Edited by Mart Min
p. cm.
ISBN 978-953-307-639-3

For EU product safety concerns:
IN TECH d.o.o., Prolaz Marije Krucifikse Kozulić 3, 51000 Rijeka, Croatia,
info@intechopen.com or visit our website at intechopen.com.

Meet the editor

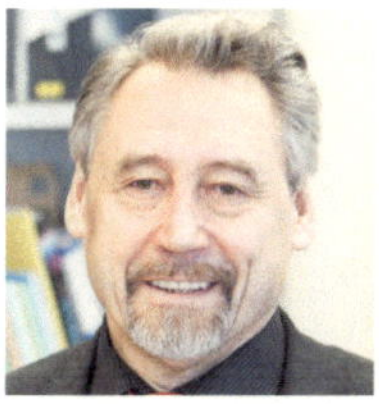

Dr. Mart Min has been with Thomas Johann Seebeck Department of Electronics of Tallinn University of Technology, Estonia, as a Professor and Lead Scientist since 1992. He received the Diploma Engineer's qualification from the same university in 1969, and the PhD degree from Kiev Polytechnic, Ukraine, in 1984. During 1992-1993 he was with the Technical University and Bundeswehr University in Munich, Germany, as a Guest Scientist and Professor. In 2007-2010 he led a research group at the Institute für Bioprozess- und Analysenmesstechnik in Heilbad Heiligenstadt, Germany. He is interested in biomedical electronics, and measurement and processing of bio-signals aimed at industrial implementation in medical devices, including collaboration with pacemaker companies St. Jude Medical and Boston Scientific/Guidant. He is a member of the IEEE Engineering in Medicine and Biology Society, International Societies of Electrocardiology and Electrical Bioimpedance. He received the Science Awards of the Republic of Estonia in 1993 and 2011, and is a nomenee for the European Inventor Award for 2011.

Contents

Preface

The use of artificial pacing has a marvellous history – clinical applications of cardiac pacing are known since 1958, when Earl Bakken, a co-founder of the company Medtronic in Minneapolis, USA, designed and produced a wearable electronic pacemaker for a patient of Dr. C. Walton Lillehei, a pioneer in open heart surgery. In October 1958, the first cardiac pacemaker was implanted at the Karolinska Institute in Solna near Stockholm, Sweden, by surgeon Dr. Åke Senning. This transistorized and battery powered pacemaker was designed by Rune Elmqvist and manufactured in Siemens-Elema, a predecessor of today's St. Jude Medical Sweden AB. Availability of miniaturized cardiac pacemakers was connected with emerging of the era of silicon based electronics – first transistors, then integrated circuits.

Nowadays pacemakers are complicated electronic devices, containing, besides a multiple-output generator of electrical pulses, sensing and computing units together with control and communication components for achieving the well-functioning demand-responsive pacing. Installed batteries can ensure about 10-years power supply. Dual-chamber synchronized pacing of both, right atrium and right ventricle, is already in common clinical use. Moreover, left ventricle pacing in cardiac synchronization therapy (CRT) is also introduced and used clinically in different ways and modes.

Further development of pacemakers as electronic devices will not stop in the near future, but this is not a straightforward subject of this book.

In **Section 1**, an alternative, biological way for development of so called biologic pacemakers on the bases of tissue engineering and studying the physiological processes taking place in living cell cultures is discussed. Self synchronization of myocites' activities is the most interesting aspect of these studies.

However, effective and safe use of versatile opportunities of modern pacemakers and pacing modes in different clinical situations requires outstandingly smart medical treatment on the bases of studying a great number of clinical cases. An important problem to be solved is the most resultant placing of pacing electrodes. Analyses of own experiences and the trials of colleagues, drawing conclusions and giving practical advices for different clinical tasks is a highly valuable contribution of authors in the **Section 2**.

Though the professional medical society has a long term experience with implementation of pacemakers, unexpected complexities and even complications in new clinical situations may arise. The authors of chapters in **Section 3** analyse the cases they have met in their own or colleagues' practice and warn about possible complications. These aspects can maybe even be acknowledged as the most valuable contributions to this book.

The book discusses practical experiences on implementation of modern pacemakers and different cardiac pacing methods in various clinical indications. A forehanded glance on the ways of further development in cardiac pacing methods and means is also presented. The approach to different clinical problems that is more pragmatic than usual, makes this book valuable for wide range of readers amongst medical professionals and biomedical engineers.

Prof. Mart Min, PhD
Thomas Johann Seebeck Department of Electronics
Tallinn University of Technology
Estonia

Part 1

Biological Aspects of Cardiac Pacing

1

Biologic Pacemaker - Role of Gene and Cell Therapy in Cardiac Arrhythmias

Hadi A.R. Hadi Khafaji[1,2]
[1]*FRCP Glasgow*
[2]*Cardiac sciences department, SKMC-Cleveland clinic,*
[1]*UK*
[2]*UAE*

1. Introduction

In mammalian heart, the sino-atrial (SA) node is the pacemaker region, which contains a family of ionic currents that contributes to the pacemaker potential. Using SA nodal cells, experiments have shown that dysrhythmias are easily elicited under conditions involving calcium overload that occur during ischemia and cardiac failure. Clinically these SA nodal dysfunctions cause bradyarrhythmias in general and are associated with syncope but rarely with death. To initiate pacemaker function an inward current (*If*) carried by sodium through a family of channels that are hyperpolarization-activated and cyclic nucleotide-gated (HCN channels) (Biel et al 2002).

Recent advances in molecular and cellular biology, specifically in the areas of stem cell biology and tissue engineering have initiated the development of a new field in molecular biology, regenerative medicine, seeks to develop new biological solutions, using the mobilization of endogenous stem cells or delivery of exogenous cells to replace or modify the function of diseased, absent, or malfunctioning tissue. As far as adult cardiomyocytes have limited regenerative capacity it represents an attractive candidate for these emerging technologies. Therefore, dysfunction of the specialized electrical conduction system may result in inefficient rhythm initiation or impulse conduction leading to significant bradycardia that may require the implantation of a permanent electronic pacemaker. Replacement of the dysfunctional myocardium by implantation of external heart muscle cells is emerging as a novel paradigm for restoration of the myocardial electromechanical properties, but has been significantly limited by the paucity of cell sources for human heart cells and by the relatively limited evidence for functional integration between grafted and host cells. Human embryonic stem cell lines may provide a possible solution for the cell sourcing problem.

Although electronic pacing is an excellent therapy, still have disadvantage like the need for monitoring and replacement, indwelling catheter-electrodes in the heart, possibility of infection, and lack of autonomic responsiveness, geometric limitations with respect to pediatric patients make it warrant a search for better alternatives (Rosen et al 2004). The biological pacemaker, a tissue that spontaneously or via engineering confers pacemaker properties to regions of the heart, is an exciting alternative. Several approaches have been taken in attempting to produce biological pacemakers. These can be considered in 3 headings: 1- The use of viral vectors to deliver genes to regions of the heart such that a pacemaker potential resulting in spontaneous impulse initiation evolves in the region of gene administration. 2- The use of embryonic stem cells grown along a cardiac lineage and manifesting the electrophysiologic properties of sinus node cells; 3- The use of mesenchymal stem cells as platforms to carry pacemaker genes to the heart, relying on gap junctional coupling such that the stem cell and a coupled myocyte form a single functional unit to generate pacemaker function (Edelberg1998, 2001, Miake et al 2002, Qu et al 2003, Plotnikovet al 2004, Kehat et al 2004, Potapova et al 2004).

2. Historical background

Till the mid-20th century, many patients with complete heart block were at risk of death. Therapy in adults was largely limited to positive chronotropic interventions, typically sublingual isoproterenol, the first mass-produced implantable pacemakers were fixed rate units featuring the attractiveness and dimensions of a sterile hockey puck, but they are life saving. Improvements in design and manufacture, insightful adaptation of computer technologies to provide programming and microcircuitry, and the imaginative approaches to a variety of cardiac pathologies have ultimately developed pacing used epicardially or endocardially to treat disorders of heart rate and rhythm and heart failure. The development of cardioverters/defibrillators and their incorporation in the pacemaker industry represent a further major development. The hardware and the methods initially applied to a very limited spectrum of heart rhythm disorders had grown into the medical device industry and into one of the most successful and effective palliative therapies in last 3 decades. (Michaelsson et al 1995, Zivin et al 2001a & b).

3. Anatomical and histological bases

The SA node region is located on the endocardial surface at the edge of the right atrium, bounded on two sides by the superior and inferior venae cavae and around the crista terminalis between the venae cavae and the right atrial muscle. Microscopically, the SA node appears as a translucent muscular region near the sino-atrial node artery. With most prominent feature is the ring bundle, which is a thin flap of tissue that extends around most of the periphery of the node and that usually appears to be the most vigorously beating part in an isolated node. On electron microscope, SA nodal cells have a relatively large nucleus and a few myofilaments. There are many caveolar invaginations along the surface membranes of these cells. The intercellular space at 20 nm is wide compared with other tissues. Isolated SA nodal cells are spindle- or spider-shaped and have a maximum length of 25–30μm, with an irregular profile in cross section and a diameter of less than 8μm. Isolated spontaneously beating SA nodal myocytes are curved and not flat on their base (Masson-Pevet 1979,Satoh Uchida 1993, Shinagawa et al 2000).

4. Physiology of natural pacing

The sinus node depolarizes spontaneously during phase 4 until membrane potential reaches threshold and an action potential is generated. (Phase 4 is initiated at the end of repolarization, when the membrane potential is very negative (about -60 mV), ion channels open that conduct slow, inward (depolarizing) Na+ currents. These currents are called

"funny" currents and abbreviated as "If". These depolarizing currents cause the membrane potential to begin spontaneous depolarization). This event occurs rhythmically and regularly for the lifetime. The slope of phase 4 depolarization results from a balance between inward and outward ion currents. The initial inward current, activated on hyperpolarization of the membrane at the end of repolarization, other currents that are inward and contribute to phase 4 depolarization are the T- and L-type Ca currents (upstroke of the sinus node action potential). Providing outward current during the same time frame are the not yet completely decayed potassium currents IKr and IKs and a weak IK1. In addition, the Na-Ca exchanger operates during phase 4 to further influence the rate of depolarization of the membrane (DiFrancesco 1981, Biel et al 2002, Bogdanov et al 2006).
The autonomic nervous system modulating the ion channel contribution to pacemaker function. Catecholamine binding to beta adrenergic receptors operates via a Gs protein-linked pathway to increase cyclic adenosine monophosphate (cAMP) synthesis and increase pacemaker rate, whereas acetylcholine binding to M2 muscarinic receptors operates via a Gi protein-linked pathway to reduce cAMP synthesis, thus reduces rate. cAMP is critical to pacemaker rate because of its action on the HCN (hyperpolarization activated cyclic nucleotide gated) channels that determine its function (Biel et al 2002). Taking in consideration, none of the ion currents described is uniquely responsible for pacemaker activity. All contribute, and marked alteration in any one can be balanced by altered function of the others, such that pacemaker activity persists, albeit at different rates. This redundancy in function is important to maintain the initiation and maintenance of the heartbeat under a variety of circumstances. A good example is the effect of ivabradine on sinoatrial rate: The latter may decrease by as much as 30%, accounting for the therapeutic effect of the drug, but effective pacemaker function is preserved (Thollon et al 2007). All currents contribute in such a way to permit the generalization that any event that increases inward current and/or decreases outward current will increase pacemaker rate.

5. Transcription factors and conduction system (Table 1)

Cardiac conduction system components work together as a functional unit to provide the rhythmic activity of the heart. Transcription factors, including homeodomain proteins and Tbox proteins, are at the core of pathways specifying the components of the cardiac conduction system. They are essential in activating or repressing a constellation of regulatory genes, most of which still remain unidentified. Together, the transcription factors and regulatory genes specify and maintain the cardiac conduction system in a normally functioning state. Mutations in genes encoding some of these transcription factors produce human disorders defined by the presence of congenital heart defects as well as associated or isolated conduction system abnormalities. In addition to the transcription factors that specify cell lineages destined to become part of the cardiac conduction system, several transcription factors regulate expression of genes encoding the ion channel proteins. Ion channels are essential in contributing to the electrophysiological properties of the conduction system by maintaining the membrane potential of myocardial cells and controlling the release of ions necessary for eliciting a muscle contraction. Dysregulation of these ion channels due to alterations in expression of their modulatory transcription factors can affect proper functioning of the conduction system and lead to the manifestation of arrhythmias. Further characterization of the molecular programs involved in cardiac conduction system specification, maintenance and function, and ion channel expression should lead to improved diagnosis and therapy of conduction system disease. (Hatcher et al 2009). Recent study report that the *Shox2* homeodomain transcription factor is restrictedly expressed in the sinus venosus region including the SA node and the sinus valves during embryonic heart development. *Shox2* null mutation results in embryonic lethality due to cardiovascular defects, including an abnormal low heart beat rate and severely hypoplastic SA node and sinus valves attributed to a significantly decreased level of cell proliferation. Genetically, the lack of *Tbx3* and *Hcn4* expression, along with ectopic activation of *Nppa, Cx40,* and *Nkx2-5* in the *Shox2*−/− SAN region, indicates a failure in SA node differentiation. Furthermore, *Shox2* overexpression in *Xenopus* embryos results in extensive repression of *Nkx2-5* in the developing heart, leading to a reduced cardiac field and aberrant heart formation. Reporter gene expression assays provide additional evidence for the repression of *Nkx2-5* promoter activity by *Shox2*. (Ramón et al 2009).

Transcription Factor	Expression in Cardiac Conduction System	Role in Cardiac Conduction System Development
Nkx2.5	AV node, AV bundle, BBs, PF	specification of AV node lineage & peripheral conduction system
Shox2	SA node, BBs	SA node specification and gene expression
Hop	AV node, His bundle, BBs	maintenance of proper CCS gene expression and function
Irx4/Irx5	none (ventricular myocardium)	regulation of ventricular ion channel expression
Tbx2	AV node, AV ring bundle	specification of AV node and AV ring bundle
Tbx3	SA node, AV node, AV bundle, proximal BBs	SA node induction, compartmentalization & maintenance, AV conduction tissue specification and patterning, suppression of myocardial gene expression in atria and ventricles
Tbx18	SA node	SA node compartmentalization
Tbx5	AV node, His bundle, BBs	postnatal maturation of AV node, AV bundle & left BB; right BB patterning
Id2	AV node, AV bundle, BBs	ventricular myocyte conduction system specification and function via cooperative regulation by Nkx2.5 & Tbx5

SA; sinoatrial node, AV; atrioventricular bundle, BB; bundle branch, PF; Purkinje fiber

Table 1. Transcription factors involved in cardiac conduction system specification, patterning, maturation & function. (Hatcher et al 2009).

6. Why biological pacemakers needed

Although electronic pacemakers reduced mortality associated with complete heart block and morbidity of sinoatrial node dysfunction, still they have disadvantages:

1. The imposed limitations on the exercise tolerance and cardiac rate-response to emotion. Despite the use of paradigms to improve heart rate response during increased physical

activity, there is no substitute currently available for the autonomic modulation of heart rate.
2. In pediatrics, patient age and size, the mass of the power pack, and the size and length of the electrode catheter are important considerations. The hardware must be tailored to the growth of the patient.
3. The placement site of the stimulating electrode in the ventricle and the resultant activation pathway may have beneficial or deleterious effects on electrophysiologic or contractile function.
4. The long-but-limited life battery expectancy, requiring testing and replacement at periodic intervals.
5. Infection may require removal and/or replacement of the pacemaker.
6. Various devices including neural stimulators metal detectors and magnetic resonance imaging equipment have been reported to interfere at times with electronic pacemaker function. (Furrer et al 2004, Martin et al 2004).

So a biological alternative that might last for the life of the patient, respond to physiologic demands for different heart rates at different times, and activate the heart via a pathway tailored to the anatomy of disease in any individual is an exciting possibility. An ideal biological pacemaker should;

1. Create relatively aceepted physiologic rhythm for the life of the individual.
2. Needs no battery or electrode, and no replacement.
3. Effectively compete in direct comparison with electronic pacemakers.
4. Have no inflammatory or infectious potential.
5. Not carcinogenic.
6. Adapt to changes in physical activity and/or emotion with appropriate rapid changes in heart rate.
7. Propagate through an optimal pathway of activation to maximize efficiency of contraction and cardiac output.
8. Not arrythmogenic.
9. Potentially curative.

7. Strategies for building a biological pacemaker

Three strategies reported till now to create biological pacemaker activity:

1. Up-regulation of adrenergic neurohumoral actions on heart rate (Edelberg1998, 2001).
2. Reduction of repolarizing current (Miake et al 2002).
3. Increasing inward current during diastole (Qu et al 2003).

All three strategies had their foundations in 20th century pharmacology and physiology. In studies of autonomic modulation, increased heart rate via beta-adrenergic catecholamines or sympathetic stimulation through an increase in pacemaker current in the sinus node and in accessory pacemakers, whereas increasing vagal tone or stimulating muscarinic receptors decreased heart rate (DiFrancesco et al 1986, Campbell et al 1989). In studies of ionic determinants of pacemaker activity, augmentation of hyperpolarizing, outward currents decreased pacemaker rate (Di Francesco et al 1995), suggesting that the opposite intervention, i.e. decreasing hyperpolarizing, outward currents, would increase rate (Miake et al 2002). Pharmacological experiments demonstrated that suppressing inward current carried by the T-type or L-type Ca channel slows pacemaker rate. (Lasker et al 1997, Robinson, Di Francesco 2001). What are needed are the tools to apply this knowledge to the molecular and genetic determinants of the pacemaker potential.

The necessary information was provided in part via the identification and cloning of the gene products that determine the beta adrenergic receptors, the inward rectifier current, and the pacemaker current. Also of central importance was the development of tools for; 1- gene therapy, wherein genes encoding the molecular subunits of interest are inserted via plasmids or viral vectors into cells of the myocardium; 2- cell therapy via the use of embryonic stem cells, whose differentiation is directed into myocardial precursors manifesting pacemaker activity, or mesenchymal stem cells used as platforms to implant channels into cardiac myocytes. A critical factor is the development of models in which to test pacemaker constructs. In vitro models of cells in culture are a standard for testing a variety of gene therapies it has been found that infecting neonatal rat ventricular myocytes with replication-deficient adenoviral constructs incorporating the gene of interest (with or without coexpression of GFP) provides a cost-effective and reproducible assay (Qu et al 2001). Using a variation on this model for testing the ability of stem cells to transmit the electrical signal of interest (Potapova et al 2004). It has been considered that a 100 times or more overexpression of current and a statistically significant effect on beating rate as standards that discriminate efficacy, More research is required to establish uniform guidelines permitting reliable correlation of in vitro and in vivo effectiveness. As an intact animal screen, the use of guinea pig (Miake et al 2002), swine (Edelberg et al 2001), and dog (Qu et al 2003, Plotnikovet al 2004, Potapova et al 2004) has been reported. The use of dog is based on its cardiac size, tractability as a chronic model, and similar electrophysiologic properties to those of man.

8. Vectors and methods of gene delivery

Gene therapy is defined as the transfer of nucleic acids to somatic cells as therapeutically useful molecules. Human genome has approximately 30,000 genes. The genetic diversity is amplified by alternate splicing of mRNA and post translational modification of proteins. The possible gene targets for arrhythmias are very large. The molecular targets of arrhythmia management are the ion channels and the modulators of ion channels like G proteins (Members of the Sicilian gambit 2001). A vector is the vehicle commonly used to introduce the gene to the target cell. It may be RNA or DNA viruses or non viral in nature. Viruses which have the capacity to incorporate themselves in the host genome are used as vectors for gene therapy. The commonly used viral vectors are genetically modified retroviruses, adenoviruses, adeno associated viruses and lentiviruses. These viral vectors are replication deficient to ensure safety, but require large amounts of vector particles for efficacy. Non viral vectors based on plasmids, DNA- lipid complexes and naked DNA are also used since they lack foreign proteins and avoid immunological problems. The feasibility of gene transfer has been demonstrated in both animals and humans. The extent of gene transfer and expression is low in clinical settings compared to experimental laboratory. The period during which a newly introduced gene is expressed is often short but variable and differs with the tissue. For example, early-generation non-viral vectors express the gene at maximum levels only for a few days (Lee et al 1996). Many adenoviral vectors express the gene for 2-3 week (Armentano et al 1997). Non viral vectors again have short duration of gene expression. This short duration of gene expression may necessitates repeat dosing, although less efficacious. In contrary, expression from adeno-associated viral vectors may not peak for several weeks, but then remain constant in some tissues for several months (Yla-Herttuala &Martin 2000). Retroviruses produce a long lasting effect by integration of the transfected gene into the host genome (Smith 1999). Various novel methods of transfection have been tried in animal models, including DNA polymer coating on inert materials and subsequent transfer to the atrial myocardium, with sustained gene activity, the classical methods of vector delivery are direct injection into the myocardium, infusion through the coronary arteries or administration to the epicardium. (Labhasetwar et al 1998). Intracoronary perfusion is another modality of gene transduction with near complete expression under optimal conditions (Donahue et al 1997). The gene transfer efficiency depends on the coronary flow rate, virus concentration, exposure time and microvascular permeability. Agents which increase the microvascular permeability have been used to enhance the delivery. Only few generalizations can be made about the vector selection and the method of gene delivery, and each disease has its own target tissue and the amount of gene product required for treatment. None of the currently available vectors satisfy the criteria of an ideal gene therapeutic system.

9. Global versus local administration

Permeabilizing agents, vasodilators and vascular endothelial growth factor (VEGF) have been used to facilitate gene delivery to large or localized regions of the heart. Cooling and aortic cross-clamping have been employed to improve gene delivery through the distribution of a coronary artery or the flooding of a chamber or chambers, Not only do these approaches appear excessive for clinical application but the best success to date seen in about 50% of cells in any region transfected, with viral transfer being diffusion-limited and especially problematic in the ventricles. (Lehnart&Donahue 2003, Roth et al 2004). Tempering interest in some viral vectors are concerns about inflammation, chronic illness or neoplasia. These issues led to exploration of hMSCs as platforms for gene delivery. That hMSCs can be loaded with specific gene constructs and delivered to the heart without eliciting inflammation or rejection and not differentiating into other cell types. But long-term stability of hMSC therapies raises concern about migration to other sites, differentiation into other cell types, and duration of expression of genes of interest. The use of various markers to trace cell location should facilitate investigators understanding of the extent of hMSC localization to sites of administration. (Potapova et al 2004, Rosen 2005, Zimmett et al 2005, Plotnikov et al 2007). Cell therapies generally have been intended to regenerate and repair myocardium rather than to be specifically antiarrhythmic. While it has been found that hMSCs to be adequate delivery platforms for ion channel generated currents, it has been followed for 6 weeks only (Plotnikov et al 2007). The question of long-term applicability will await long-term studies of hMSC survival as well as comparison with gnomically-incorporated viral constructs.

Somatic gene therapy provides a conceptually attractive strategy for modifying the global cardiac electrophysiological substrate in disease states such as the inherited and acquired long QT syndromes. Another attractive target for local gene therapy may be to selectively modify the conduction properties of the AV node. This may be of value in the treatment of atrial fibrillation. (Nattel 2002). The feasibility of using gene therapy for AV nodal modification in an attempt to control the ventricular rate during atrial fibrillation demonstrated by using adenoviral gene delivery selectively to the AV nodal region via the coronary circulation; the AV nodal conduction properties could be modified by overexpression of an inhibitory G protein (G alpha i2). G alpha i2 overexpression in the AV nodal cells suppressed baseline atrioventricular conduction and slowed the ventricular rate during atrial fibrillation without producing complete heart block, thus mimicking the effects of beta-adrenergic antagonists (Donahue 2000). More appealing targets in the short term may be arrhythmias in which localized manipulation of the electrophysiological substrate may be sufficient to allow effective treatment.

Recent study, investigated the effect of overexpression of the cardiac potassium channel missense mutation Q9EhMiRP1. This gene mutation is one of the known causes of the long QT syndrome and results in diminished potassium currents following clarithromycin administration. In vitro transfection of the Q9E-hMiRP1gene resulted in a clarithromycin induced reduction of the potassium outward current in the transfected cells when compared to wild-type hMiRP1 overexpression. With the utilization of a novel gene delivery technique, both plasmids were injected locally into the pig's atrial myocardium with 15% of the atrial cells being transfected. This study conclude that overexpression of this mutated channel gene may have an inducible localized class III-like antiarrhythmic effect on the atrial tissue that may be used in the future for the treatment of reentrant atrial arrhythmias (Burton et al 2003). Viral vector-based therapies are not yet applied clinically to arrhythmia management but have been effective in proof-of-concept experiments suggesting that gene therapy can be of use.

10. Cell therapy for the treatment of cardiac arrhythmias (Table 2&3)

An alternative approach to overcome the shortcomings of gene therapy may be the use of genetically modified cell grafts that can be initially transfected ex vivo with excellent long-term efficiency and then transplanted to the in vivo heart. This will require the following:

1. Establish the proper cell sources for transplantation.
2. Assessment of the phenotypic structural and functional properties of the cell grafts, in vitro.
3. Establish transplantation strategies to deliver the cells to the desired locations.
4. Achieve the desired in vivo effect by assuring the survival of the cell grafts, their integration and interactions with host tissue, and their proper function.

Cell therapy can be applied for the treatment of cardiac arrhythmias at three different levels:

1. Replace absent or malfunctioning cells of the conduction system.
2. Modify the myocardial electrophysiological substrate by using cell grafts genetically engineered to express specific ionic channels, which can couple and modify the electrophysiological properties of host tissue through electrotonic interactions.
3. Modify the myocardial environment by local secretion of specific recombinant proteins.

A major limitation for the development of such cell replacement strategies is the paucity of cell sources for human cardiomyocytes. The use of the recently described human embryonic stem cell lines may be solution to this cell-sourcing problem (Gepstein 2002). These unique cell lines have the capability to be propagated in vitro in the undifferentiated state in large quantities and to be coaxed to differentiate to a plurality of cell lineages, including cardiomyocytes (Kehat et al 2001a). This differentiating system is not limited to the generation of isolated cardiac cells, but rather a functional cardiac syncytium is generated with a stable pacemaker activity and electrical propagation (Kehat et al 2002). that can also respond to adrenergic and cholinergic stimuli. The ability to generate, ex vivo, different subtypes of human cardiomyocytes (with pacemaking-, atrial-, ventricular-, or Purkinje-like phenotypes) (Mummery et al 2003) that could lend themselves to genetic manipulation may be of great value for future cell therapy strategies aiming to regenerate or to modify the conduction system.

The ability of the grafted cells (pacemaker cells or conductive tissue) to integrate structurally and functionally with host tissue is a sole requirement. The human ES cell derived cardiomyocytes were able to integrate ex vivo both structurally and functionally with preexisting cardiac tissue and to generate a single functional syncytium (Kehat et al 2001 b). Whereas it is not surprising that cardiomyocyte cell grafts can form intercellular connections with host cells (Isner 2002). Recent studies have demonstrated that other cell types such as fibroblasts (Rook et al 1992, Fast et al 1996, Gaudesius et al 2003) are also capable of forming gap junctions with host cardiomyocytes and that specific electrotonic interactions can be generated between these cells. The feasibility of using genetically engineered fibroblasts, transfected to express the voltage-gated potassium channel Kv1.3, to modify the electrophysiological properties of cardiomyocyte cultures have been examined, in a study, using a high-resolution multi-electrode array mapping technique to assess the electrophysiological and structural properties of primary neonatal rat ventricular cultures. The transfected fibroblasts were demonstrated to significantly alter the electrophysiological properties of the cardiomyocyte cultures. These changes were manifested by a significant reduction in the local extracellular signal amplitude and by the appearance of multiple local conduction blocks (Feld et al 2002). The location of all conduction blocks correlated with the spatial distribution of the transfected fibroblasts as assessed by vital staining and all of the electrophysiological changes were reversed following the application of a specific Kv1.3 blocker.

Genetically engineered cell grafts, transfected to express potassium channels, can couple with host cardiomyocytes and alter the local myocardial electrophysiological properties by reducing cardiac automaticity and prolonging refractoriness. Investigators studied the ex vivo, in vivo, and computer simulation studies to determine the ability of transfected fibroblasts to express the voltage-sensitive potassium channel Kv1.3 to modify the local myocardial excitable properties. Co-culturing of the transfected fibroblasts with neonatal rat ventricular myocyte cultures resulted in a significant reduction (68%) in the spontaneous beating frequency of the cultures compared with baseline values and co-cultures seeded with naive fibroblasts. In vivo grafting of the transfected fibroblasts in the rat ventricular myocardium significantly prolonged the local effective refractory period from an initial value of 84 +/-8 ms (cycle length, 200 ms) to 154+/-13 ms (P<0.01). Marga toxin partially reversed this effect (effective refractory period, 117 +/-8 ms; P <0.01). In contrast, effective refractory period did not change in nontransplanted sites (86+/-7 ms) and was only mildly increased in the animals injected with wild-type fibroblasts (73+/-5 to 88+/-4 ms; P<0.05). Similar effective refractory period prolongation also was found during slower pacing drives (cycle length, 350 to 500 ms) after transplantation of the potassium channels expressing fibroblasts (Kv1.3 and Kir2.1) in pigs. (Yankelson et al 2008).

The possible utilization of cell grafts (fibroblasts, different stem cell derivatives, or other cell sources) that can be genetically manipulated ex vivo to display specific electrophysiological characteristics and then grafted to the in vivo heart may possess a number of theoretical advantages over direct gene therapy. These advantages may be related to a better efficiency and control of the transfection process ex vivo, the ability to screen the phenotypic properties of the cells before transplantation, and the possible achievement of long-term effect because cardiac cell grafts were demonstrated to survive for prolonged periods following transplantation (Muller-Ehmsen et al 2002). Yet, determining the optimal way for the delivery of the cells, controlling their survival following transplantation, assuring appropriate integration of the cells with host tissue, and developing means to control the

required electrophysiological effect are all important obstacles for the future use of this approach as a therapeutic strategy.
Ischemic heart disease represents one of the most important conditions predisposing to arrhythmias. A variety of preclinical and clinical studies have demonstrated the potential utility of gene therapy in the management of chronic ischemic patients through the local secretion of angiogenic growth factors such as vascular endothelium growth factor (VEGF) and fibroblast growth factor (Isner 2002). Cell therapy strategies may similarly play a dual role in promoting angiogenesis. First, cells transfected ex vivo may be used for sustained local release of recombinant proteins with angiogenic properties following in vivo grafting. Second, transplantation of specific cell types such as endothelial progenitor cells may contribute directly to the neovascularization process. The improved understanding of the molecular pathways involved in the development of heart failure allow definition of several molecular targets for gene therapy to improve systolic and diastolic properties of failing myocytes . To focus on modulating calcium homeostasis, manipulating the beta-adrenergic receptor signaling pathways, and improving cardiomyocyte resistance to apoptosis need to be looked for in future strategies. Similarly, cellular cardiomyoplasty and tissue engineering approaches to regenerate functional myocardium also represent a novel approach for the treatment of heart failure (Reinlib & Field L 2000, Hajjar et al 2000, Kehat et al 2001 b).

11. Gene therapy for the treatment of bradyarrhythmias (table 2)

Implanted pacemakers have become the preferred treatment for sinus node dysfunction and high-grade AV block with excellent results with very low morbidity (Kusumoto & Goldschlager 1996). Nonetheless, the ideal therapy for these disorders may be the development of a biological solution allowing reconstitution of the physiological electrical activity of the cardiac conduction system with the same plasticity and adaptability to the human body and to the physiology of the cardiovascular system. Recently; investigators hypothesized that overexpression of an engineered HCN construct via somatic gene transfer offers a flexible approach for fine-tuning cardiac pacing in vivo. Using various electrophysiological and mapping techniques, the authors examined the effects of in situ focal expression of HCN1- *DeltaDeltaDelta*, the S3-S4 linker of which has been shortened to favor channel opening, on impulse generation and conduction. Porcine models of sick-sinus syndrome by guided radiofrequency ablation of the native SA node were generated followed by implantation of a dual-chamber electronic pacemaker to prevent bradycardia-induced hemodynamic collapse. Interestingly, focal transduction of Ad-CGI-HCN1-*DeltaDeltaDelta* in the left atrium of animals with sick-sinus syndrome reproducibly induced a stable, catecholamine-responsive in vivo "bioartificial node" that exhibited a physiological heart rate and was capable of reliably pacing the myocardium, substantially reducing electronic pacing (Tse Hung et al 2006).
Overexpression of the pacemaker-specific current is an interesting strategy for the generation of a biological pacemaker. Investigators assessed the ability of localized overexpression of the hyperpolarization-activated, cyclic nucleotide-gated (HCN-2) isoform pacemaker current to generate stable pacemaking activity in vivo. Four days after the injection of adenoviral constructs of the mouse HCN2 into the canine left atrium, the emergence of a new atrial pacemaking activity during vagal stimulation-induced sinus arrest were seen. Electrophysiological mapping localized the source of this activity to the injection site at the left atrium. Whole cell electrophysiological recordings from transfected

myocytes demonstrated the presence of a relatively high-magnitude pacemaker current. (Qu et al 2001).

Enhancement of the chronotropic response of the native pacemaking cells is another strategy proposed to regulate the normal pacemaking activity of the heart by local gene delivery (Edelberg 1998, 2001). Aiming to enhance the responsiveness of the native atrial pace making cells to adrenergic input through up regulation of the Beta 2-adrenergic receptors. Using detailed ex vivo and in vivo studies, the authors demonstrate a significant positive chronotropic effect following overexpression of the human beta 2-adrenergic receptor in atrial tissue.

The above studies demonstrated the ability of local gene delivery to alter the chronotopic properties of the heart; it mainly focused on modifying the function of existing and abnormal pacemaking cells rather than actually creating a new biological pacemaker.

Another strategy for the creation of a biological pacemaker in vivo was described is based on the production of dominant negative inhibition of the Kir2-encoded inward rectifier potassium channels (Ik1) in ventricular myocytes (Kir2.1AAA). The Ik1 current, which is intensely expressed in atrial and ventricular myocytes but not in the pacemaking nodal cells, maintains the negative resting membrane potential of ventricular myocytes and thereby, suppresses any spontaneous diastolic activity. The investigators hypothesized that dominant negative inhibition of this current could restore the latent pacemaking activity in these cells and convert the quiescent ventricular myocytes into pacemaking cells. adenoviral gene delivery of Kir2.1AAA into the left ventricular cavity of guinea pigs was performed. In some of the animals studied, electrocardiogram recordings demonstrated the emergence of a new ventricular source of impulse initiation. In vitro electrophysiological recordings from the transfected myocytes demonstrated, electrophysiological properties and spontaneous activity resembling those of genuine pace making cells. (Kubo et al 1993, Miake et al 2002).

Biological pace maker for Brady arrhythmias	**Gene therapy** -Enhancement of chronotropic response of native pace maker cells by up regulating the B2 adrenergic receptors. (Edelberg1998, 2001). -Shifting the balance between excitatory & inhibitory current using dominant negative inhibition of the Kie2- encoded inward rectifier K channels in cardiac myocytes. (Miake et al 2002). -Over expression of the activated HCN -2 isoform pace maker current in the atria (Qu et al 2003). - Focal expression of HCN1- DeltaDeltaDelta. (Tse Hung et al 2006).
	Cell therapy Grafting of engineered tranfected fibroblast to express specific K channels to modulate the electrical activity of the cardiac tissue (Yankelson et al 2008).

Table 2. Possible approach for biological pace maker for treatment of Bradyarrhythmias .

12. Gene therapy for the treatment of tachyarrhythmias (Table 3)

Different mechanisms underlying various cardiac tachyarrhythmias (reentry, triggered activity, and abnormal automaticity) result from abnormalities in the myocardial electrophysiological or structural substrate. That may be anatomic or functional and may be localized to a specific area within the myocardium or affect the heart globally. These abnormalities may be inherited (different monogenic ion channel mutations in the congenital long QT syndrome, Brugada syndrome, etc.) or acquired in a variety of clinical conditions (ischemic heart disease and heart failure leading to ventricular tachyarrhythmias or diseased atria leading to atrial fibrillation) (Keating & Sanguinetti 2001, Marban 2002, Roberts & Brugada 2003).

Understanding of the electrophysiological abnormalities leading to the development of the different rhythm disorders is needed to target specific genes that will either reverse the abnormal phenotype or modify the excitable properties of the myocardial substrate in a favorable way. An attractive target for this type of somatic gene therapy may be to correct the abnormal global electrophysiological substrate in the inherited or acquired long QT syndromes, which can be familial, or inherited (autosomal recessive or dominant trait), or acquired in a variety of clinical conditions, is characterized by the prolongation of the QT interval in the electrocardiogram and by an increased risk for the development of ventricular arrhythmias and sudden cardiac death (Keating & Sanguinetti 2001, Marban 2002).

Heart failure represents a prototype of an acquired long QT condition, which predisposes the patients to the development of ventricular arrhythmias. Experimental evidence have shown that such increased propensity for ventricular arrhythmias may originate partly from the downregulation of K+ currents (namely Ito and Ik1) in failing myocytes leading to significant prolongation of the action potential duration (APD) (Beuckelmann et al 1993, Marban 1999). Action potential duration prolongation in failing myocytes may initially be an adaptive response because it increases the time available for excitation-contraction coupling thereby augmenting myocardial contractility. But such process may be maladaptive, predisposing the ventricle to early afterdepolarizations (EADs), inhomogeneous repolarization, and the development of lethal ventricular arrhythmias on the long term bases.

Electrical alternans has been linked to the development of ventricular arrhythmias. Increasing the rapid component of the delayed rectifier current (IKr) may suppress electrical alternans and may be antiarrhythmic. IKr in isolated canine ventricular myocytes were increased by infection with an adenovirus containing the gene for the pore-forming domain of IKr [human ether-a-go-go gene (HERG)]. The voltage at which peak IKr occurred were significantly less negative in HERG-infected myocytes, thereby shifting the steady-state voltage-dependent activation and inactivation curves to less negative potentials (HuaF et al 2004). This has supported the idea that increasing IKr may be a viable approach to suppressing electrical alternans and arrhythmias.

Recent study has pursued a novel gene transfer approach to modulate electrical conduction by reducing gap junctional intercellular communication (GJIC) and hence potentially modify the arrhythmia substrate. With ultimate goal of developing a nondestructive approach to uncouple zones of slow conduction by focal gene transfer. Lentiviral vectors encoding connexin43 (Cx43) internal loop mutants were produced and studied in vitro. Transduction of neonatal rat ventricular myocytes (NRVMs) revealed the expected sub-cellular localization of the mutant gene product. Fluorescent dye transfer studies showed a significant reduction of GJIC in NRVMs that had been genetically modified. Additionally, adjacent mutant gene-modified NRVMs displayed delayed calcium transients, indicative of electrical uncoupling. Multi-site optical mapping of action potential (AP) propagation in gene-modified NRVM mono-layers revealed a 3-fold slowing of conduction velocity (CV) relative to non transduced NRVMs. In conclusion; lentiviral vector–mediated gene transfer of Cx43 mutants reduced GJIC in NRVMs. Electrical charge transfer was also reduced as evidenced by delayed calcium transients in adjacent NRVMs and reduced CV in NRVM

monolayers. These data validate a molecular tool that opens the prospect for gene transfer targeting gap junctions as an approach to modulate cardiac conduction (Eddy et al 2007).
Because heart failure is characterized by both depressed contractility and delayed repolarization, the unopposed correction of the latter by the strategies described above may further aggravate the already depressed mechanical properties. In vivo, this dual gene therapy approach resulted in abbreviation of the QT interval with preservation of contractility this has been shown by a group of investigators designed a novel dual gene strategy aiming to offset the loss of contractility due to the potassium current-induced action potential duration shortening with the overexpression of the calcium ATPase sarcoplasmic reticulum Calcium ATPase (SERCA). Using a bicistronic adenoviral vector allowing a single promoter to drive the co expression of two genes, the authors co expressed in guinea pig hearts the Kir2.1 cardiac inward rectifier potassium channel together with SERCA1. Myocytes isolated from these hearts demonstrated shortened action potential durations when compared with controls but also displayed larger calcium transients. (Ennis et al 2002). The rational for using SERCA in the dual gene therapy strategy, originates from previous studies showing the ability of SERCA overexpression to augment cardiac contractility by increasing sarcoplasmic reticulum calcium loading (Hajjar et al 2000). Overexpression of SERCA alone also resulted in a favorable electrophysiological effect manifested by shortening of action potential duration and a significant reduction in the incidence of after contractions in the transfected myocytes (Davia et al 2001, Terracciano et al 2002).

Biological pacemaker for Tachyarrhythmia	**Gene therapy** ***Localized approach ;*** - Delivering a dominant negative HERG mutant (HERGG628S) via vascular infusion to a peri-infarct zone of pigs (Sasano et al 2006). -AV nodal modification by Gαi 2 (Donahue et al 2000). -Local atrial prolongation of ADP by overexresion of of Q9E –hMi RP1(Burton et al 2003). ***global approach ;*** ADP shorting for heart failure &prolonged QT; -Overexpression of Dorsophilia shakers B K channels in cultured ventricular myocytes.(Nuss et al 1996) - Oveexpresion of human K+ channels HERG encoding the Ikr current (Nuss et al 1999). -Oveexpresion of the Ca++ ATPase SERCA (Davia et al 2001, Terracciano et al 2002). -Oveexpresion of the Ca++ ATPase SERCA with kir 2.1(Ennis et al 2002). -Oveexpresion the accessory subunit KCNE 3 to increase the activity of KCNQ1 channel. (Mazhari et al 2002). -Lentiviral vectors encoding connexin43 to modulate electrical conduction by reducing gap junctional intercellular communication (GJIC) (Eddy et al 2007). **Cell therapy** Grafting of engineered tranfected fibroblast to express specific K channels to modulate the electrical activity of the cardiac tissue (Yankelson et al 2008).

Table 3. Possible approach for biological pace maker for treatment of Tachyarrhythmia.

13. Ventricular tachycardia & fibrillation

Whereas myocardial infarct-induced arrhythmias might respond to local therapy, variations in anatomy from patient to patient require extensive mapping to determine sites at which to localize therapy. Using mapping to identify sites for local radiofrequency ablation reduced the need for defibrillation in patients who had devices implanted for secondary prevention. Using mapping to identify the border zone of an infarct in a canine model ablation were replaced with intramyocardially-administered gene therapy in preliminary studies and without destroying tissue - achieved a reduction in VT/VF incidence (Reddy et al 2007, Lau et al 2009).

14. Specific gene therapies for ischemic arrhythmias

14.1 Speeding conduction via connexins or Na channels

The importance of connexins and hence gap junctions in arrhythmias has been shown in many studies. the overexpression of Cx45 results in ventricular tachycardia in mice (Betsuyaku et al 2006) while mutations of Cx40 are associated with atrial fibrillation in humans.(Gollob et al 2006) Studies of the epicardial border zone of healing canine myocardial infarcts have demonstrated altered connexin distribution and density in regions of generation of reentrant ventricular tachycardia.(Peters et al 1997) The modulation of gap junctions as an anti-arrhythmic strategy initially attempted to block conduction. However, the gap junctional blockers used to date have not been channel specific neither isoform-specific and in disrupting coupling between cells have been found to cause potentially fatal arrhythmias. On the positive side, antiarrhythmic peptides have been used to increase junctional conductance. One such peptide, rotigaptide, appears to target Cx43 specifically, and may be antiarrhythmic (Dhein et al 2003).

At least 10 different Na channel genes encode alpha subunits in the mammalian genome; these have been cloned from brain, spinal cord, skeletal and cardiac muscle, uterus, and glia (Allessie et al 1977). Since slow conduction is an essential feature of reentrant cardiac arrhythmias, other mammalian Na channels that might have more favorable properties than the cardiac Na channel in circumstances that favor slow conduction were looked for (Lau et al 2009). One such circumstance is membrane depolarization, as in myocardial infarction in such circumstances the voltage dependence of steady state Na channel inactivation is of interest. The midpoint of the cardiac Na channel (SCN5A) is negative to −73mV. This is important because in infarcted tissue when myocytes are depolarized to −65mV virtually all SCN5A-derived cardiac Na channels are inactivated. In contrast, skeletal muscle (SkM1) Na channels have an inactivation midpoint of −68mV and almost half of these channels would be available to open during an action potential in a depolarized cell. This suggests that Na channels such as SkM1 with more favorable biophysical properties than SCN5A might be a useful antiarrhythmic therapy. The effectiveness of this approach has been shown in a canine model in which the incidence of inducible polymorphic VT was 75% of controls and 17% of SkM1-administered dogs 5 days postinfarction. Moreover, SkM1 administration reduced electrogram fragmentation and increased Vmax of phase 0 (consistent with more rapid conduction), as had been predicted for SkM1 (Lau et al 2009).

14.2 Targeting diastolic membrane potential

In ventricular tachycardia in the setting of a partially healed infarct, the viable but depolarized tissue in the border zone provides the substrate for a reentrant arrhythmia (Allessie et al 1977). a logical approach to enhance conduction in these circumstances is to hyperpolarize diastolic membrane potential, thereby making more Na current available. In normal myocytes the diastolic membrane potential is largely set by the inward rectifier IK1 (generated by Kir2.1 with some contribution from Kir2.2) (Zaritsky 2001). Studies overexpressing these channels are needed.

14.3 Enhancing rate responsiveness and/or refractoriness

Reentrant arrhythmias require reexcitation of tissue by a propagating waveform. an intervention that facilitates recovery of excitability in the pathway may restore antegrade activation and forestall retrograde invasion of that path by the reentering waveform. Alternatively, it may speed propagation of the reentering waveform such that it encounters tissue that remains refractory. Recent study showed that 6-fold overexpression of native hERG eliminates T wave alternans in isolated canine ventricular myocytes and in computer simulations (Hua et al 2004). Using a different approach, delivering a dominant negative HERG mutant (HERGG628S) via vascular infusion to a peri-infarct zone of pigs. Monomorphic ventricular tachycardia (VT) had been consistently inducible in infarcted animals before gene transfer, but one week later all HERGG628S- transferred pigs showed no such arrhythmia. This result emphasizes the therapeutic potential of yet a different local approach to VT therapy in chronic infarcts (Sasano et al 2006).

15. Long QT syndromes (LQTS)

Since 1991, 7 LQTS genes have been discovered and more than 300 mutations have been identified to account for the disease. Gene therapy has been suggested as a possible way to reverse the electrophysiological changes associated with the acquired or congenital long QT syndromes. Studies following short-term in vivo transfection in small animals or in isolated cultured cardiomyocytes demonstrated that overexpression of the KV4.3 gene encoding the Ito can significantly shorten the action potential durations (APD) in myocytes having a normal APD at baseline (Johns et al 1995, Hoppe et al 1999, 2000).

Blockage of the IKr prolongs the QT interval and increases the dispersion of repolarization predisposing to torsades de pointes. Molecular genetic analysis could be useful to solve subclinical mutations or polymorphisms. Individuals with cardiac potassium channel missense mutation, Q9E-hMiRP1 are predisposed to develop QT prolongation after clarithromycin administration. Experimental studies have demonstrated that cells transfected with plasmid DNA containing Q9E-hMiRP1 have reduced potassium currents on exposure to clarithromycin. Site specific gene therapy for arrhythmias by transfecting cell clones with the K+ channel genes is a feasible approach to the management of LQTS (Burton et al 2003). Mutated K+ channels resulting in loss of function have been implicated in LQT 1 and 2. The potassium channel alpha subunit genes KCNH2 [HERG] and KCNQ1 [KvLQT1] responsible for Ikr and Iks respectively are mutated in LQTS. In normal epithelia, KCNE3 [E3] interacts with the KVQT1 [Q1] thereby augmenting the potassium currents. E3 subunit can be genetically expressed in cardiac tissues, which is normally scarce, to abbreviate the action potential duration and enhance the potassium current. This potentially prevents arrhythmias in LQTS. Adenovirus encoded E3 introduced into guinea pig ventricles shortened QT interval on homogenous transduction, but could be potentially arrhythmogenic if transduction is heterogenous (Mazhari et al 2002). Overexpression of a foreign potassium channel can also effectively abbreviate the prolonged action potential duration (APD) in failing cardiomyocytes. By adenoviral delivery of the inactivated defective Drosophila shaker B potassium channel (ShK) to cultured ventricular myocytes isolated from the rapid-pacing heart failure canine model resulted in significant shortening of the prolonged APDs in these cells. A low level of ShK expression was sufficient to modify the action potential waveform of the failing myocytes to resemble that of normal ventricular myocytes. However, the importance of adequate control of the level of transgene expression became apparent because higher levels of ShK expression resulted in the generation of bizarre-shaped and overly shortened action potentials leading to significant impairment of the contractile properties of the transfected myocytes. (Nuss et al 1996). An alternative strategy to Ito or Ikr was suggested (Mazhari et al 2002) by over expression of the accessory subunit KCNE3 (E3, encoding MiRP2), a well-known positive regulator of the KCNQ1 (Q1, encoding KvLQT1) channel in different cell types (Schroeder et al 2000) that is not normally expressed in the heart. Ectopic expression of the KCNE3 subunit in ventricular mocytes both ex vivo and in vivo lead to its co-assembly with Q1 and to a significant increase in the slowly activating delayed rectifier potassium (Iks) current. This in turn resulted in significant shortening of APD at the cellular level and of the QT interval when delivered in vivo.

Another candidate current that can be used to shorten the action potential duration is the human ether-a-go-go (HERG) encoding the Ikr rapid component of the delayed rectifier potassium current. Ikr is believed to play an important role in normal repolarization (Trudeau et al 1995). and both naturally occurring mutations as well as pharmacological blockade of this current may result in QT prolongation and induction of ventricular arrhythmias in predisposed individuals (Keating et al 2001). Adenoviral delivery of the HERG gene to cultured rabbit myocytes (which usually develop action potential duration prolongation and increased incidence of early afterdepolarizations after a few days in culture) resulted in significant action potential duration abbreviation, a significant increase in the relative refractory period, and a more than fourfold decrease in the incidence of early afterdepolarizations (Nuss et al 1999).

16. Current problems with gene therapy

Gene therapy is in stage of infancy. Majority of trials to date are experimental, Except for a few human trials. The key to success in gene therapy is primarily dependent on the selection of a number of essential elements; an "ideal vector" that can be used to deliver the desired transgene to the relevant tissue with goal of transgene expression in the required quantity, location, and period to exert its beneficial effects. The choice of the specific vector will determine the above properties. It is important to note that only a few vectors, namely recombinant adenoviruses, adeno-associated viruses, and perhaps lentiviral vectors can achieve efficient, high-level transgene expression in post mitotic cells such as cardiomyocytes (Robbins et al 1998). Using the appropriate route of delivery is the next step for success. Intracoronary artery catheter delivery, retroinfusion through the coronary veins, direct injection into the myocardium using an epicardial or endocardial catheter approach, intra-pericardial release, and intra-cavitary catheter delivery during transient cross-clamping of the aorta were applied till today (Hajjar et al 2000).

The expected ideal result from gene therapy is a permanent cure of arrhythmias with a single stage treatment with minimal or no adverse effects. Clearly we are far from the ideal. Problems with vectors include variability in transfection capabilities, inefficient delivery at site, limited period of gene expression, and immunogenicity. The level and efficiency of expression of many trans genes are suboptimal. The tissue expression of many genes is transient. Many viral vectors are potentially immunogenic and carcinogenic.

Successful transfer of the therapeutic gene to all the myocytes at the target site is not fully achieved experimentally. The receptors for many viral vectors are present in many tissues thereby limiting the specificity of gene delivery. The interaction between vector and host genome can result in the vector being rendered replicant and lose the therapeutic gene. Traditional vectors need to be engineered to increase their affinity for the target tissue or cell and prevent transduction to other cells (Baker 2004). In atrial fibrillation gene needs to be delivered to a wide area, the transfer methods like direct injection into myocardium fails to deliver the gene a short distance from the injection site. Gene therapy for arrhythmia treatment may itself being arrhythmogenic. As well as the incomplete restoration. In a non linear system like biological organisms, making an isolated change in a specific aberration will result in restoration of normal function only if the defect is truly isolated and is the direct cause of the phenotypic response. The long term response of a genetic modification in the myocardium is unknown, continued research and time is needed to solve these problems with certainty. studies described in the previous sections established the feasibility of gene delivery to modify the excitable properties of the myocardial tissue but also raise several limitations, include those that are inherent to other gene therapy strategies such as the possible expression of the transgene in non target organs, the potential to trigger autoimmunity, potential toxic effect of the vector or transgene, and host immune response. In addition the use of gene therapy for the treatment of cardiac arrhythmias may be hampered by a number of specific limitations; 1) limited knowledge of the molecular mechanisms underlying many of the cardiac arrhythmias and complexity of ion channel expression in various regions of the hearts may preclude the utilization of a single ion channel transgene. 2) successful antiarrhythmic gene therapy treatment strategies would require, in most cases, sustained long-term expression of the transgene (months or years). Such option is not feasible with current vector technologies. 3) limitations is related to the inability to adequately control several other key parameters such as the level of transgene expression within the cells, the number of transfected myocytes, their transmural distribution, and their regional distribution within the heart. In vivo myocardial expression using currently available viral vectors is not predictable, is relatively short-lived, is inhomogeneous, may lead to increased dispersion of different electrophysiological properties, and may actually facilitate the generation of arrhythmias.

17. Future prospective

Improvement in the understanding of the mechanisms underlying many of cardiac arrhythmias and the development of molecular and cellular tools suggest a future role for gene and cell therapies for treatment of different cardiac arrhythmia. Bridging the gap between the proof-of-concept and the clinical application will require important methodological developments as well as extensive animal experiments. Newer refinements in vector development and design are needed to have better transduction in cardiovascular tissue. Cell specific regulatory elements and promoters to selectively target the cardiac tissue is a potential area of interest (Beck et al 2004). Bacterial gene delivery as an alternative to viral vectors has been proposed (Palffy et al 2006). Hybrid vectors, gutted vectors and new generation non viral vectors may hold the key to future. Evidence from both viral and stem cell approaches state that proof of concept is there. Trials can be designed that permit us to test biological versus electronic pacemakers in relative safety in patients who are protected from failure of the biological unit. Tandem pacing is the proposed way to proceed clinically (patients with chronic atrial fibrillation and complete heart block); i.e. implant both a biological pacemaker and an electronic demand pacemaker in the same individual , this has been tested in dogs in complete heart block an adenoviral HCN2 construct (into the left bundle-branch system) were delivered and an electronic demand unit, the electrode of which was placed in the right ventricular endocardial apex (Bucchi et al 2006). The biological pacemaker fired 70% of the time and was catecholamine responsive. Moreover, when the biological unit slowed, the electronic unit took over; similarly, the electronic unit sensed the biological unit well and discontinued its function when the biological function emerged, the memory function of the electronic unit can track the function of the biological unit, providing a record for the cardiologist.

Given the imperfections that still reside with electronics, the possibility of a system with no wires, no hardware, and a software that is of the body's own ion channels and autonomic nervous system offers something more appealing, if it can be made to function at the level needed and for the time required. As mentioned above, rate responsiveness is here, and improved and leadless systems have arrived as well. Therefore, there are two competitive approaches evolving. Which will dominate, traditional electronics upgraded to achieve still newer levels of success or biologics, is unknown, and the future will answer.

18. References

Allessie MA, Bonke FIM, Schopman FJG. 1977. Circus movement in rabbit atrial muscle as a mechanism of tachycardia. III. The "leading circle" concept: a new model of circus movement in cardiac tissue without the involvement of an anatomical obstacle. *Circ Res*; 41:9–18.

Armentano D, Zabner J, Sacks C, et al. 1997. Effect of the E4 region on the persistence of transgene expression from adenovirus vectors. *J Virol*; 71:240816.

Baker AH. 2004. Designing gene delivery vectors for cardiovascular gene therapy. *Progs biophys mol* 2004; 84; 279-99.

Beck C, Uramoto H , Jan Boren,et al . 2004. Tissue specific targeting for cardiovascular gene transfer. Potentials vectors and future challenges. *Curr Gene Therapy*; 4; 457-67.

Betsuyaku T, Nnebe NS, Sundset R, et al. 2006. Overexpression of cardiac connexin45 increases susceptibility to ventricular tachyarrhythmias in vivo. *Am J Physiol Heart Circ Physiol*; 290(1):H163–H171.

Beuckelmann DJ, Nabauer M, Erdmann E. 1993. Alterations of K+ currents in isolated human ventricular myocytes from patients with terminal heart failure. *Circ Res* 73: 379–385, 1993.

Biel M, Schneider A, Wahl C. 2002. Cardiac HCN channels: Structure, function, and modulation. *Trends Cardiovasc Med*; 12:202–216.

Bogdanov KY, Maltsev VA, Vinogradova et al .2006. Membrane potential fluctuations resulting from submembrane Ca2_ releases in rabbit sinoatrial nodal cells impart an exponential phase to the late diastolic depolarization that controls their chronotropic state. *Circ Res.*; 99:979 –987.

Bucchi A, Plotnikov AN, Shlapakova I, et al. 2006. Wild-type and mutant HCN channels in a tandem biological-electronic cardiac pacemaker. *Circulation*. 114:992–999.

Burton DY, Song C, Fishbein I, et al. 2003 . The incorporation of an ion channel gene mutation associated with the long QT syndrome (Q9E-hMiRP1) in a plasmid vector for site-specific arrhythmia gene therapy: in vitro and in vivo feasibility studies. *Human Gene Ther;*; 14:907-22.

Campbell GD, Edwards FR, Hirst GDS, et al 1989. Effects of vagal stimulation and applied acetylcholine on pacemaker potentials in the guinea pig heart. *J Physiol (Lond)*; 415:57–68.

Davia K, Bernobich E, Ranu HK, et al 2001. SERCA2A overexpression decreases the incidence of after contractions in adult rabbit ventricular myocytes. *J Mol Cell Cardiol* 33: 1005- 1015.

Dhein S, Larsen BD, Petersen JS, et al. 2003. Effects of the new antiarrhythmic peptide ZP123 on epicardial activation and repolarization pattern. *Cell Commun Adhes*; 10(4–6):371–378.

DiFrancesco D. 1981. A study of the ionic nature of the pacemaker current in calf Purkinje fibres. *J Physiol.*; 314:377–393.

Di Francesco D, Mangoni D, Maccaferri M. 1995. The pacemaker current in cardiac cells. In: Zipes DP, Jalife J, editors. *Cardiac electrophysiology: from cell to bedside*. 2nd ed. Philadelphia: WB Saunders; p. 96–103.

Donahue JK, Heldman AW, Fraser H, et al. 2000. Focal modification of electrical conduction in the heart by viral gene transfer. *Nat Med* 6: 1395- 1398.

Donahue JK, Kikkawa K, Johns DC, et al 1997. Ultrarapid, highly efficientviral gene transfer to the heart. *Proc Natl Acad Sci U S A.*; 94:4664-8.

Eddy Kizana, Connie Y. Chang, et al. 2007. Gene Transfer of Connexin43 Mutants Attenuates Coupling in Cardiomyocytes Novel Basis for Modulation of Cardiac Conduction by Gene Therapy. *Circ Res.*; 100:1597-1604.

Edelberg JM, Aird WC, Rosenberg RD. 1998. Enhancement of murine cardiac chronotropy by the molecular transfer of the human β2-adrenergic receptor cDNA. *J Clin Invest*; 101:337–343.

Edelberg JM, Huang DT, Josephson ME, et al. 2001. Molecular enhancement of porcine cardiac chronotropy. *Heart*; 86:559–562.

Ennis IL, Li RA, Murphy AM, et al .2002. Dual gene therapy with SERCA1 and Kir2.1 abbreviates excitation without suppressing contractility. *J Clin Invest* 109: 393–400.

Fast VG, Darrow BJ, Saffitz JE, et al. 1996. Anisotropic activation spread in heart cell monolayers assessed by high-resolution optical mapping. Role of tissue discontinuities. *Circ Res* 79: 115–127, 1996.

Feld Y, Melamed-Frank M, Kehat I, et al. 2002. Electrophysiological modulation of cardiomyocytic tissue by transfected fibroblasts expressing potassium channels: a novel strategy to manipulate excitability. *Circulation* 105: 522–529.

Furrer M, Naegeli B, Bertel O. 2004. Hazards of an alternative medicine device in a patient with a pacemaker. *N Engl J Med*; 350(16): 1688- 90.

Gaudesius G, Miragoli M, Thomas SP, et al. 2003. Coupling of cardiac electrical activity over extended distances by fibroblasts of cardiac origin. *Circ Res* 93: 421–428.

Gepstein L. 2002. Derivation and potential applications of human embryonic stem cells. *Circ Res* 91: 866–876.

Gollob MH, Jones DL, Krahn AD, et al. 2006. Somatic mutations in the connexin 40 gene (GJA5) in atrial fibrillation. *N England J Med*; 354(25):2677–2688.

Hajjar RJ, del Monte F, Matsui T et al 2000. Prospects for gene therapy for heart failure. *Circ Res* 86: 616–621.

Hatcher CJ, Basson CT. 2009. Specification of the Cardiac Conduction System by Transcription Factors *Circ Res*. September 25; 105(7): 620–630.

Hoppe UC, Johns DC, Marban E, t al. 1999. Manipulation of cellular excitability by cell fusion: effects of rapid introduction of transient outward K+ current on the guinea pig action potential. *Circ Res* 84: 964–972.

Hoppe UC, Marban E, Johns DC. 2000. Molecular dissection of cardiac repolarization by in vivo Kv4.3 gene transfer. *J Clin Invest* 105: 1077- 1084.

Hua F, Johns DC, Gilmore RF Jr. 2004. Suppression of electrical alternans by overexpression of HERG in canine ventricular myocytes. *Am J Physiol Heart Circ Physiol;* 286:H2342–H2352.

Isner JM.(2002) Myocardial gene therapy. *Nature* 415: 234–239.

Johns DC, Nuss HB, Chiamvimonvat N, et al .1995. Adenovirus-mediated expression of a voltage-gated potassium channel in vitro (rat cardiac myocytes) and in vivo (rat liver). A novel strategy for modifying excitability. *J Clin Invest* 96: 1152–1158.

Keating MT and Sanguinetti MC. 2001. Molecular and cellular mechanisms of cardiac arrhythmias. *Cell* 104: 569–580.

Kehat I, Amit M, Gepstein A, et al 2001b. Functional integration of human embryonic stem cell derived cardiomyocytes with preexisting cardiac tissue: Implication for myocardial repair. *Circulation* 104, Suppl. II: 618.

Kehat I, Gepstein A, Spira A, et al 2002. High-resolution electrophysiological assessment of human embryonic stem cell-derived cardiomyocytes: a novel in vitro model for the study of conduction. *Circ Res* 91: 659–661.

Kehat I, Kenyagin-Karsenti D, Snir M, et al. 2001a. Human embryonic stem cells can differentiate into myocytes with structural and functional properties of cardiomyocytes. *J Clin Invest* 108: 407–414.

Kehat I, Khimovich L, Caspi O, et al. 2004. Electromechanical integration of cardiomyocytes derived from human embryonic stem cells. *Nat Biotechnol;* 22:1282–2389.

Kubo Y, Baldwin TJ, Jan YN, et al 1993. Primary structure and functional expression of a mouse inward rectifier potassium channel. *Nature* 362: 127–133.

Kusumoto FM and Goldschlager N. 1996 . Cardiac pacing. *N Engl J Med* 334: 89–97.

Labhasetwar V, Bonadio J, Goldstein S, et al 1998. A DNA controlled-release coatingfor gene transfer: transfection in skeletal and cardiac muscle. *J Pharm Sci.;* 87:1347-50.

Lasker SM, Han D, Kline RP. 1997. Zatebradine slows ectopic ventricular rhythms in canine heart 2 hours after coronary artery ligation. *J Cardiovasc Pharmacol;* 29 (5):662- 9.

Lau DH, Clausen C, Sosunov EA, et al. 2009. Epicardial border zone overexpression of skeletal muscle sodium channel, SkM1, normalizes activation, preserves conduction and suppresses ventricular arrhythmia: an in silico, in vivo, in vitro study. *Circulation*. Jan 6; 119 (1):19-27.

Lee ER, Marshall J, Siegel CS, et al. 1996. Detailed analysis of structures and formulations of cationic lipids for efficient gene transfer to the lung. *Hum Gene Ther;* 7: 170117.

Lehnart SE, Donahue JK. 2003. Coronary perfusion cocktails for in vivo gene transfer. *Methods Mol Biol;* 219:213–218.

Marban E. 2002 . Cardiac channelopathies. *Nature* 415: 213–218.

Marban E. 1999. Heart failure: the electrophysiologic connection. *J Cardiovasc Electrophysiol* 10: 1425–1428.

Martin ET, Coman JA, Shellock FG, et al. 2004. Magnetic resonance imaging and cardiac pacemaker safety at 1.5- Tesla. *J Am Coll;* 43 (7):1315- 24.

Masson-Pevet, M. 1979 . The Fine Structure of Cardiac Pacemaker Cells in the Sinus Node and in Tissue Culture (thesis). Amsterdam, University of Amsterdam.

Mazhari R, Nuss HB, Armoundas AA, et al 2002 . Ectopic expression of KCNE3 accelerates cardiac repolarization and abbreviates the QT interval. *J Clin Invest.* ; 109:1083-90.

Members of the Sicilian gambit. 2001. New approaches to antiarrhythmic therapy, partII; *Circulation;* 104: 2990-2994.

Miake J, Marbán E, Nuss HB. 2002. Gene therapy: biological pacemaker created by gene transfer. *Nature;* 419:132–133.

Michaelsson M, Jonzon A, Riesenfeld T. 1995. Isolated congenital complete heart block in adult life: a prospective study. *Circulation*; 92: 442-9.

Muller-Ehmsen J, Peterson KL, Kedes L,et al . 2002. Rebuilding a damaged heart: long-term survival of transplanted neonatal rat cardiomyocytes after myocardial infarction and effect on cardiac function. *Circulation* 105: 1720–1726.

Mummery C, Ward-van Oostwaard D, Doevendans P, et al. 2003. Differentiation of human embryonic stem cells to cardiomyocytes: role of coculture with visceral endoderm-like cells. *Circulation* 107: 2733–2740.

Nattel S. 2002. New ideas about atrial fibrillation 50 years on. *Nature* 415: 219–226.

Nuss HB, Johns DC, Kaab S, et al .1996. Reversal of potassium channel deficiency in cells from failing hearts by adenoviral gene transfer: a prototype for gene therapy for disorders of cardiac excitability and contractility. *Gene Ther* 3: 900–912.

Nuss HB, Marban E, and Johns DC. Et al .1999. Overexpression of a human potassium channel suppresses cardiac hyperexcitability in rabbit ventricularmyocytes. *J Clin Invest* 103: 889–896.

Palffy R, Gadlik R, J Hodosy, M Behuliak. 2006. .Bacteria in gene therapy; Bactofection versus alternative gene therapy. *Gene Therapy* (13) 101-105.

Peters NS, Coromilas J, Severs NJ, Wit AL. 1997. Disturbed connexin43 gap junction distribution correlates with the location of reentrant circuits in the epicardial border zone of healing canine infarcts that cause ventricular tachycardia. *Circulation; 95*(4):988–996.

Plotnikov AP, Shlapakova I, Szabolcs MJ, et al. 2007. Xenografted adult human mesenchymal stem cells provide a platform for sustained biological pacemaker function in canine heart. *Circulation*; 116:706–713.

Plotnikov AN, Sosunov EA, Qu J, et al. 2004. Biological pacemaker implanted in canine left bundle branch provides ventricular escape rhythms that have physiologically acceptable rates. *Circulation*; 109:506–512.

Potapova I, Plotnikov A, Lu Z, et al. 2004. Human mesenchymal stem cells as a gene delivery system to create cardiac pacemakers. *Circ Res.* Apr 16; 94(7):952-9.

Qu J, Barbuti A, Protas L, et al 2001. HCN2 overexpression in newborn and adult ventricular myocytes: distinct effects on gating and excitability. *Circ Res*; 89:E8– E14.

Qu J, Plotnikov AN, Danilo P Jr, et al. 2003. Expression and function of a biological pacemaker in canine heart. *Circulation*; 107:1106–1109.

Ramón A. Espinoza-Lewisa, Ling Yua, et al 2009.*Shox2 is essential for thedifferentiation of cardiac pacemakercells by repressing Nkx2-5Dev Biol. March 15; 327(2): 376–385.

Reddy VY, Reynolds MR, Neuzil P, et al. 2007. Prophylactic catheter ablation for the prevention of defibrillator therapy. *N Engl J Med*; 357:2657–65.

Reinlib L and Field L. 2000. Cell transplantation as future therapy for cardiovascular disease? a workshop of the National Heart, Lung, and Blood Institute. *Circulation* 101: E182–E187.

Robbins PD, Tahara H, and Ghivizzani SC. 1998. Viral vectors for gene therapy. *Trends Biotechnol* 16: 35–40.

Roberts R and Brugada R. 2003. Genetics and arrhythmias. *Annu Rev Med* 54: 257–267.

Robinson RB, DiFrancesco D. 2001. Sinoatrial node and impulse initiation. In: Spooner PM, Rosen MR, editors. *Foundations of cardiac arrhythmias*. New York: Marcel Dekker; p. 151- 70.

Roth DM, Lai NC, Gao MH, et al. 2004. Indirect intracoronary delivery of adenovirus encoding adenylyl cyclase increases left ventricular contractile function in mice. *Am J Physiol Heart Circ Physiol*; 287:H172–177.

Rosen M. 2005. Biological pacemaking: In our lifetime? *Heart Rhythm*; 2:418–428.

Rook MB, van Ginneken AC, de Jonge B, et al.1992. Differences in gap junction channels between cardiac myocytes, fibroblasts, and heterologous pairs. *Am J Physiol Cell Physiol* 263: C959–C977.

Rosen MR, Brink PR, Cohen IS, et al. 2004. Genes, stem cells and biological pacemakers. *CardiovasRes*; 64:12–23.

Sasano T, McDonald AD, Kikuchi K, et al. 2006. Molecular ablation of ventricular tachycardia after myocardial infarction. *Nature Med*; 12:1256–1258.

Satoh, H. and Uchida, T. 1993. Morphological and electrophysiological changes induced by calciumionophores (A23187 and X-537) in spontaneously beating rabbit sino-atrial node cells. *Gen. Pharmacol.* 24: 49–87.

Schroeder BC, Waldegger S, Fehr S, et al .2000. A constitutively open potassium channel formed by KCNQ1 and KCNE3. *Nature* 403: 196–199.

Shinagawa, Y., Satoh, H. and Noma, A. 2000. The sustained inward current and inward rectifier K+ current in pacemaker cells dissociated from rat sinoatrial node. *J. Physiol. (Lond.)* 523: 593–605.

Smith AE. 1999. Gene therapy--where are we? *Lancet*. 354 Suppl 1:SI1-4.

Terracciano CM, Hajjar RJ, Harding SE. 2002. Overexpression of SERCA2a accelerates repolarisation in rabbit ventricular myocytes. *Cell Calcium* 31: 299–305.

Thollon C, Bedut S, Villeneuve N, et al. 2007. Use-dependent inhibition of hHCN4 by ivabradine and relationship with reduction in pacemaker activity. *Br J Pharmacol;* 150:37- 46.

Trudeau MC, Warmke JW, Ganetzky B, et al 1995. HERG, a human inward rectifier in the voltage-gated potassium channel family. *Science* 269: 92–95.

Tse Hung-Fat ,Tian Xue, PhD; Chu-Pak Lau et al .2006. Bioartificial Sinus Node Constructed via In Vivo Gene Transfer of an Engineered Pacemaker HCN Channel Reduces the Dependence on Electronic Pacemaker in a Sick-Sinus Syndrome Model *,Circulation* ; 114:1000-1011.

Yankelson, Yair Feld, MD, Tal Bressler-Stramer et al. 2008. Cell Therapy forModification of the Myocardial Electrophysiological Substrate *Circulation*;117:720-731.

Yla-Herttuala S, Martin JF. 2000 .Cardiovascular gene therapy. *Lancet;* 355; 213-222.

Zimmett JM, Hare JM. 2005. Emerging role for bone marrow derived mesenchymal stem cells in myocardial regenerative therapy. *Basic Res Cardiol;* 100:471–481.

Zaritsky JJ, Redell JB, Tempel BL, et al. 2001.The consequences of disrupting cardiac inwardly rectifying K+ current (IK1) as revealed by the targeted deletion of the murine Kir2.1 and Kir2.2 genes. *J Physiol; 533.3:697*–710.

Zivin A, Bardy GH, Mehra R. 2001, Cardiac pacemakers. In: Spooner PM, Rosen MR, editors. *Foundations of cardiac arrhythmias*. New York: Marcel Dekker; p. 571– 98.a

Zivin A, Bardy GH, Mehra R. 2001. Implantable cardioverter defibrillators. In: Spooner PM, Rosen MR, editors. *Foundations of cardiac arrhythmias*. New York: Marcel Dekker; p. 599–619.b

2

Coherent Resonant Properties of Cardiac Cells

A. Chorvatova and D. Chorvat Jr
International Laser Centre, Bratislava, Slovakia

1. Introduction

Despite significant advancements in understanding cardiac cell biology, we still lack a clear insight into precise mechanisms that are responsible for the cell functionality. It is becoming increasingly evident that this information does not reside exclusively in the genome or in individual proteins, as no real biological functionality is expressed at these levels. Instead, to comprehend the true functioning of a biological system, it is essential to understand the integrative physiological behaviour of the complex molecular interactions in their natural environment and precise spatio-temporal topology. As more information is available about the living cells, we are uncovering more and more analogies between biological structures and artificially engineered nano/micro devices. We believe that these resemblances are not just coincidence, but that they reflect deep structural and functional relationships of these entities at the mesoscale level.

In this chapter, a new concept for the description of electrically excitable living cardiac cells is presented. Based on an analogy with a laser-like quantum resonator, in this concept each cardiac cell can be represented by a network of independent nodes, having discrete energy levels and certain transition probabilities. The interaction between these nodes is given by a threshold-limited energy transfer in a state analogical to the population inversion, leading to the "laser-like" behaviour of the whole system.

To explain the new concept, we draw a larger picture of the description of living systems, based on their oscillatory behaviour. We present a phenomenon of resonance and debate its eventual role in the synchronisation of the coherent oscillatory behaviour in living systems. We then detail coherent resonant properties of cardiac cells and discuss pulse-generation in the heart based on these properties from an engineering point of view. In the presented framework, the heart is viewed as a coherent network of synchronously firing cardiac cells behaving as pulsed laser-like amplifiers, coupled to pulse-generating pacemaker master-oscillators.

The presented concept emphasizes the study of integrative cellular states and their communication systems from the "engineering" point of view, rather than the simple quantification of protein cascades involved in cell regulation. In parallel, a concept similar to the one described in this chapter can easily be applied to other cell types, such as rhythmically-firing neurones. In light of the novel view of cardiac cells derived from the concept of biological quantum resonators, it is increasingly important to look at cells by assessing their functionality at mesoscopic level, in addition to knowing their composition and structure. Gathered knowledge can also serve for improving existing optoelectronic detection technologies used for biomedical investigation.

2. Resonance and living systems

2.1 Physiology: Understanding the logic of life

Physiology, which in Greek means "study of the logic of life", is, in its pure form, an extraordinary discipline which studies the true behaviour of components of complex living systems - such as the coherent functioning of our own heart, capable of pumping blood every second of your life, often for 70 years or more. But what really the life is? What makes human body different from a rock? These questions hunt people for thousands of years and yet, even with recent advancements in the research and technology that brought an outstanding level of knowledge on living systems, we still lack precise definition of what the life really is. In biology, it is generally accepted that the system has to preserve five main features to be considered alive:

1. First, a living system has to have capacity to maintain differences with its environment and thus keep inequality by remaining in a constant movement (example being the electro-chemical gradient guarded by the membrane complexes in living cells).
2. To maintain these differences in a dynamic way, the system needs to insure efficient energy management by constant exchange of energy and materials with the system's environment, leading to the energy transfer and capture (insured, in living cells, by a process known as metabolism).
3. To efficiently minimize energy requirements of a system as a whole, each living system needs to search for appropriate tools to organize its components: in other words, the system needs to compartmentalize its components into sub-systems and specialise their functions (done by creation of organelles and organs).
4. Once compartmentalized, the system has to insure efficient communication between the created specialized sub-systems of the system as a whole, which is secured by advanced information management, in other words by insuring the flow of information within the system's energy-producing units. This extremely important feature of a living system is achieved by efficient stocking and usage of the gathered information (stored in the genetic code of DNA and translated using signalling pathways in cells).
5. Finally, the functioning of a living system requires the ability of an adaptation to a constantly changing environment and therefore its permanent re-engineering. This is guaranteed by the processes of development, reproduction and evolution, which are, in fact, advanced optimization tools used to lower the energy needs required for the system survival (example being genetic mutations).

In this interpretation, living system is a highly energetically-advantageous dynamic disequilibrium of coherently behaving components organized in efficiently communicating sub-systems, which has capacity to adapt to changing environment and reproduce. In other words, in order to stay alive, each system needs to maintain differences with its environment, using wisely its energy by compartmentalization of its tasks and by efficient communication, perpetuating itself by evolutive reproduction. To understand how is such dynamic disequilibrium created and maintained in cells, it is important to comprehend that to keep a system alive, several tools need to be used - the most important of all being an appropriate energy and information management tools. This includes, on one hand, minimization of energy by the permanent search for diversified energy sources and, on the other hand, the transfer of information about the existing energy state, while ensuring a highly orderly behaviour of the network of its subsystems.

In the modern history, one of the first who tried to uncover the relationship between the life and the laws of Physics was Erwin Schrödinger (apart of being a pioneer in the quantum mechanics of light) in "What is life?" book (Schrödinger, 1944). In this work, Schrödinger proposed that life is based on an unconventional application of the 2nd thermodynamic law. This principle states that in a non-living world, the entropy of each isolated system which is not in equilibrium will tend to increase over time, while approaching its maximal value in the equilibrium. That is the reason why a wine glass would never spontaneously re-generate from the sand, but if you break it on the beach, it will disintegrate into pieces, which will be shaped by wind and sea, and will eventually turn to sand. In other words the disorder - the entropy - of what was originally the wine glass will increase. In this way, the world is going constantly towards an increase in chaos.

However, while non-living systems are characterized by an increase in entropy that leads to increase in chaos, this principle does not seem to apply to living systems. Instead, these are rather in contrast with the 2nd law of thermodynamics by their effort to always improve their organization and therefore to create an efficient state based on minimal entropy. But what seems to be a paradox at a first sight can actually be explained in a simple way, as living systems always exist as a quasi-opened ones in a much bigger environment, to which the 2nd thermodynamic principle does apply and hence in which the total entropy increases. So, despite the fact that for the period of its lifetime the relative entropy of a living system is decreasing, in the instant of death the system re-equilibrates its electrochemical differences with its environment, reaching a permanent state of thermodynamic equilibrium of "maximum entropy".

To maintain its differences with the environment in a dynamic way, a living system needs to keep its own entropy low in an environment in which entropy is constantly rising and this is done by efficient energy management. Described "paradox" thus explains why every living system has a constant need for energy, as it continuously needs to "fight" against increasing entropy in its environment, which is driving it to engage into a bigger chaos, resulting in death. Maintaining low entropy and therefore high order is a dynamic life-long battle of each and every living creature, which demands efficient energy and information management, leading to synchronous behaviour of its components in harmony with each other in the precise environment.

A system considered alive is characterized by a coherent synchronization of a complex non-linear behaviour of its subsystems, providing the most advantageous energy efficiency. To achieve this aim, it is undeniable that dynamically behaving living systems do function as oscillators: from cell division, circadian cycle to heartbeat, clocklike rhythms are at the bases of functioning of each and every living organism. This means that if we want to keep a system alive, we need to insure that all of its oscillatory components behave coherently in a dynamic disequilibrium and, at the same time, such synergic character of the components of a non-linear living system has to be based on the synchronization of their own non-linear oscillatory behaviour. To understand how a coherent behaviour of a complex oscillatory system is guaranteed, it is necessary to comprehend what drives cyclic behaviour of its components at a first place. Study of synchronous oscillations (described by S. Strogatz (Strogatz, 2003;Strogatz & Stewart, 1993)) indicates that a coherent behaviour of the system does not grow gradually, but instead it breaks out cooperatively when the number of connections or couplings (even weak ones) between its components suddenly exceeds the threshold. And in the array of different possibilities how to affect such coupling between oscillating components, there is one particular feature: the phenomenon of resonance.

2.2 Phenomenon of resonance

The phenomenon of resonance is known for centuries. It was originally observed in music by the father of music, Ernst Chladni (1756 - 1827), who has done an extensive research on vibrating plates (Chladni, 1787) and, by showing various modes of vibration in a mechanical surface, improved large number of musical instruments. One of the most prominent scientists interested in the phenomenon of resonance was Nikola Tesla (1856-1946), who described its electrical, as well as mechanical versions (Valone, 2002). He ended up obsessed with it, creating resonant lightning storms, artificial earthquakes, or near collapse of a Manhattan skyscraper, which also lead to several inventions, such as the radio prototype. The phenomenon of resonance of light was described by Erwin Schrödinger (Schrödinger, 1933), based on the quantum mechanical principle of electromagnetic propagation in the form of a wave and of a particle, as an eventual "catastrophe" that can happen under certain conditions in the light beam.

Resonance (schematically represented at **Fig. 1**) is a physical phenomenon, characteristic of oscillatory phenomena and/or systems, such as harmonic oscillators (Bloch, 1997;Bohm, 1951). It is a tendency of an oscillatory system to oscillate at maximum amplitude at specific frequency. Resonance is an abnormally large vibration at moments (and only at the moments) when the frequency of the stimulus is the same, or nearly the same as the natural vibrational frequency of the system. As a result, the system is driven to pick its natural resonance frequency out from a complex excitation, e.g. what we do when we tune a radio to a specific frequency, and it often does it while searching for the best energy efficiency. Consequently, resonance can force systems to take specific shapes and forms, as demonstrate the powerful example of standing wave Chladni figures (Chladni, 1787).

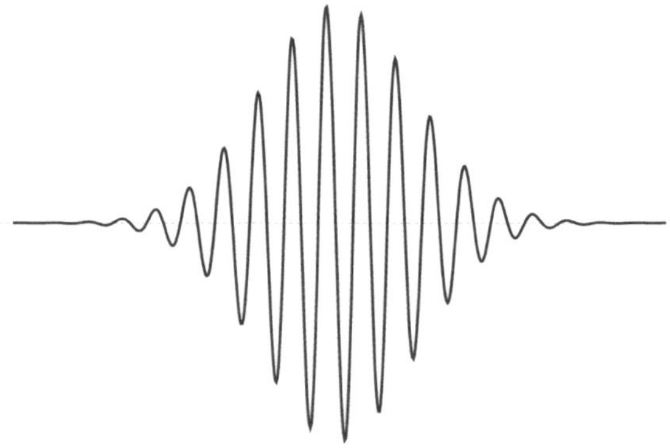

Fig. 1. The pattern of resonance (x axis: time, y axis: amplitude)

Without even realizing it, we often use resonances in our everyday life. Each time you are swinging your child at a swing you do, unconsciously, choose the natural resonance frequency of the system in order to do this task with the smallest effort; each time you tune to your favourite radio, or play an acoustic instrument, you take advantage of resonances. But this phenomenon can also be dangerous, as it can be translated into a non-amortized oscillation reaching the critical frequency of the system and in such a case, the power inside the system rises exponentially. This can lead to oscillating bridges (such as the case of the London Millennium Bridge, phenomenon observed on the day of its opening) (Eckhardt *et al.*, 2007), or even their collapse (such as the case of the Tacoma-Narrows bridge) and/or breaking glasses by opera singers.

Resonance can happen in three principal conditions (Bohm, 1951). First, in a specific object, when this object is disturbed at its natural frequency, or the resonance frequency. This situation can happen in mechanical devices, electric circuits, or acoustic instruments. Second, the resonance can build up in an object under conditions when a forcing is done at the same frequency as the natural frequency of the oscillating system. This is an example of the resonance in a pendulum (used when swinging a child on a swing). Finally, third condition arises in the situation of lack of damping or energy loss.

In medicine, resonance technologies are frequently used for the detection of human body alterations during disease, namely the nuclear magnetic resonance (NMR) is well known. Described in 1937, in the theoretical work of I.I. Rabi (Rabi *et al.*, 1992), the method was later applied by Felix Bloch and Edward M. Purcell, who were awarded a Noble Prize of Physics in 1952 for the discovery of new methods for nuclear magnetic precision measurements. This discovery revolutionized medicine by greatly improving non-invasive functional imaging of human body, including the brain and, in 2003, Paul C. Lauterbur and Peter Mansfield were awarded Nobel Prize in Physiology and Medicine for their discoveries in magnetic resonance imaging (MRI).

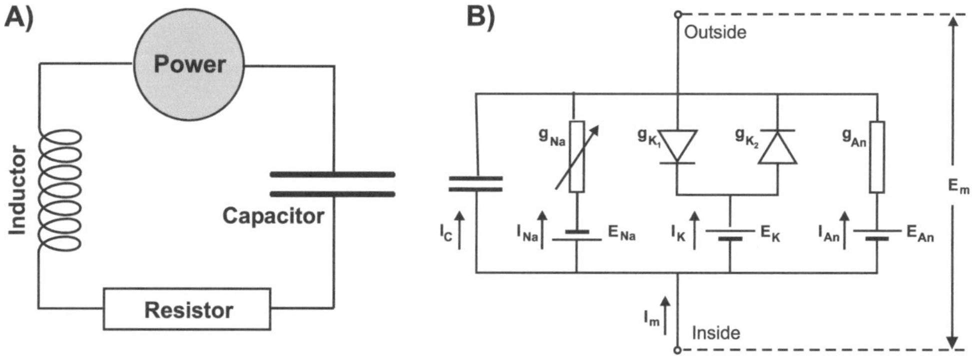

Fig. 2. Comparison of the resonating electric circuit (A) and the equivalent electrical circuit of a cardiac cell (B); I: current, g: conductance, C: capacitance, E: Electric voltage, Na: sodium ions,. K: potassium ions, An: Anions, m: membrane.

Importantly, resonance can happen in any system that uses energy, as each force we know in physics has a resonant representation (Bohm, 1951). Whether it is kinetic, rotational and gravitational energy (the case of pendulum), or electromagnetic one (the case of electrical circuits and lasers), or mechanical and elastic one (the case of resonating bridges), each time when the resonance occurs in a system, the resulting action concerns an energy accumulation. Resonance also occurs in oscillating electrical circuits (**Fig. 2A**). Each electrical circuit can be described as a resistor-inductor-capacitor (RLC) circuit. If the frequency of power supply of such circuit matches exactly the natural frequency of the circuit's LC combination, the resonance can happen and in such case, the circuit enters the state of resonance. In resonance, the series impedance is minimal and therefore the voltage for a given current is at its minimum. Or, in other words, at resonance, the electric current for a given voltage is at its maximum. It was the original and extraordinary work of Tesla that

showed us the truly incredible power of resonance in an electrical circuit and can be demonstrated by Tesla electric lightning experiments (Valone, 2002). These experiments, today known as Tesla coils, use conductive bars to direct the lightning and thus can be used to conduct, i.e. to direct the electric signal.
Most of the times, resonance is described in oscillating systems when the oscillator is subjected to periodic forcing as the energetically most efficient state, matching the system's natural frequency of oscillations. Case of a pendulum (**Fig. 3**) is an example of the resonance using kinetic, elastic, mechanical, gravitational and rotational force.

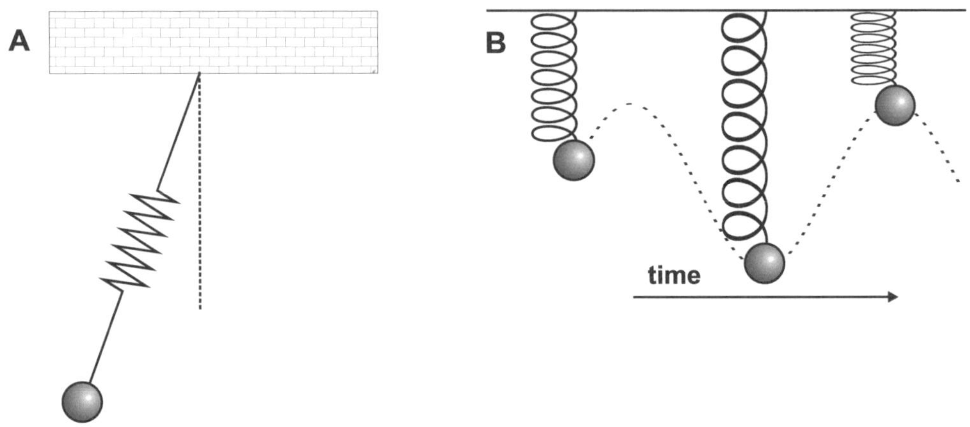

Fig. 3. Schematic representation of a pendulum (A) and its movement in time (B).

Resonance is a state where minimal energy is necessary to induce maximum effect. In other words, when the force that drives an oscillatory system (or its driving force) matches the system's natural frequency of vibrations (also called its resonance frequency), the amplitude of the steady state response will be greatest in proportion to the amount of the driving force. Induced phenomenon of resonance is therefore translated into a tendency of a system to absorb more energy. As a result, resonance state is energetically most efficient state. Consequently, for a system to secure most advantageous energy efficiency, it needs to enter the state of resonance by coherent behaviour of its components.

2.3 Symphony of life: Resonance in living systems

The concept of the "symphony of life", based on an idea that life is being played comparably to musical instruments and therefore that there are similarities between the music and functioning of living systems has been known for more than a century. Indeed, already hundred years ago William Bateson used musical analogy to make some evolutionary genetic points clearer and easier to understand as he pointed out that an eight-petal form is the same to a four-petal form as one octave is to another (Bateson, 1894;Bateson, 1913) and there are many other examples. In this understanding, recognition of dynamic patterning process has an important implication for evolutionary thinking. Modularity, segmentation and repetition, observed in living systems, are comparable to measures and tones in music, as pointed out in the Dr Ken Weiss 2002 review on "Good vibrations: the silent symphony of life" (Weiss, 2002). Other researchers identified similarities between Chladni-like simulation and hair-colour patterning (Murray, 1993). Dr Weiss also revealed that chemical "vibration" is harmonious to the organism and has properties similar to those of music (Weiss, 2002).

Among others, he demonstrated that a small amount of mutational change might have sufficed to reconfigure silent background variation to jump teosine to maize form, creating its most important cultivar - just as Chladni figure can jump when the sound frequency changes.

Another example of comparison between the living system and music was done by Denis Noble in "Music of life" book (Noble, 2006). In this interpretation, functioning of an organ of our body, such as the heart, can be compared to the musical harmony. The book discusses how to reconstruct, at an integrative level, rhythm and more specifically the heart beat, the most obvious of biological oscillators, while analysing how to create a new, higher hierarchical level using regulatory network of interactions at each level of the system organization. Noble's extensive work on the modelling of the beating heart (Noble, 2004) demonstrated that, to understand a complex phenomenon such as the heart rhythm, it is necessary to apply biology that goes beyond the genome. There is no "single gene module" that can explain creation of complex functions such as circadian rhythms, but more gene and protein components appear to be involved.

If life can be described as being played comparably to musical instruments to create a harmonious symphony, it is largely because, as tones of music, all known living systems have oscillatory behaviour. Great majority of processes that are obsered in the living systems function at the bases of an ON - OFF (0 - 1) "switch-like" states, like musical tonality. This suggests that each system oscillates between these two states at a certain rate, or in other words, with a defined frequency. It can pass from one dynamic state to another at a very short time-base (oscillating frequency-dependent states). Most activities of any known living system (including cells, humans, or populations) work in such a cyclical way. For example, most proteins oscillate between specific states: such as bound/unbound state (for many enzymes), or opened and closed one (for ionic channels, for example), in a synchronous way. And most biochemical regulatory proteins and their ligands interact with other proteins as a lock and a key. Furthermore, we also find oscillatory behaviour at the level of our cells : one of the best examples being cardiac cells, with their capacity to produce periodic oscillations at the frequency of our heart beat. But, in fact, all cells and organisms are subjected to cycles, as nicely described by Arthur T. Winfree in "The Geometry of Biological Time" (Winfree, 1980) or Foster & Kreitzman in "Rhythms of Life" (Foster R & Kreitzman L, 2004). We can retrieve such increase-decrease patterns in the functioning of the living system at every of its levels, as demonstrated in **Table 1**.

Biological effect		
biochemical enzymatic reactions	association	dissociation
membrane ionic channels	opening	closing
skeletal muscle movement	acceleration	stopping
neuronal networks	stimulation	inhibition
cardiac cells during heart beat	contraction	relaxation (expansion)
vessels	constriction	dilatation
endocrine system	synthesis	degradation
respiration	oxygenation (O_2 utilization)	reduction (CO_2 utilization)

Table 1. Oscillatory phenomena in living systems

In the last decades, lot of work was done in understanding complex oscillations. Theory that derives from these observations, also referred to as "synchronized chaos", revealed that it is the synergic character of non-linear oscillating systems that make them so rich and powerful. As pointed out by Strogatz (Strogatz, 2003), tendency to synchronize is one of the most general drives in the universe, extending from atoms to animals, from people to planets. Sync is one of the oldest and most elementary parts of non-linear sciences. In this context it is particularly important to understand that it is the synchronization of the chaotic behaviour of oscillatory components which constitutes a complex non-linear dynamic (living) system, and is crucial for the decision-making in choosing the most energetically advantageous interactions of such system with its environment, or between its sub-systems.

As living systems clearly have an oscillatory behaviour and are composed of many sub-systems, such oscillatory sub-systems have therefore capacity to generate resonances between themselves. What are scientific proofs that resonance can also occur in living systems? The idea has been around for years: since Georges Lakhovski, who proposed in the "Secret of Life" (Lakhovsky, 1929) that cells can find their resonance frequency of oscillations in an array of multiple vibrations, to a controversial Luc Montagnier, a 2008 Nobel price winner for Medicine for the discovery of HIV virus, who proposed in his disputed article (Montagnier *et al.*, 2009) a surprising idea that resonance can help living systems to recover the memory of events, this issue is now debated for nearly a century. However, this issue remains largely unexplored scientifically and thus still rather debatable with little direct scientific evidence or experimental proof at others than atom and/or molecular levels.

At the molecular level, scientists were clearly able to demonstrate the presence of the resonance energy transfer between atoms and molecules in our cells. In fact, the capacity of Föster resonance energy transfer (FRET) (Lakowicz, 2006;Periasamy, 2001) between atoms and molecules is frequently employed as an imaging method to enhance knowledge on the molecular structure of cellular proteins. Based on visualization of fluorescence which lights up when a resonance transfer occurs between two very close atoms of specific proteins, researchers were capable to establish ultra-structure of great number of proteins, or protein machines (Periasamy *et al.*, 2008). It is also noteworthy that with its ionic channels allowing transmission of ions and creation of the cell membrane potential, each cell in our body is also an electric circuit (Junge, 1992). With an example being the heart cells (see schematic representation of an equivalent electrical circuit for a cardiac cells at **Fig. 2B**), cell is often an oscillatory electric circuit - and, as described in previous chapters and illustrated at **Fig. 2A**, resonance can occur in oscillatory electric systems. In addition, a well documented example of the use of resonance in living systems has been found in neuronal networks. This research demonstrated that a living cell has the capacity to generate what is called "stochastic resonance" which is in fact the capability of the cell to extract a specific signal from a large noise (McDonnell & Abbott, 2009;Wiesenfeld & Jaramillo, 1998). Stochastic resonance is a cooperative event in which coupling of the oscillatory events of small amplitude and noisy responses improves the system's sensitivity to discriminate weak signals (Moss *et al.*, 2004); thus, the system exhibiting this phenomenon behaves as a kind of detector, trying to extract a weak periodic signal. Presence of resonance in such network makes a difference by allowing a highly efficient extraction of specific signal from a mix of others.

2.4 Life as propagator of resonances

Resonance has all the attributes to act as the driving force in living systems, capable to generate and maintain the highly energetically advantageous dynamic disequilibrium of coherently behaving components crucial for each living system or, more precisely, for the life itself. Examples listed in the Section 2.3 demonstrate the presence of resonance at a molecular level and also suggest that this phenomenon can play a role in the synchronisation of functions in living systems. Taking into consideration the five main features which describe living systems (Section 2.1), resonance can occur in each of them: 1) resonance can happen in oscillating objects with a coherent behaviour that are in constant movement, it therefore allows to maintain differences between the resonating object and its environment in a dynamic way; 2) resonance is a phenomenon directly linked to energy use and maximization, thus allowing efficient energy management; 3) confinement of resonance into a distinct space - resonance cavity - pushes each system that employs resonances to compartmentalize and to specialize energy use. 4) The use of resonances is a highly efficient way to retrieve information about the observed system while using minimum energy, as demonstrated by resonance-based sensors and detectors, and thus it also insures an advanced information management. 5) By entering into resonance, oscillating components evolve into a completely new state, based on adaptation with their environment.

Resonance insures highest energy efficiency and helps to understand how the living system can pass from one hierarchical level to another - two fundamental requirements of the living system. As a non-linear effect, resonance has a capacity to energetically boost the synchronized coupling between these components in a precisely determined space. It is a specific state where the system can create maximum energy or, in other words, a state where the system can function with minimum energy. As a result, it can promote cooperativity and thus coherent behaviour of the whole system. In this way, resonance has the ability to push living systems to choose their shape, form, or size (as it is capable to do it in non-living matter when creating standing wave Chladni figures for example) and may thus be a potential decision-maker for these systems. In addition, resonance can only happen between (at least) two coherently oscillating entities – one unit cannot generate resonance. It is a completely new equilibrium, exactly as the creation of a new hierarchical level. As noted by Schrödinger (Schrödinger, 1933), the new state created when two oscillating systems enter the state of resonance is very different form the original states in which these systems were before entering resonance. In this context, resonance is a unique force allowing synchronization of the system, leading to its energetically most efficient coherent behaviour.

In this interpretation, life can be understood as based on propagation of resonances, where the life of eukaryotes starts with a resonance between the ovule and the sperm, which then propagates from one cell to another, from one component to another every day of our lifetime, until the resonance transfer weakens and eventually stops. In the latter situation, the system would require much higher amounts of energy to function, engaging in a non-linear use of energy, leading to a diseased state characterized by an energy collapse and, finally, once the system's natural resonance frequency is perturbed and the system lacks energy to function, the life ends - or, in other words, the living system dies.

3. Resonant properties of the heart

3.1 Coherent resonant properties of cardiac cells

Previously, our group introduced basic framework for the description of the harmonious behaviour of the heart based on synchronous oscillations of cardiac myocytes, each behaving as a pulsed biological "laser-like" quantum resonator/amplifier (Chorvat, Jr. & Chorvatova, 2008). Already, several other groups emphasized quantum and/or wave features of the behaviour of living biological systems, including studies on conduction pathways in microtubules (Hameroff *et al.*, 2002;Penrose, 2001), DNA mutagenesis (McFadden, 2000;McFadden & Al Khalili, 1999) and/or information processing (Davies, 2005;Davies, 2004) and its synchronization (Strogatz & Stewart, 1993). In our concept, each cardiac cell is understood as an ensemble of independent functional units acting analogically to the network of atoms in laser active medium, constituted of a network of independent nodes, each node involving a set of discrete energy levels and transition probabilities between them. Quantum-like behaviour of the whole network is based on the interaction between the neighbouring nodes, which is given by the threshold-limited energy transfer leading to quantum-like behaviour of the whole network.

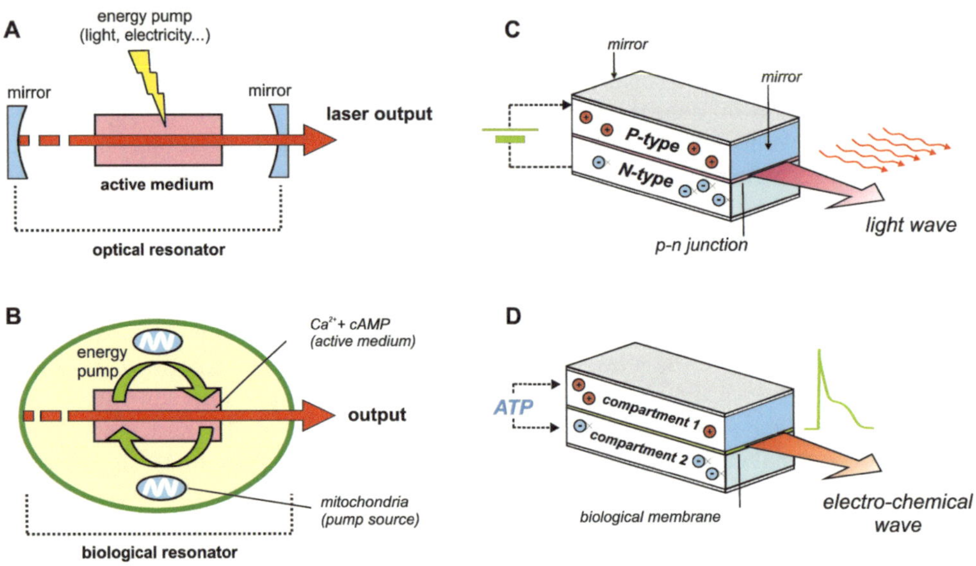

Fig. 4. Comparison of the function principle of the laser (A,C) and the cardiac pacemaker cell (B,D).

We have based this new concept of coherent resonant properties of the heart cells on an analogy with lasers - practical implementations of quantum resonators (**Fig. 4**) - in order to underline its advantages for the best energy efficiency of these cells. The LASER (Light Amplification by Stimulated Emission of Radiation) is a well-known device producing an intense monochromatic beam of coherent light, engineered on the principles of the quantum mechanics. The device uses a resonant cavity to induce light amplification and produce a coherent light output. First laser was constructed by Theodore Maiman in 1960, based on the original work of Albert Einstein and the groups of Townes/Basov and Prokhorov (reviewed in (Hecht, 2010)). Electromagnetic waves (such as its best known representation – light) have proven capacity to resonate according to the original work of Schrödinger (Schrödinger, 1933). When properly used, resonant cavity can generate coherent light waves, allowing creation of the laser.

In lasers, the presence of an active lasing medium is a key factor in their functioning (**Fig. 4A, C**). The particles of such lasing medium become progressively excited under continual optical pumping, resulting in their increasing number residing in higher-energy quantum states (described in details in (Chorvat, Jr. & Chorvatova, 2008)). Consequently, when the number of particles in the excited state exceeds the number of particles in the ground state, the state of population inversion is achieved. In this case, the active medium acts as an optical amplifier, where the intensity of the light passing through it rises, instead of being absorbed. In addition to the requirements for a defined atomic or molecular structure of the laser's active medium, carefully-designed geometry (an optical resonator) needs to be employed to effectively combine the processes of spontaneous emission and light amplification by stimulated emission. As a result, in the active medium, a spontaneous emission of photons followed by the phenomenon of light amplification based on the process of stimulated emission takes place - which represents the basis of the laser. The resulting light output has unique properties which include directionality, monochromaticity, high power and coherence.

In cardiomyocytes, we believe that "active medium" of a biological laser-like resonator (**Fig. 4B**) results from stochastic behaviour of ionic channels (Chorvat, Jr. & Chorvatova, 2008), namely the voltage-gated calcium ones (Junge, 1992). Opening of these channels in response to an action potential (AP) in a small microdomain between the transverse (T)-tubule and a sarcoplasmic reticulum (SR), also called a dyad, triggers process of calcium-induced calcium release (CICR), which underlies excitation-contraction coupling in cardiac cells (Bers, 2002;Niggli & Egger, 2002) and is responsible for the contraction of the heart cell. In an analogy with the laser, the process of energy "absorption" is related to pushing the biological system into a higher energy state, while "emission" can be understood as return from such disequilibrium. In cardiac cells, we believe that the "absorption" relates to the active transport of ions - their removal from the cytosol. This process happens as active extrusion of ions such as calcium through the membrane out of the cytosol, using effective means of transportation such as Na/Ca exchanger (Kimura *et al.*, 1986) on one hand and, on the other hand, the compartmentalization of calcium ions into SR intracellular stores using adenosine trisphosphate (ATP)-powered SR calcium pumps (SERCA). This allows creation of a 10,000-fold calcium gradient between the intracellular stores and the cytosol (Lehnart *et al.*, 2004), thus constituting a thermodynamically-unstable disequilibrium. Once this dynamic disequilibrium is in place, the process of "emission" can take place, which represents, in fact, an active process of return from such disequilibrium. In cardiac cells, this process can be understood either as a "spontaneous emission" process, witnessed by unitary calcium release (calcium sparks), or as "stimulated emission", triggered by stochastic opening of calcium channels and leading to CICR.

In this setting, the "population inversion"-like phenomena would take place in one node of a cardiac cell, which corresponds to several dyadic spaces between two t-tubules and the contractile apparatus, once the number of nodes in the "ready-to-fire" state becomes greater than the number of nodes with equilibrated calcium concentration. In this state only, the cardiac cell can achieve the capacity to sequentially amplify the calcium response occurring in one node to neighbouring nodes, and thus over to the whole cell and/or to the cardiac tissue. This process, macroscopically described as a continuous calcium wave, can be seen as sequential "stimulated emission" phenomena, with interaction between neighbouring nodes driven by threshold-limited energy transfer of a quantum nature.

In brief, our concept implies that in contractile cardiac myocytes, stochastic calcium release and the unitary properties of ionic channels stimulated during each excitation-contraction coupling cycle create "population inversion" and "spontaneous emission" phenomena, analogical to laser active medium (Chorvat, Jr. & Chorvatova, 2008). Such medium, when powered by an incoming threshold-reaching voltage discharge in the form of an AP, responds to the calcium influx through L-type calcium channels by stimulated emission of Ca^{2+} ions in a coherent, synchronized and amplified CICR process. In this setting, molecular amplification stimulated by phosphorylation in protein cascades adds tuneable features to cardiac cells. The energy thus generated in cardiac cells is used for the mechanical work - change in the conformation of a cell contractile apparatus - that results in the cell shortening and thus the whole heart contraction. Consequently, we propose that the heart functions as a coherent network of synchronously-firing cardiac myocytes behaving as amplifying blocks, coupled to pulse-generating pacemakers, acting as master-oscillators, all cooperating in a coherently-resonating cellular network under the hormonal control of the brain – the central regulator and control system, thus acquiring capacity to behave as a highly efficient pump expulsing the blood with smallest energy requirements. Advantages of the concept of a cardiac cell as a quantum resonator include high energy efficiency, robustness and self-control.

3.2 Pacemakers: Pulse generation based on coherent resonant properties of heart cells

To design a pulse-generating system from an engineering point of view, precise interplay between several nonlinear effects must be reached, leading to the creation of short pulses, stable operation and high power efficiency. For example, in a laser, different techniques can achieve pulse generation, two of the most common being mode-locking and quality-switching. We have previously described these processes in details (Chorvat, Jr. & Chorvatova, 2008), where we also draw an analogy between different pulse-generating modes in a laser and those in the heart (**Fig. 4B,D**). Overall, no precise protein is responsible for cardiac rhythm; this mechanism is rather integrated at the cellular level (Noble, 2006). Cardiac tissue is known to be a highly non-linear medium that can support various complex rhythmic activities. To synchronize propagation between different cells in the heart, coherence of this firing is crucial, which means that it needs to be synchronous, but also delayed in time.

The rhythmic electrical activity - an inherent property of the heart - is initiated by the pacemakers in the sino-atrial (SA) node (Boyett *et al.*, 2000). Pacemakers are the only cells in the heart that are capable of generating endogenous pulsed oscillations, thanks to spontaneous changes in membrane ionic permeability and specialized currents, particularly, pacemaker "funny" I_f current (Brown *et al.*, 1979;DiFrancesco, 1993;DiFrancesco, 2006), thus governing heart-beating frequency (Noble, 2006). From an engineering point of view, I_f current seems an ideal candidate for a quality-switching (Q-switch), which – in a laser – is based on a preventive feedback into the active medium while the laser medium is pumped. Consequently, as laser power increases, population inversion is generated, but without triggering the stimulated emission and increasing energy is stored in the active medium. At the opportune moment, the Q-switch device switches on, allowing an efficient extraction of the stored energy by highly-power pulse generation. Control of membrane depolarization via presence of high levels of basal cAMP and its attendant protein kinase A (PKA) phosphorylation (Bridge *et al.*, 2006) point to their possible role in medium saturation and thus the control of firing properties of pacemakers in analogy with the creation of a "saturable absorber". In pacemakers, in contrast to ventricles, phosphorylation levels control the firing properties, with calcium having rather the tuning role allowing better internal control and flexibility. Thereby, the inherent, pulse-generating, pacemaking mechanism of the heart SA node can be regarded as a pulse-generating "master-oscillator".

Pulse-generating, pacemaker "master-oscillators" synchronize functioning of ventricular cells, which behave as a network of resonating structures constituted from a series of multi-pass amplifier components using energetically-efficient synchronisation tools, which allow the heart to function as a cell network, such as phase-locking. Phase-locking is an effect when several subunits are synchronized together in oscillatory behaviour with a coherent phase. Indeed, phase-locking, period-doubling bifurcations were previously proposed for a cardiac oscillator (Glass, 1991). To translate the signal towards neighbouring cells, cardiac myocytes employ electrically coupled junctional channels, permeable to small cytoplasmic molecules and ions, such as calcium, called gap junctions and/or narrow junctional clefts. Electrical field and gap junctional mechanisms act in concert to improve and stabilize the propagation of cardiac muscles (Sperelakis, 2003), resulting in synchronized responsiveness of the entire network of cells. Gap junctions are thereby important contributors to the unidirectionality of wave propagation as well as its synchronization between cells. Strong gap-junctional coupling has been proposed to synchronize the electrical oscillations of cells, while weak coupling has instead the capacity to phase-lock two cells (Sherman & Rinzel, 1992). The heart has also been proposed to be a network of dynamically-coupled nonlinear oscillators from the metabolic point of view (Aon *et al.*, 2006).

In the heart, pulse-generating pacemaker cells are electrically connected to neighbouring cells, thus allowing the synchronized propagation of oscillations within heart tissue. Once the pulse is generated in pacemaker cells, cardiac myocytes are then synchronized during each heart beat by voltage discharges in the form of AP, based on the flow of electric current (Junge, 1992), which induces depolarization and subsequent contraction of cardiac myocytes. AP is a threshold process, result of a careful interplay between voltage-sensitive sodium and potassium ionic channels (Junge, 1992;Nerbonne & Kass, 2005;Noble, 1962), which can be viewed in an analogy to an electronic design known as gain switching, which is at the basis of the creation of pulsed lasers. In this process, optical gain is negative when carrier density or pump intensity in the active region of the device is below the threshold, and switches to a positive value when the lasing threshold is exceeded. These characteristics are very comparable to the properties of APs, which switch the cell membrane potential from negative values (of around -75 mV, when the cell is at its resting potential, below the threshold for AP activation) to positive values (to about +40 mV, the Nernst equilibrium potential of sodium ions).

In addition, a number of molecular mechanisms perform regulatory tuning functions in the heart adding tunability features to cardiomyocyte "resonators". One of the most important is the hormonal control of ATP-powered protein phosphorylation, a well-recognized mode of signalling (Hata & Koch, 2003) by protein cascades, initiated by G-protein stimulation. One example of such tuning in the heart is highly important β-adrenergic sympathetic regulation, which enhances cardiac function during stress and exercise performance (Movsesian, 1999). In pacemaker cells this regulation causes increases in cAMP production within cells, which, in turn, enhances "funny" I_f current (DiFrancesco, 2006) and phosphorylates calcium channels, thus leading to an increase in the frequency of AP generation in these cells and, therefore, of heart beat. The modulation of calcium cycling by β-adrenergic receptor stimulation controls the strength of ventricular myocyte contraction and cardiac contractile reserves (Movsesian, 1999). Hormonal regulation acts as a general cell "tuning" mechanism with subsequent protein cascades as fine attenuators adjusting cell resonant properties.

Presented novel view of cardiac cells and pacemaker pulse-generation derived from the engineering-driven concept of biological quantum resonator opens new insights into understanding of heart functioning, thus allowing to comprehend several interrelated phenomena and their alteration in cardiovascular diseases. The concept brings a new viewpoint on cardiac diseases as possible alterations of cell resonant properties. In disease, disturbance of these features will first lead to adaptive remodelling, trying to restore the biological resonator, followed by the replacement of individual functions. However, if the repair mechanisms are not sufficient, the system will reach a state with distorted lasing properties, culminating in a non-linear energy collapse. It also points to the fact that to achieve efficient pharmaceutical treatment in such a complex environment, investigating the effects of medications on cell resonant properties is desirable as a signature of their energy efficiency. Last, but not least, deeper knowledge of cellular properties can thus be further translated into conceptual guidelines for the development of new emerging laser and optoelectronic technologies.

3.3 Heart disease from the viewpoint of alteration of coherent resonant properties of cardiac cells

Proposed concept of cardiac cells behaving as biological resonators brings a new viewpoint on cardiac diseases as possible alterations of their coherent resonant properties. Normal heart function can be seen as precisely-tuned, highly energetically-effective synchronous firing of the network of cardiomyocytes, each behaving as a biological resonator. In this setting, each cardiac cell functions with minimum energy to perform the required work. Consequently, the description of the heart functioning is based on the principle of harmony, as suggested previously for complex biological systems such as the heart (Noble, 2006), which emphasizes that some features, such as the pacemaker, are only observable in the state of precise balance of its components. At the same time, functioning involving precise resonant balance implicates that even a slight misalignment of components constituting the resonating system results in a significant drop in the system's energy efficiency, often in a complete loss of resonating properties.

In this regard, life-threatening conditions such as abnormal cardiac cell enlargement (hypertrophy) can be easily understood in the context of hypertrophy changing the size of the resonant cavity, preventing cells to sustain their resonant properties, leading to an increase in energy needs, loss of effectiveness and eventually heart failure (HF). For example, same set of proteins present in a cardiac cell, but with modified 3-dimensional topology could substantially alter its functioning. We have previously analyzed in details (Chorvat, Jr. & Chorvatova, 2008), how can the HF - a cardiac disease touching large populations of patients - be described from the viewpoint of modifications of cardiac resonant properties.

We pointed out that typical features which accompany this disease can be understood as a failure of the biological resonator to achieve the "population inversion" state. Indeed, cardiac disease in general, and HF in particular, has been associated with increased occurrence of spontaneous calcium sparks, decreased cytosolic calcium transients and often diminished SR calcium load (Bers *et al.*, 2003) due to reduced function of SERCA pumps, enhanced Na/Ca exchange function and increased calcium leakage. These alterations have been proposed to lead to alteration of CICR. In addition, metabolic flexibility (Taegtmeyer *et al.*, 2004), allowing the heart to switch from one substrate to another is severely reduced, leading to higher energy requirements in disease. Finally, synchronisation parameters are also affected: prolongation of AP duration is a characteristic feature of myocytes from diseased hearts (Hart, 1994) due to modifications of K^+ currents and Ca^{2+} handling. Cardiac hypertrophy or thickened heart muscle is a common hallmark of the progression of the disease. After adaptive myocardial remodeling (Gerdes, 2002), cardiac hypertrophy develops (Tamura *et al.*, 1999), leading to congestive HF.

These findings suggest that cardiac cell in a failing heart exhibit features of 1) a rising "spontaneous emission" phenomena, vs. lowered "stimulated emission" ones; 2) the higher energy need, and 3) the overall loss of resonant and synchronisation properties. In this understanding, adaptive properties of cardiac muscles are put in place to restore the biological resonator capabilities of cells in their new environment, while maladaptive properties rather point to the incapacity of such restoration.

3.4 Towards intelligent sensing of the dynamics in living systems: Resonance as a detection principle

Resonance has a wide range of applications in technologies, particularly mass-media and other communication systems, but also nanotechnologies and information technologies. Radio is the oldest and to this day probably the best-known mass-media device which construction is based on resonance. Nikola Tesla was the first to demonstrate the feasibility of wireless communications in 1893, yet it was Guglielmo Marconi who developed the first workable radio communication and sent and received the first radio signal in Italy in 1895. Indeed, tuning to a preferred station equals choosing a resonance frequency. To this day, resonance remained a key technology governing the mass communication: in the last decades, nanoscale MicroElectroMechanical Systems (MEMS) oscillator/resonator technology has been greatly advanced and is now started to be employed in the cell phone and the consumer electronics industry (Saliterman, 2006). Its advantages are numerous, including small fabrication size and improved integration, possibility of simultaneous multi-frequency use and finally the low power consumption; all these features predestine RF MEMS resonators to be used in portable applications.

Technologies based on resonance strongly advanced biomedical studies in the last decades. The extraordinary nature of resonance where the maximum response can be induced by minimum energy is indeed a holy-grail aim for any experimental method, promising ultra-high sensitivity and specificity with minimum disturbance of the system under study. The resonance principle can be found in the roots of many macroscopic real-time 3D visualization techniques with one of the brightest examples being MRI (magnetic resonance imaging), which is exploiting the resonance of a nucleus of atoms absorbing energy from the magnetic field and is often used to image internal organs in medical diagnosis. On the other hand, resonance of light waves is mostly used for investigation of living cells and tissues and provide foundation of techniques such as optical tomography, speckle-interferometry, non-linear optical microscopy or FRET (Lauterborn *et al.*, 2003;Periasamy & Diaspro, 2003;Lakowicz, 2006;Verbiest *et al.*, 2009;Sun *et al.*, 2011). All these technologies take profit from a special capacity of resonance to improve the signal recognition from the studied phenomena while minimizing sample damage. Consequently they are now used daily in medicine and medical practice, although utilization of the resonance principle takes place in many cases unwittingly.

In the future it is expected that resonance-based detection will be more and more widely used in study of living systems. In recent years, MEMS resonance biosensors are being implemented in the analytical laboratories to analyze the presence of molecules at a nanometric scale (Hillberg *et al.*, 2005;Rosen & Gurman, 2010). These are now used to isolate and identify stem cells, perform sensitive fingerprint sensor applications and are even intended to repair failing hearts (cardioMEMS, bioMEMS) (Gupta *et al.*, 2010). Indeed, MEMS resonance biosensors have a wide range of applications from neural probes, blood analysis, to fabrication of endoscopes, as well as data storage. Another example is development of ultra sensitive biochemical sensors, based on surface plasmon resonance and resonant waveguide gratings, used to determine e.g. the affinities and kinetics of target analytes in a sample binding to the biological receptors immobilized on the sensor surface (Fang *et al.*, 2006).

To improve the study of complex phenomena in living cells that we observe at the cellular and multicellular levels - such as the pacemaker - we now need to expand detection technologies and create resonance detectors capable of sensing resonance alterations in living systems at higher hierarchical levels. Currently, we apply deterministic approach in this investigation, which means that we characterize all entities from which such system is built. In other words, we cut the system into pieces and examine each piece in details (determining its anatomical design, or protein mapping). However, modelling of complex living systems, such as the heart, revealed fundamental limitations of such scientific investigations. Denis Noble (Noble, 2006) detailed serious limitations that are attached to the use of such "bottom-up" or "top-down" approach in the study of living systems and their functions, mainly linked to the failure of these approaches to examine what does create the bond between sub-systems to generate a new, higher hierarchical level. As a result, this approach is proving not to be enough: as an example, it is becoming clear that despite knowing the whole genome, we still cannot understand why a healthy system suddenly, in the middle of an (apparently healthy) lifetime, changes into a diseased one. We now start to understand that, instead of dissecting individual components of a complex living system, we rather need to study the system as a whole from its "centre" to comprehend the casual chain in the system.

Recent technologies, described above, allow detection of resonance states at the level of atoms and molecules. However, at the moment there are no such appropriate detection systems working at the level of whole cells or organs. More specifically, in the future we will need to design a new type of intelligent detectors, capable of deciphering the natural resonance frequencies and their changes in physiological and pathophysiological conditions to monitor complex phenomena, such as the pacemaker physiology. We need devices capable of capturing coherent behaviour resulting from interplay of each of its sub-components at every hierarchical level. Search for new, multi-dimensional intelligent detection systems that would have capacity to observe the system and its behaviour in an observer-independent way, is the future of recording tools that would account for the complexity of the studied system and would therefore become sensors of its functionality, as well as of its alterations in diseased states.

4. Conclusion

Understanding complex phenomena in living systems is the challenge of the 21st century. Despite searching for centuries for the best description of what life really is, we still lack

precise understanding of this extraordinary phenomenon. Living systems function at a basis of a highly energetically-advantageous dynamic disequilibrium of oscillating components, organized in sub-systems. To create and maintain such system, it is therefore highly important that its components behave coherently. To achieve such behaviour, it is necessary to strengthen synchronized coupling between these components. We propose that the phenomenon of resonance can contribute to this synchronisation in a highly effective way. Fundamental for all oscillating systems, resonance is closely linked to energy usage and, with each force having resonant representation, this phenomenon has all the attributes to play a fundamental role in driving coherent behaviour in living systems. It can therefore also help us to comprehend such complex phenomena in living systems as is the pacemaker. Monitoring harmonious behaviour of the heart based on synchronous oscillations of cardiac cells, each functioning as a pulsed biological quantum resonator/amplifier, opens a new insight into understanding of pacemaking and thus of heart functioning at a synch. We are now beginning to understand, with heart beat being the first such example, that some cell features, such as its resonant properties, are only observable in the state of precise balance - in a physiological state. This concept also incorporates the role of genes in re-creating, in the new environment, a state with the most appropriate biological resonant properties by tuning the cell resonator via the expression of precise protein clusters. Investigation of resonance properties can allow to comprehend not only the normal functioning of living cardiac cells, but also their alterations in a disease. Understanding cell resonant properties as a signature of their energy efficiency can also help to achieve an efficient pharmaceutical treatment by investigating effects of medications in such complex environment. We are convinced that resonant features are not likely to be unique to cardiac cells, but that resonance is a more generalized feature in living systems.
Nowadays, it is crucial to add an engineering point of view to the analysis of physiological phenomena. We have developed tools that allow us to decipher every component of the living system individually. Now we need to design new advanced tools that would allow to study functioning of the coherent behaviour of the living system in its dynamic complexity: detectors that would be able to monitor resonances in living systems at their different hierarchical levels. In parallel, deeper knowledge of cellular properties as biological quantum resonator can be further translated into design of new emerging resonance-based optoelectronic detection technologies.

5. Acknowledgment

We would like to acknowledge support from the EC's Seventh Framework Programme LASERLAB-EUROPE, grant agreement n° 228334, and Research grant agency of the Ministry of Education, Science, Research and Sport of the Slovak Republic VEGA No. 1/0530/09.
We would specially like to thank Jan Kodon (www.reasonance.org) for fruitful discussion.

6. References

Aon, M. A., Cortassa, S., & O'Rourke, B. (2006). The fundamental organization of cardiac mitochondria as a network of coupled oscillators. *Biophys.J* 91, 4317-4327.

Bateson, W. (1894). *Materials for the study of variation*, reprinted 1992 ed. Johns Hopkins Press, Baltimore.

Bateson, W. (1913). *Problems of genetics*, reprinted 1979 ed., Yale University Press, New Haven.

Bers, D. M. (2002). Cardiac excitation-contraction coupling. *Nature* 415, 198-205.

Bers, D. M., Eisner, D. A., & Valdivia, H. H. (2003). Sarcoplasmic reticulum Ca2+ and heart failure: roles of diastolic leak and Ca2+ transport. *Circ.Res.* 93, 487-490.

Bloch, S. C. (1997). *Introduction to classical and quantum harmonic oscillators*, reprinted 2001 ed., pp. 1-363. A Wiley-Interscience, NY, U.S.A.

Bohm, D. (1951). *Quantum Theory*, reprinted 1989 ed., pp. 1-646. Dover Publications, NY, U.S.A.

Boyett, M. R., Honjo, H., & Kodama, I. (2000). The sinoatrial node, a heterogeneous pacemaker structure. *Cardiovasc.Res.* 47, 658-687.

Bridge, J. H., Davidson, C. J., & Savio-Galimberti, E. (2006). A novel mechanism of pacemaker control that depends on high levels of cAMP and PKA-dependent phosphorylation: a precisely controlled biological clock. *Circ.Res.* 98, 437-439.

Brown, H. F., DiFrancesco, D., & Noble, S. J. (1979). How does adrenaline accelerate the heart? *Nature* 280, 235-236.

Chladni, E. (1787). *Entdeckungenu¨ber die Theorie des Klanges [Discoveries concerning the theory of sound]*, pp. 1-100. Leipzig.

Chorvat, D., Jr. & Chorvatova, A. (2008). Cardiac cell: a biological laser? *Biosystems* 92, 49-60.

Davies, P. (2005). A quantum recipe for life. *Nature* 437, 819.

Davies, P. C. (2004). Does quantum mechanics play a non-trivial role in life? *Biosystems* 78, 69-79.

DiFrancesco, D. (1993). Pacemaker mechanisms in cardiac tissue. *Annu.Rev.Physiol* 55, 455-472.

DiFrancesco, D. (2006). Serious workings of the funny current. *Prog.Biophys.Mol.Biol.* 90, 13-25.

Eckhardt, B., Ott, E., Strogatz, S. H., Abrams, D. M., & McRobie, A. (2007). Modeling walker synchronization on the Millennium Bridge. *Phys.Rev.E Stat.Nonlin.Soft.Matter Phys.* 75, 021110.

Fang, Y., Ferrie, A. M., Fontaine, N. H., Mauro, J., & Balakrishnan, J. (2006). Resonant waveguide grating biosensor for living cell sensing. *Biophys.J* 91, 1925-1940.

Foster R & Kreitzman L (2004). *Rhythms of Life*, pp. 1-276. Profiles Books, Ltt, London.

Gerdes, A. M. (2002). Cardiac myocyte remodeling in hypertrophy and progression to failure. *J.Card Fail.* 8, S264-S268.

Glass, L. (1991). Nonlinear dynamics of physiological function and control. *Chaos.* 1, 247-250.

Gupta, K., Kim, D. H., Ellison, D., Smith, C., Kundu, A., Tuan, J., Suh, K. Y., & Levchenko, A. (2010). Lab-on-a-chip devices as an emerging platform for stem cell biology. *Lab Chip.* 10, 2019-2031.

Hameroff, S., Nip, A., Porter, M., & Tuszynski, J. (2002). Conduction pathways in microtubules, biological quantum computation, and consciousness. *Biosystems* 64, 149-168.

Hart, G. (1994). Cellular electrophysiology in cardiac hypertrophy and failure. *Cardiovasc.Res.* 28, 933-946.

Hata, J. A. & Koch, W. J. (2003). Phosphorylation of G protein-coupled receptors: GPCR kinases in heart disease. *Mol.Interv.* 3, 264-272.

Hecht, J. (2010). A short history of laser development. *Appl.Opt.* 49, F99-122.

Hillberg, A. L., Brain, K. R., & Allender, C. J. (2005). Molecular imprinted polymer sensors: implications for therapeutics. *Adv.Drug Deliv.Rev.* 57, 1875-1889.

Junge, D. (1992). *Nerve and muscle excitation*, 3 ed., pp. 1-263. Sinauer Associates, Inc. U.S.A., Sunderland, Massachusetts.

Kimura, J., Noma, A., & Irisawa, H. (1986). Na-Ca exchange current in mammalian heart cells. *Nature* 319, 596-597.

Lakhovsky, G. (1929). *The Secret of Life*, reprinted in 2007 ed., pp. 1-201. A Digireads.com Publishing, Stilwell, U.S.A.

Lakowicz, J. R. (2006). *Principles of Fluorescence Spectroscopy*, 3 ed., pp. 1-923. Springer, New York.

Lauterborn, W., Kurz, T., & Wiesenfeldt, M. (2003). *Coherent Optics: Fundamentals and Applications*, pp. 1-333. Springer-Verlag, Berlin Heidelberg.

Lehnart, S. E., Wehrens, X. H., Kushnir, A., & Marks, A. R. (2004). Cardiac ryanodine receptor function and regulation in heart disease. *Ann.N.Y.Acad.Sci.* 1015, 144-159.

McDonnell, M. D. & Abbott, D. (2009). What is stochastic resonance? Definitions, misconceptions, debates, and its relevance to biology. *PLoS.Comput.Biol.* 5, e1000348.

McFadden, J. (2000). *Quantum Evolution*, pp. 1-338. Norton&Company Ltd., NY, U.S.A.

McFadden, J. & Al Khalili, J. (1999). A quantum mechanical model of adaptive mutation. *Biosystems* 50, 203-211.

Montagnier, L., Aissa, J., Ferris, S., Montagnier, J. L., & Lavallee, C. (2009). Electromagnetic signals are produced by aqueous nanostructures derived from bacterial DNA sequences. *Interdiscip.Sci.* 1, 81-90.

Moss, F., Ward, L. M., & Sannita, W. G. (2004). Stochastic resonance and sensory information processing: a tutorial and review of application. *Clin.Neurophysiol.* 115, 267-281.

Movsesian, M. A. (1999). Beta-adrenergic receptor agonists and cyclic nucleotide phosphodiesterase inhibitors: shifting the focus from inotropy to cyclic adenosine monophosphate. *J.Am.Coll.Cardiol.* 34, 318-324.

Murray, J. (1993). *Mathematical biology*, 2 ed., Springer-Verlag, Berlin.

Nerbonne, J. M. & Kass, R. S. (2005). Molecular physiology of cardiac repolarization. *Physiol Rev.* 85, 1205-1253.

Niggli, E. & Egger, M. (2002). Calcium quarks. *Front Biosci.* 7, d1288-d1297.

Noble, D. (1962). A modification of the Hodgkin--Huxley equations applicable to Purkinje fibre action and pace-maker potentials. *J Physiol* 160, 317-352.

Noble, D. (2004). Modeling the heart. *Physiology (Bethesda.)* 19, 191-197.

Noble, D. (2006). *The music of life. Biology beyond the genome.*, 1 ed., pp. 1-153. Oxford University Press, Inc., New York, U.S.A.

Penrose, R. (2001). Consciousness, the brain, and spacetime geometry: an addendum. Some new developments on the Orch OR model for consciousness. *Ann.N.Y.Acad.Sci.* 929, 105-110.

Periasamy, A. (2001). Fluorescence resonance energy transfer microscopy: a mini review. *J Biomed.Opt.* 6, 287-291.

Periasamy, A. & Diaspro, A. (2003). Multiphoton microscopy. *J Biomed.Opt.* 8, 327-328.

Periasamy, A., Wallrabe, H., Chen, Y., & Barroso, M. (2008). Chapter 22: Quantitation of protein-protein interactions: confocal FRET microscopy. *Methods Cell Biol.* 89, 569-598.

Rabi, I. I., Zacharias, J. R., Millman, S., & Kusch, P. (1992). Milestones in magnetic resonance: 'a new method of measuring nuclear magnetic moment'. 1938. *J Magn Reson.Imaging* 2, 131-133.

Rosen, Y. & Gurman, P. (2010). MEMS and microfluidics for diagnostics devices. *Curr.Pharm.Biotechnol.* 11, 366-375.

Saliterman, S. S. (2006). *Fundamentals of BioMEMS and Medical Microdevices*, pp. 1-608. SPIE Press Book, London, UK.

Schrödinger, E. (1933). *Mémoires sur la mécanique ondulatoire*, reprinted 1988 ed., pp. 1-234. Jacques Gabay, Paris.

Schrödinger, E. (1944). *What is life?*, reprinted 2006 ed., pp. 1-184. Cambridge University Press, Cambridge.

Sherman, A. & Rinzel, J. (1992). Rhythmogenic effects of weak electrotonic coupling in neuronal models. *Proc.Natl.Acad.Sci.U.S.A* 89, 2471-2474.

Sperelakis, N. (2003). Combined electric field and gap junctions on propagation of action potentials in cardiac muscle and smooth muscle in PSpice simulation. *J Electrocardiol.* 36, 279-293.

Strogatz, S. H. (2003). *Sync: the emerging science of spontaneous order*, pp. 1-338, Penguin Books, London, UK.

Strogatz, S. H. & Stewart, I. (1993). Coupled oscillators and biological synchronization. *Sci.Am.* 269, 102-109.

Sun, Y., Wallrabe, H., Seo, S. A., & Periasamy, A. (2011). FRET Microscopy in 2010: The Legacy of Theodor Forster on the 100th Anniversary of his Birth. *Chemphyschem.* 12, 462-474.

Taegtmeyer, H., Golfman, L., Sharma, S., Razeghi, P., & van Arsdall, M. (2004). Linking gene expression to function: metabolic flexibility in the normal and diseased heart. *Ann.N.Y.Acad.Sci.* 1015, 202-213.

Tamura, T., Said, S., & Gerdes, A. M. (1999). Gender-related differences in myocyte remodeling in progression to heart failure. *Hypertension* 33, 676-680.

Valone, T. (2002). *Harnessing the Wheelwork of Nature: Tesla's Science of Energy*, pp. 1-288. Adventures Unlimited Press, Kempton, U.S.A.

Verbiest, T., Clays, K., & Rodriguez, V. (2009). *Second-order Nonlinear Optical Characterization Techniques: An Introduction*, pp. 1-192. CRC Press Online.

Weiss, K. (2002). Good vibrations: the silent symphony of life. *Evolutionary Anthropology* 11, 176-182.

Wiesenfeld, K. & Jaramillo, F. (1998). Minireview of stochastic resonance. *Chaos.* 8, 539-548.

Winfree, A. T. (1980). *The Geometry of Biological Time*, reprinted 2001 ed., pp. 1-777. Springer-Verlag, NY, Berlin, Heidelberg.

Part 2

Pacemakers in Clinical Practice

3

Clinical Applications of Pacemakers in Patients with Bradycardia and Other Specific Conditions

Guillermo Llamas-Esperón, Vitelio Mariona,
Santiago Sandoval-Navarrete and Rocío Muñoz-Sandoval
Hospital Cardiológica Aguascalientes,
Mexico

1. Introduction

This chapter explains the foundations for permanent pacing and proposes a rational and critical approach about the indications for stimulation which are supported by current scientific evidence. We also review stimulation mode selection in different clinical scenarios, technical aspects of implantation, and outline a follow-up program for patients who carry stimulation devices.

We consider convenient mentioning the initials used to designate the stimulation mode for pacemakers. The first letter refers to the paced chamber (could be 0=none, A=atrium, V=ventricle, D=dual), the second letter refers to the sensed chamber (could be 0=none, A=atrium, V=ventricle, D=dual), and the third letter to the type of response the pacemaker will have when detecting an intrinsic beat (could be 0=none, I=inhibitory, T=trigger, D=dual). There is a forth letter which confirms the presence of a sensor which modulates heart rate in to response physical activity (R=rate response). Thus, a VVI mode pacemaker paces and senses only the right ventricle, and it is inhibited if sensing an intrinsic beat. A DDD pacemaker paces and senses both chambers (right atrium and ventricle) and both leads can be inhibited by an intrinsic beat.

2. Main clinical indications for pacing

Cardiac stimulation through permanent pacing is a therapy that currently is clearly established for the treatment of patients with symptomatic bradycardia due to function alterations in the sinus and atrioventricular (AV) node. There are some indications in asymptomatic patients, which in general, are more controversial, with less scientific evidence in its favour.

2.1 Sinus node dysfunction (SND)

In 1923 Wenckebach described the electrocardiographic characteristics of SND, and in 1968 Ferrer published the manifestations considering it as a clinical entity.[1]

The node is formed, from a cytologic point of view, by P cells and transitional cells. P cells are responsible for the pacemaker function and present as groups of 3 or 4 cells. Transitional cells have two varieties: some connect P cells with the atria and the others form links between the groups of P cells. Sinus node pacemaker activity is widely distributed and its automaticity is modulated by the autonomic function. Parasympathetic stimulation depresses automaticity and favors impulse propagation towards the lower part of the right atrium; on the contrary, sympathetic stimulation increases its automaticity and atrial activation starts in the upper part of the atrium.[2]

The sinus node has a central portion responsible for the origin of the stimulus, and another which is peripheral, in charge of the conduction towards the atria; the last one is separated from the atrial myocardium by a band of connective tissue. Aging is associated with structural changes in the sinus node: increase in the amount of collagen, decrease in connexin (Cx43) expression, and possibly decrease in I_{Na} flow in the node periphery (the center of the node does not express that flow). [3] These alterations, either in the formation and/or propagation of the atrial impulse, condition a broad variety of presentations such as:

- Persistent sinus bradycardia
- Chronotropic incompetence without identifiable causes
- Paroxysmal or persistent sinus arrest compensated by escape rhythms in the ventricular myocardium, in the AV junction and in some cases as paroxysmal or persistent atrial fibrillation (AF).

The bradycardia-tachycardia syndrome is the association between sinus bradycardia and/or sinus arrest and AF.[4] In this case tachycardia events depress node automatism by a suppression mechanism secondary to overstimulation. This way when tachycardia ceases abruptly, arrest or asystole supervene due to failure in the inferior pacemakers to rescue the heart rate. [5]

2.1.1 Epidemiology

SND presents in the elderly, usually between the sixth and seventh decades of life.[6,7] Although it can present at any age as a secondary phenomenon due to any alteration that implies sinus node cell destruction, such as heart surgery, inflammation or ischemia. It conditions an annual complete AV block incidence of 0.6%, with 2.1% prevalence. [7,8]

2.1.2 Clinical ma ions

Clinical manifestations are variable and can go from an asymptomatic stage, to subtle symptoms like dyspnea due to chronotropic incompetence (an inadequate response of heart rate to physical activity), to dizziness, to the most dramatic which is syncope. [9]

2.1.3 Diagnosis

The following are tests which can be helpful to diagnose SND:

- An electrocardiogram should be the initial test, although due to the briefness it may not completely correlate with the symptoms.
- A treadmill test is useful to evaluate chronotropic response, it should be considered positive when the patient cannot reach 70% of the expected heart rate according to the age. [10]
- 24-hour holter monitoring is recommended when symptoms are regular; when the symptoms are sporadic an implantable loop recorder is an excellent alternative. [11]

Electrophysiological studies evaluate sinus function through two methods: 1) sinus node recovery time, which analyzes node automaticity after a suppression period after overstimulation; 2) sinoatrial conduction time, which analyzes the conduction time to the sinus node and from the sinus node to the atrium as a response to atrial extrastimuli.[12]

2.1.4 Treatment

For SND indications as for the rest of the chapter we refer to the classification of recommendations and level of evidence established by different cardiology societies. Currently the only effective method for the treatment of symptomatic SND is the implantation of a permanent pacemaker. See Table 1 for complete recommendations.

Class I	
1.	Is indicated for SND with documented symptomatic bradycardia, including frequent sinus pauses that produce symptoms. (Level of Evidence: C)
2.	Is indicated for symptomatic chronotropic incompetence. (Level of Evidence: C)
3.	Is indicated for symptomatic sinus bradycardia that results from required drug therapy for medical conditions. (Level of Evidence: C)
Class IIa	
1.	Is reasonable for SND with heart rate less than 40 bpm when a clear association between significant symptoms consistent with bradycardia and the actual presence of bradycardia has not been documented. (Level of Evidence: C)
2.	Is reasonable for syncope of unexplained origin when clinically significant abnormalities of sinus node function are discovered or provoked in electrophysiological studies. (Level of Evidence: C)
Class IIb	
1.	May be considered in minimally symptomatic patients with chronic heart rate less than 40 bpm while awake. (Level of Evidence: C)
Class III	
1.	Is not indicated for SND in asymptomatic patients. (Level of Evidence: C)
2.	Is not indicated for SND in patients for whom the symptoms suggestive of bradycardia have been clearly documented to occur in the absence of bradycardia. (Level of Evidence: C)
3.	Is not indicated for SND with symptomatic bradycardia due to nonessential drug therapy. (Level of Evidence: C)

Table 1. Recommendations for permanent pacing in sinus node dysfunction[7]

2.2 Hypersensitive carotid sinus syndrome

It is defined as presyncope or syncope caused by an extreme reflex response to the stimulation of the carotid sinus. This hyperactive response is manifested as asystole equal or greater to 3 seconds, secondary to an AV block and an important decrease on systolic pressure.[13,14] It has two components:

3. Cardioinhibitory: resulting from an increase in the parasympathetic tone and manifested by a decrease in the sinus rate or prolongation of the PR interval, an advanced AV block, alone or in combination.
4. Vasopressor: conditioned by a reduction in the sympathetic activity, resulting in loss of vascular tone and hypotension. This effect is independent of the changes in the heart rate.

For the definite diagnosis it is important to rule out other potentially fatal causes such as ventricular tachycardia and/or ventricular fibrillation. Ultimately, the treatment for symptomatic patients is permanent pacing. See Table 2 for complete recommendations.

Class I
1. Is indicated for recurrent syncope caused by spontaneously occurring carotid sinus stimulation and carotid sinus pressure that induces ventricular asystole of more than 3 seconds. (Level of Evidence: C)
Class IIa
1. Is reasonable for syncope without clear, provocative events and with a hypersensitive cardioinhibitory response of 3 seconds or longer. (Level of Evidence: C)
Class IIb
1. May be considered for significantly symptomatic neurocardiogenic syncope associated with bradycardia documented spontaneously or at the time of tilt-table testing. (Level of Evidence: B)
Class III
1. Is not indicated for a hypersensitive cardioinhibitory response to carotid sinus stimulation without symptoms or with vague symptoms. (Level of Evidence: C) 2. Is not indicated for situational vasovagal syncope in which avoidance behavior is effective and preferred. (Level of Evidence: C)

Table 2. Recommendations for permanent pacing in hypersensitive carotid sinus syndrome and neurocardiogenic syncope[7]

2.3 Acquired atrioventricular block

Patients with abnormalities in the AV conduction can vary from asymptomatic, to having episodes directly related to bradycardia, ventricular arrhythmias or both. It is vitally important to do an adequate clinical evaluation of symptomatic patients, and of the findings in the different diagnostic tests available. Identifying the different degrees of AV block is mandatory to make a satisfactory correlation and consequently an assertive therapeutic decision, which historically has been demonstrated to be a permanent pacemaker when there are symptoms conditioned by this alteration.[15-18] See Table 3 for complete recommendations.

The following is the classification of AV blocks:

4. Anatomically, it is defined as supra-, intra-, or infra-His.
5. AV block is classified as first-, second-, or third-degree (complete) block.
   a. First-degree AV block is defined as abnormal prolongation of the PR interval (greater than 0.20 seconds).
   b. Second-degree AV block is subclassified as type I and type II.
      i. Type I second-degree AV block is characterized by progressive prolongation of the interval between the onset of atrial (P wave) and ventricular (R wave) conduction (PR) before a nonconducted beat and is usually seen in conjunction with QRS. Is characterized by progressive prolongation of the PR interval before a nonconducted beat and a shorter PR interval after the blocked beat.
      ii. Type II second-degree AV block is characterized by fixed PR intervals before and after blocked beats and is usually associated with a wide QRS complex. When AV conduction occurs in a 2:1 pattern, block cannot be classified unequivocally as type I or type II, although the width of the QRS can be suggestive, as just described. Advanced second-degree AV block refers to the blocking of 2 or more consecutive P waves with some conducted beats, which indicates some preservation of AV conduction. In the setting of AF, a prolonged pause (e.g., greater than 5 seconds) should be considered to be due to advanced second-degree AV block.
   c. Third-degree AV block (complete heart block) is defined as absence of AV conduction.

Class I	
1.	Is indicated for third-degree and advanced second-degree AV block at any anatomic level associated with bradycardia with symptoms (including heart failure) or ventricular arrhythmias presumed to be due to AV block. (Level of Evidence: C)
2.	Is indicated for third-degree and advanced second-degree AV block at any anatomic level associated with arrhythmias and other medical conditions that require drug therapy that result in symptomatic bradycardia. (Level of Evidence: C)
3.	Is indicated for third-degree and advanced second-degree AV block at any anatomic level in awake, symptom-free patients in sinus rhythm, with documented periods of asystole ≥3.0 seconds or any escape rate less than 40 bpm, or with an escape rhythm that is below the AV node. (Level of Evidence: C)
4.	Is indicated for third-degree and advanced second-degree AV block at any anatomic level in awake, symptom-free patients with AF and bradycardia with 1 or more pauses of at least 5 seconds or longer. (Level of Evidence: C)
5.	Is indicated for third-degree and advanced second-degree AV block at any anatomic level after catheter ablation of the AV junction. (Level of Evidence: C)
6.	Is indicated for third-degree and advanced second-degree AV block at any anatomic level associated with postoperative AV block that is not expected to resolve after cardiac surgery. (Level of Evidence: C)
7.	Is indicated for third-degree and advanced second-degree AV block at any anatomic level associated with neuromuscular diseases with AV block, such as myotonic muscular dystrophy, Kearns-Sayre syndrome, Erb dystrophy (limb-girdle muscular dystrophy), and peroneal muscular atrophy, with or without symptoms. (Level of Evidence: B)
8.	Is indicated for second-degree AV block with associated symptomatic bradycardia regardless of type or site of block. (Level of Evidence: B)
9.	Is indicated for asymptomatic persistent third-degree AV block at any anatomic site with average awake ventricular rates of 40 bpm or faster if cardiomegaly or LV dysfunction is present or if the site of block is below the AV node. (Level of Evidence: B)
10.	Is indicated for second- or third-degree AV block during exercise in the absence of myocardial ischemia. (Level of Evidence: C)
Class IIa	
1.	Is reasonable for persistent third-degree AV block with an escape rate greater than 40 bpm in asymptomatic adult patients without cardiomegaly. (Level of Evidence: C)
2.	Is reasonable for first- or second-degree AV block with symptoms similar to those of pacemaker syndrome or hemodynamic compromise. (Level of Evidence: B)
3.	Is reasonable for asymptomatic second-degree AV block at intra- or infra- His levels found at electrophysiological study. (Level of Evidence: B)
4.	Is reasonable for asymptomatic type II second-degree AV block with a narrow QRS. When type II second-degree AV block occurs with a wide QRS, including isolated right bundle-branch block, pacing becomes a Class I recommendation. (Level of Evidence: B)
Class IIb	
1.	May be considered for neuromuscular diseases such as myotonic muscular dystrophy, Erb dystrophy, and peroneal muscular atrophy with any degree of AV block (including first-degree AV block), with or without symptoms, because there may be unpredictable progression of AV conduction disease. (Level of Evidence: B)
2.	May be considered for AV block in the setting of drug use and/or drug toxicity when the block is expected to recur even after the drug is withdrawn. (Level of Evidence: B)
Class III	
1.	Is not indicated for asymptomatic first-degree AV block. (Level of Evidence: B)
2.	2. Is not indicated for asymptomatic type I second-degree AV block at the supra-His (AV node) level or that which is not known to be intra- or infra-Hisian. (Level of Evidence: C)
3.	Is not indicated for AV block that is expected to resolve and is unlikely to recur (e.g., drug toxicity, Lyme disease, or transient increases in vagal tone or during hypoxia in sleep apnea syndrome in the absence of symptoms). (Level of Evidence: B)

Table 3. Recommendations for acquired atrioventricular block in adults[7]

2.4 Congenital atrioventricular block

Indications for permanent pacemaker implantation in patients under 18 year, are in general the same as for adults, there are only a few considerations. 1) There must be clinical correlation between the AV conduction alteration and the symptoms of the patient; 2) bradycardia

Class I	
1.	Is indicated for advanced second- or third-degree AV block associated with symptomatic bradycardia, ventricular dysfunction, or low cardiac output. (Level of Evidence: C)
2.	Is indicated for SND with correlation of symptoms during age-inappropriate bradycardia. The definition of bradycardia varies with the patient's age and expected heart rate. (Level of Evidence: B)
3.	Is indicated for post-operative advanced second- or third-degree AV block that is not expected to resolve or that persists at least 7 days after cardiac surgery. (Level of Evidence: B)
4.	Is indicated for congenital third-degree AV block with a wide QRS escape rhythm, complex ventricular ectopy, or ventricular dysfunction. (Level of Evidence: B)
5.	Is indicated for congenital third-degree AV block in the infant with a ventricular rate less than 55 bpm or with congenital heart disease and a ventricular rate less than 70 bpm. (Level of Evidence: C)
Class IIa	
1.	Is reasonable for patients with congenital heart disease and sinus bradycardia for the prevention of recurrent episodes of intra-atrial reentrant tachycardia; SND may be intrinsic or secondary to antiarrhythmic treatment. (Level of Evidence: C)
2.	Is reasonable for congenital third-degree AV block beyond the first year of life with an average heart rate less than 50 bpm, abrupt pauses in ventricular rate that are 2 or 3 times the basic cycle length, or associated with symptoms due to chronotropic incompetence. (Level of Evidence: B)
3.	Is reasonable for sinus bradycardia with complex congenital heart disease with a resting heart rate less than 40 bpm or pauses in ventricular rate longer than 3 seconds. (Level of Evidence: C)
4.	Is reasonable for patients with congenital heart disease and impaired hemodynamics due to sinus bradycardia or loss of AV synchrony. (Level of Evidence: C)
5.	Is reasonable for unexplained syncope in the patient with prior congenital heart surgery complicated by transient complete heart block with residual fascicular block after a careful evaluation to exclude other causes of syncope. (Level of Evidence: B)
Class IIb	
1.	May be considered for transient postoperative third-degree AV block that reverts to sinus rhythm with residual bifascicular block. (Level of Evidence: C)
2.	May be considered for congenital third-degree AV block in asymptomatic children or adolescents with an acceptable rate, a narrow QRS complex, and normal ventricular function. (Level of Evidence: B)
3.	May be considered for asymptomatic sinus bradycardia after biventricular repair of congenital heart disease with a resting heart rate less than 40 bpm or pauses in ventricular rate longer than 3 seconds. (Level of Evidence: C)
Class III	
1.	Is not indicated for transient postoperative AV block with return of normal AV conduction in the otherwise asymptomatic patient. (Level of Evidence: B)
2.	Is not indicated for asymptomatic bifascicular block with or without first-degree AV block after surgery for congenital heart disease in the absence of prior transient complete AV block. (Level of Evidence: C)
3.	Is not indicated for asymptomatic type I second-degree AV block. (Level of Evidence: C)
4.	Is not indicated for asymptomatic sinus bradycardia with the longest relative risk interval less than 3 seconds and a minimum heart rate more than 40 bpm. (Level of Evidence: C)

Table 4. Recommendations for permanent pacing in children, adolescents, and patients with congenital heart disease[7]

without associated symptoms is not a justification for permanent device implantation; 3) it is fundamental to consider the implantation site according to the size of the device and the height of the patient, keeping in mind alternatives such as the epicardic.

The most common indications for permanent pacing in this group of patients are:
a) advanced second-degree AV block; b) third-degree AV block; c) bradycardia-tachycardia syndromes, and d) symptomatic sinus bradycardia.[19,20] As always diagnosis should be done correlating clinical and tests findings. Exhaustive search of causes that could be triggering this disease should always be considered. See Table 4 for complete recommendations.

2.5 Chronic bifascicular block

Syncope is the most common manifestation in patients with bifascicular block, fortunately despite the recurrence, is not associated with increase on sudden death. [21,22] That cannot be stated for patients with third-degree AV block, in this case if they present syncope there is an increase in the incidence of sudden death.[23] It is important to consider an electrophysiological study to evaluate and treat ventricular arrhythmias.[24] Bifascicular block refers to ECG evidence of impaired conduction below the AV node in the right and left bundles. Alternating bundle-branch block (also known as bilateral bundle-branch block) refers to situations in which clear ECG evidence for block in all 3 fascicles is manifested on successive ECGs.

All of these considerations oblige us to make a certain diagnosis to give the optimal treatment to these patients. See Table 5 for complete recommendations.

Class I	
1.	Is indicated for advanced second-degree AV block or intermittent third- degree AV block. (Level of Evidence: B)
2.	Is indicated for type II second-degree AV block. (Level of Evidence: B)
3.	Is indicated for alternating bundle-branch block. (Level of Evidence: C)
Class IIa	
1.	Is reasonable for syncope not demonstrated to be due to AV block when other likely causes have been excluded specifically ventricular tachycardia. (Level of Evidence: B)
2.	Is reasonable for an incidental finding at electrophysiological study of a markedly prolonged HV interval (greater than or equal to 100 milliseconds) in asymptomatic patients. (Level of Evidence: B)
3.	Is reasonable for an incidental finding at electrophysiological study of pacing-induced infra-His block that is not physiological. (Level of Evidence: B)
Class IIb	
1.	May be considered in the setting of neuromuscular diseases such as myotonic muscular dystrophy, Erb dystrophy, and peroneal muscular atrophy with bifascicular block or any fascicular block, with or without symptoms. (Level of Evidence: C)
Class III	
1.	Is not indicated for fascicular block without AV block or symptoms. (Level of Evidence: B)
2.	Is not indicated for fascicular block with first-degree AV block without symptoms. (Level of Evidence: B)

Table 5. Recommendations for permanent pacing in chronic bifascicular block[7]

2.6 Pacing for atrioventricular block associated with Acute Myocardial Infarction

Pharmacological and mechanical reperfusion therapies have favored decrease in the incidence of AV block associated to acute myocardial infarction (AMI). [25] Indications for permanent pacing in patients with AMI depend on the intraventricular conduction defect, which does not necessarily depends on the symptoms or on the fact that the patient required transitory pacing. When an AV block or an intraventricular conduction block appears after an AMI, the localization of the AMI and the type of conduction alteration should be considered for permanent pacing.[26, 27] See Table 6 for complete recommendations.

Class I	
1.	Is indicated for persistent second-degree AV block in the His-Purkinje system with alternating bundle-branch block or third-degree AV block within or below the His-Purkinje system after ST-segment elevation MI. *(Level of Evidence: B)*
2.	Is indicated for transient advanced second-or third-degree infranodal AV block and associated bundle-branch block. If the site of block is uncertain, an electrophysiological study may be necessary. *(Level of Evidence: B)*
3.	Is indicated for persistent and symptomatic second- or third-degree AV block. *(Level of Evidence: C)*
Class IIb	
1.	May be considered for persistent second- or third-degree AV block at the AV node level, even in the absence of symptoms. (Level of Evidence: B)
Class III	
1.	Is not indicated for transient AV block in the absence of intraventricular conduction defects. *(Level of Evidence: B)*
2.	Is not indicated for transient AV block in the presence of isolated left anterior fascicular block. *(Level of Evidence: B)*
3.	Is not indicated for new bundle-branch block or fascicular block in the absence of AV block. *(Level of Evidence: B)*
4.	Is not indicated for persistent asymptomatic first-degree AV block in the presence of bundle-branch or fascicular block. *(Level of Evidence: B)*

Table 6. Recommendations for permanent pacing after the acute phase of myocardial infarction[7]

3. Indications for pacing in other specific conditions

There are other specific conditions in which stimulation through pacemakers can achieve beneficial clinical effects, with more or less scientific evidence in its favor.

3.1 Neurocardiogenic syncope

Syncope can be defined as a transitory loss of conscience related with the loss of posture (eventually falling to the floor). Frequently is referred as fainting, and can be the cause of hospitalization in 6% of patients admitted to a general hospital. Neurocardiogenic syncope is a frequent clinical entity in children and adults, generally associated to a benign prognosis. The concept known as neurally mediated syncopal syndrome can be represented by the hypersensitive carotid sinus syndrome, vasovagal syncope also known as neurocardiogenic syncope, and recently related with autonomic dysfunction and positional syncope. This is the origin in more than half of unexplained syncope at any age. Neurocardiogenic syncope has prevalence in general population of 22%[28] and it is conditioned by a triggering stimulus of a neural autonomic reflex, usually self-limited, which conditions arterial hypotension secondary to peripheral vasodilatation and/or important bradycardia or transitory asystole.

The majority of patients can be satisfactorily treated with drugs such as beta-blockers (atenolol), selective serotonin reuptake inhibitors (paroxetine), water retention drugs (fludrocortisone) and some vasoconstrictors (midodrine) as well as dietary measures, such as high salt intake, exercise and lifestyle modifications. Nevertheless a small group of patients is affected by frequent fainting that can disturb daily living, and others can present episodes similar to sudden death which does not improve with the usual therapeutic measures. Some authors have called this type of manifestations as "malignant" neurocardiogenic syncope, because of recurrent falls and even physical trauma.[29] Some of these patients can have prolonged asystole or important bradycardia during the neurocardiogenic syncope, that is why the placement of a pacemaker has been proposed and could be justified, although this is highly controversial. Various randomized trials have shown important reduction in the number of syncopal events in selected patients, although in the first studies, the patients were assigned at random to receive or not cardiac stimulation and this could be related to a placebo effect.[30,31,32] Afterwards, in two trials the pacemaker was placed on all the patients and then randomized to have it "on" or "off" to avoid the placebo effect. Neither study demonstrated significant difference on a 6 month follow up. However one of the studies showed that the most benefited patients with this therapeutic where those with asystole, compared to those with marked bradycardia.[33,34,35] We must remember that up to 25% of patients with neurocardiogenic syncope have a dominant vasodepressor component without significant bradycardia, and most likely those patients have the least benefit with a pacemaker. It is estimated that approximately one third of the patients have bradycardia or asystole as cause of syncope in the tilt-table test or during the spontaneous syncopal episodes. The SYMPACE trial established that the recurrence of syncope was prolonged even more in the patients with asystole than the patients with bradycardia (91 days vs. 11 days).[35] Some studies demonstrated a beneficial effect on induced syncope during the tilt-table test.[36,37]

Seventy-seven patients included in 3 studies which had syncope during the tilt-table test, improved substantially after placement of a dual-chamber pacemaker.[38,39,40] However, other studies were not able to demonstrate the ability to avoid syncope, in some patients (82%) after placement of the pacemaker a tilt-table test was repeated and they only had presyncope. Thus it was possible to demonstrate that 80 to 90% of patients had marked symptomatic improvement reducing up to 90 to 95% the number of expected syncopal events.[13] Three randomized controlled studies commented nevertheless, that in selected patients it is possible to demonstrate benefits in most of them.[30,31,32] In the Second Vasovagal Pacemaker Study (VPS II), 100 patients were included and received a pacemaker. Then they were randomized to pacing with rate drop sensing, or sensing without pacing. The cumulative risk of syncope at 6 months was 40% for the control group and 31% for the actively paced group. The relative risk reduction in time to syncope with pacing was 30% (1 $p = 0.14$).[33] Nonetheless they concluded that pacemaker placement should not be used as a first line therapy in these patients.

Although since the 90s it has been accepted by the Therapeutic Guidelines of the Cardiac Stimulation British Group and the AHA/ACC, the use of pacemakers for the treatment of severe neurocardiogenic syncope, should not be considered as first line treatment. However it can be considered in those patients with recurrent syncope despite optimal medical treatment, mainly in patients without prodromal symptoms that allow them to have precautions at the beginning of the episode. Also, in those in which pacing can reduce the frequency of syncope and/or prolong the time since the beginning of symptoms to the loss of conscience episode, thus facilitating necessary measures to avoid falling, like sitting or lying down.

In the other hand we must have in mind that the symptoms in the patient with neurocardiogenic syncope are partially secondary to bradycardia, which can be prevented by pacing, but greatly peripheral vasodilatation is the producing mechanism. It is important to stress the fact that although prolonged asystole, provoked or spontaneous, can be worrying, usually the prognosis is benign in those patients even without pacemaker.41

In the patient with an intense cardioinhibitory response in the tilt-table test, placement of dual-chamber pacemaker can be an alternative to the medical therapy, especially in the highly symptomatic patient, and primarily when other therapeutic alternatives have failed.

Early detection of imminent neurocardiogenic syncope by the sensing system of the pacemaker is an important factor when defining the best strategy of stimulation, as it is the optimal method of stimulation. We must remember that the drop in the heart rate is usually insidious and not abrupt and it is usually accompanied by peripheral vasodilatation. Ammirati et al compared rate drop responsiveness and rate hysteresis. They demonstrated a benefit for those with rate drop responsiveness (0/12 fainted) compared with rate hysteresis (3/8 fainted).[42] Mc Leod et al compared three groups of symptomatic patients: 1) without pacemaker, 2) single-chamber pacemaker and, 3) dual-chamber pacemaker. They established that both pacing modes were equivalent, and more effective than no pacing, in preventing syncope. Dual-chamber pacing was superior to VVI pacing in preventing presyncope.[43] Some authors think that high stimulating frequency (120 beat per minute), can be superior to standard stimulating frequency (80 beats per minute) to improve symptoms and avoid syncopal episodes.[44]

Most of the patients with a pacemaker placed to correct the cardioinhibitory component of cardioneurogenic syncope, can also receive complementary medical therapy to inhibit the peripheral vasodilatation component. Patient-activated drug delivery systems using phenylephrine have been used to abort syncopal episodes with encouraging preliminary results.[45]

We can conclude that although pacing is not the first line therapy in patients with neurocardiogenic syncope, in some cases in which frequency and intensity of fainting deteriorates quality of life, and mainly in those in which the cardioinhibitory effect during the tilt-table test, could benefit with placement of dual-chamber pacemaker programmed with a drop response algorithm with high stimulating frequencies (120 beats per minute). For complete recommendations see Table 2.

3.2 Neuromuscular diseases

In some neuromuscular diseases such as myotonic dystrophy and Emery-Dreifuss muscular dystrophy, some patients can develop ventricular arrhythmias and atrioventricular disorders which can progress to complete AV block. In these patients permanent pacing will possibly be required.[47] Some authors have demonstrated disappearance of Stokes-Adams episodes through pacemaker implantation.[48] In these cases the recommendations will be those indicated for AV block.

3.3 Long-QT syndrome

In patients with congenital long-QT syndrome, therapy with ß-adrenergic blockers should be consider the first line of treatment, will be continued for life and should be supplemented with implantation of a permanent pacemaker only in cases where bradycardia or AV block is an important characteristic of the syndrome.[49] The use of oral ß-adrenergic blockers, is

considered the standard therapy and are usually successful in the long-term preventive treatment of important arrhythmias, however is has been demonstrated that in some patients a permanent pacing is fundamentally necessary, and even so the implantation of a cardioverter-defibrillator.
It is recommendable that besides the implantation of a pacemaker, ß-Adrenergic blocker therapy be continued.[50] Some consider that because of the availability of the cardioverter-defibrillator with dual-chamber pacing capabilities, and given the high risk in some patients it could be adequate to use it as first line therapy in symptomatic patients with high risk of sudden death. But since cardioverter-defibrillators do not prevent torsade de pointes, these patients should also continue with ß-adrenergic blockers.[51] See Table 7 for complete recommendations.

Class I
1. Is indicated for sustained pause-dependent VT, with or without QT prolongation. (Level of Evidence: C)
Class IIa
1. Is reasonable for high-risk patients with congenital long-QT syndrome. (Level of Evidence: C)
Class IIb
1. May be considered for prevention of symptomatic, drug-refractory, recurrent AF in patients with coexisting SND. (Level of Evidence: B)
Class III
1. Is not indicated for frequent or complex ventricular ectopic activity without sustained VT in the absence of the long-QT syndrome. (Level of Evidence: C)
2. Is not indicated for torsade de pointes VT due to reversible causes. (Level of Evidence: A)

Table 7. Recommendations for pacing to prevent tachycardia[7]

3.4 Hypertrophic Obstructive Cardiomyopathy (HOCM)

HOCM is a primary myocardial disease, characterized by asymmetric hypertrophy of the interventricular basal septum, conditioning reduction between the posterior wall of the left ventricle (LV) and the septum, leading to abnormal systolic anterior motion of the anterior mitral leaflet, which generates dynamic obstruction of the LV outflow tract (LVOT). This obstruction causes significant gradient with important symptoms, predominantly during effort, such as dyspnea, angina, syncope, or even sudden death. Most of the patients with HOCM have normal or above normal systolic LV function. It is common to find stiffness of the LV due to hypertrophy, conditioning considerable diastolic dysfunction that generates a high LV end-diastolic pressure with reduced diastolic volumes, contributing to the symptoms (dyspnea). The clinical evolution is extremely variable, great proportions are asymptomatic, but 25% have important obstruction with abundant symptoms and bad prognosis. HOCM is considered the most frequent cause of effort-induced syncope or sudden death in people younger than 30 years.
Treatment has the primordial purpose of reducing LVOT gradient, facilitating systolic flow and improving diastolic filling, which also improves symptoms. The mayor conditioners of LVOT obstruction are systolic septal bulging, malposition of the anterior papillary muscle, drag forces, and hyperdynamic LV contraction conditioning the Venturi effect. Some investigators have demonstrated that afterload reduction with vasodilator agents, such as nitroglycerin, increases the gradient, as do positive inotropic drugs like digoxin, β-agonists, and exercise which also has positive inotropic effect.

The management of patients with HOCM comprises different areas: a) activity restriction to avoid volume depletion, b) improvement of symptoms and quality of life, c) improvement of survival rate and prevention of sudden death, d) to prevent and correct complications (syncope and arrhythmias), and finally e) screening of relatives.

Medical treatment has been used for chronic symptomatic HOCM patients, but in a small percentage (10%) of cases surgical options can be justified, if symptoms or an important LVOT gradient persist. Dual-chamber pacing (DDD) has been used in patients with HOCM without response to medical treatment.[52,53,54,55] In the early 90s permanent pacing was proposed not only as an alternative, but as a substitute of myectomy. The principle that explained the beneficial effect of DDD pacing was by achieving pre stimulation of the right ventricle apex, that way the LV empties before the basal portion contracts and conditions dynamic obstruction. It requires a precise adjustment on the ventricular stimulation (AV interval), that way at rest or exertion the pacemaker stimulates the apex and the distal septal region, without compromising ventricular filling or cardiac output. It improves the gradient and symptoms by 25%, although in most cases improvement has been measured based on the patient´s perception, which in most cases is only for short periods of time. Some think that pacing can condition deterioration of diastolic function[56], gradient decrease can be associated to important ventricular filling alterations and fall on the cardiac output, and LVOT gradient reduction can be quite modest and less than the one obtained by surgical myectomy.[53,54] Improvement on functional ability has not been demonstrated by pacing. Some authors even think that the perceived improvement after the pacemaker placement can be a placebo effect.[57,58,59,60,61]

Pacemakers have not demonstrated reduction in the risk of sudden death, nor conditions favourable LV remodelling. Some have suggested that DDD pacing can remodel and attenuate the hypertrophic septum as years goes by[54], but it has not been confirmed in prospective studies. There are three prospective randomized studies that analyzed the benefits of permanent pacing in the HOCM patient, without demonstrating the clinical or functional benefit. In fact, in one of the patients, after 9 months the LVOT gradient was similar to the one before surgery.[59,60]

The ACC/AHA guidelines for pacing consider it as class IIb in patients with symptomatic HOCM, and unresponsive to medical treatment, and class III in the patients that improve with β-blockers or calcium channel blockers. Even though the indications are clear, some studies in which the main objective is to define pacemaker utility, have included mildly symptomatic patients or even cases in which resting obstruction is not demonstrable, and only appears with provocation maneuvers[59] or even with dobutamine infusion.[62] Pacemaker implantation can be influenced by: a) implantation is simple and less invasive compared to myocardial ablation, b) common method, most cardiologists are familiarized with the technique, c) commonly used drugs are employed, without side effects like bradycardia, d) surgical myectomy or percutaneous transluminal septal myocardial ablation (PTSMA) can be done at a later time, e) it can be withdrawn or inactivated at any time. A useful strategy can be to place a temporary pacemaker and do hemodynamic measurements. If the gradient is not lowered, there will not be any benefit by placing a permanent pacemaker.[63,64,65] Some authors think that in patients over 65 years, pacing may condition clinical and hemodynamic improvement[60] and represents less risk than surgical myectomy and PTSMA. In patients with pacemakers we have the advantage of being able to increase β-blockers or verapamil doses, since they are protected from the deleterious effects like bradycardia. On the other hand, we can delay AV nodal conduction and facilitate synchronization and ventricular apex pre stimulation.

In 1995, a group of investigators placed a DDD pacemaker on a group of paediatric patients with non obstructive asymptomatic hypertrophic cardiomyopathy, in an attempt to interfere with genetic forces that later on, could develop LVOT obstruction. This was deeply criticized and nowadays is not considered as a therapeutic option in these patients.[66,67,68] Maron et al demonstrated in a group of patients older than 65 years, objective improvement of symptoms after DDD pacing. Yufu et al analyzed results in one patient, after placement of one apical epicardial electrode on the LV, with apparent improvement. Komsuoglu et al reported the case of one patient with resting LVOT gradient of 130 mmHg, that reduced to 100 mmHg with DDD pacing with synchronized right auricular and ventricular stimulation, and reduced it to 20 mmHg after the placement of a biventricular pacemaker (atrial sensing and synchronous right and left ventricular pacing), placing percutaneously the LV electrode on the distal segment of the cardiac veins to have an early stimulation of the posterolateral LV wall. Unlike Yufu, they did not found improvement by stimulating only the LV.

In patients with high risk of severe ventricular arrhythmias or even on survivors of sudden death, the use of an implantable automatic defibrillator has been recommended. Results have been variable in these patients. In patients with ventricular tachycardia usefulness of an implantable defibrillator has been analyzed. In patients with high LVOT gradient in which an implantable cardioverter defibrillator (ICD) is indicated, we can obtain larger benefit if we use the DDD or biventricular component of the ICD.

4. Selecting the stimulation mode

The main issues to take into account in the decision-making process to determine the optimal pacing mode are: the diagnosis that is causing the permanent cardiac stimulation indication, the need to maintain AV synchrony and the presence of chronotropic incompetence that demands to implant a device with rate response sensor. Other special features can influence the pacemaker type and the stimulation mode selection, for example: devices with capability to deliver atrial therapies (AF prevention or antitachycardia stimulation), prolonged longevity battery, automatic capture verification, etc.

4.1 Sinus Node Dysfunction (SND)

The algorithm in Figure 1 synthesizes the critical path in pacing mode selection for SND. Given the fact that in a patient with SND and normal AV conduction, the cardinal problem is sinus impulse generation, at least theoretically, ideal pacing mode is AAI. However, other methods have been studied, namely right ventricular pacing (VVI) and DDD. The current evidence that helps to guide the decision in this aspect is exposed in the next sections.

4.1.1 Risk of AV block development

An important matter is the concern about the risk of AV block in the following years after pacemaker implantation. In the Danish study directed by Nielsen et al, (atrial vs. dual-chamber pacing), the incidence of symptomatic AV block after a follow-up period of 2.9 years, was 1.9% per year.[69]

4.1.2 Atrial based versus ventricular pacing protocols

There is little information comparing atrial stimulation with other modalities. The only major randomized trial that included a true atrial pacing arm (AAI) compared with VVI was the reported by Andersen and colleagues. They found a beneficial effect of atrial pacing sustained over time (8 years of follow-up), with improvement in survival, less atrial fibrillation, fewer thromboembolic complications, less heart failure, and a low-risk of atrioventricular block.[70,71]

In the Danish study, when atrial pacing was compared with dual-chamber stimulation, DDDR pacing caused increase in left atrium diameter and AF resulted significantly less common during AAIR pacing.[69]

Furthermore, there are few doubts about the obtained benefits by aiming to preserve the intrinsic ventricular activation. The MOST substudy linked the RV pacing rate with the risk of hospitalization due to heart failure and the probability to develop AF.[72] Moreover, in the DAVID study (patients with implantable defibrillator), primary outcome of death or heart failure (HF) hospitalization was less common (13.3 vs. 22.6%) in the group that maintained intrinsic ventricular rhythm in comparison with patients with predominant ventricular paced rhythm.[73]

A meta-analysis of the five main trials showed a significant reduction in the AF incidence and, possibly, ictus incidence, when selected pacing mode was an atrial based protocol (AAI/DDD) against ventricular single-chamber protocols.[74]

4.1.3 Algorithms to reduce ventricular stimulation in SND

Assuming the fact that ventricular stimulation has deleterious effects in cardiac function, stimulation protocols have been conceived attempting to reduce right ventricular pacing. Basically, there are two modalities: those who include AV interval (AVI) lengthening, and the minimal ventricular pacing (MVP) protocol. The first consist in programming a prolonged basal AV interval or an algorithm of AV hysteresis. AV hysteresis consists basically in a gradual lengthening of the programmed AV interval to determine if an intrinsic ventricular depolarization occurs within certain interval. In the MVP protocol, a DDDR stimulation mode changes to AAIR when spontaneous AV conduction is detected. When AV block occurs persistently, then AAIR mode turns into DDDR. This protocol has demonstrated to reduce ventricular stimulation rate in a larger proportion than other algorithms. In fact, the SAVEPACE trial, that included 1070 patients with dual chamber pacemaker, with and without MVP protocol, reported that patients without MVP showed 99.1% of ventricular pacing, while MVP patients had 9.1%. AF incidence was 7.9% in the MVP group and 12.7% in the other.[75]

4.1.4 Summary

In isolated SND, in absence of AV node conduction abnormalities, seems reasonable to choose an atrial based stimulation mode (AAI or DDD), while programming algorithms favoring intrinsic ventricular activation. This approach appears to be related with a reduction in the incidence of AF, HF related hospitalizations, and possibly, in the occurrence of stroke. Moreover, since AF is not infrequent in patients with SND, is essential to implant a pacemaker with automatic mode switching (AMS).[69-76]

4.2 Atrioventricular block

In most patients with AV block it is desirable to maintain AV synchrony, but mainly in those with LV dysfunction. As has been mentioned before, single-chamber RV stimulation eliminates cardiac activation synchrony, with negative effects in the risk of AF, LV failure,

and mitral regurgitation development.[69,70,71,75] That pathophysiological changes lead to negative clinical outcomes: increase in the incidence of death, HF hospitalizations and ictus.[72,73,74]
On the other hand, advanced age is sometimes advocated as a reason to prefer single-chamber stimulation. At this point, it is noteworthy to mention that almost every main trial was conducted in old people (the population at higher risk of conduction disturbances).[69-75]
When selecting the pacing mode in a patient with AV block, the first question to answer is if there is the desire to maintain the AV synchrony (if patient maintains sinus impulse generation and has no atrial arrhythmias precluding atrial sensing/pacing). The next aspect is to look for chronotropic incompetence, to evaluate the need of a rate response sensor. Then, one can ask if atrial stimulation is desired (for example to prevent AF or to treat supraventricular tachyarrhythmias).
The algorithm in Figure 2 shows a decision tree diagram to determine pacing mode for AV block.

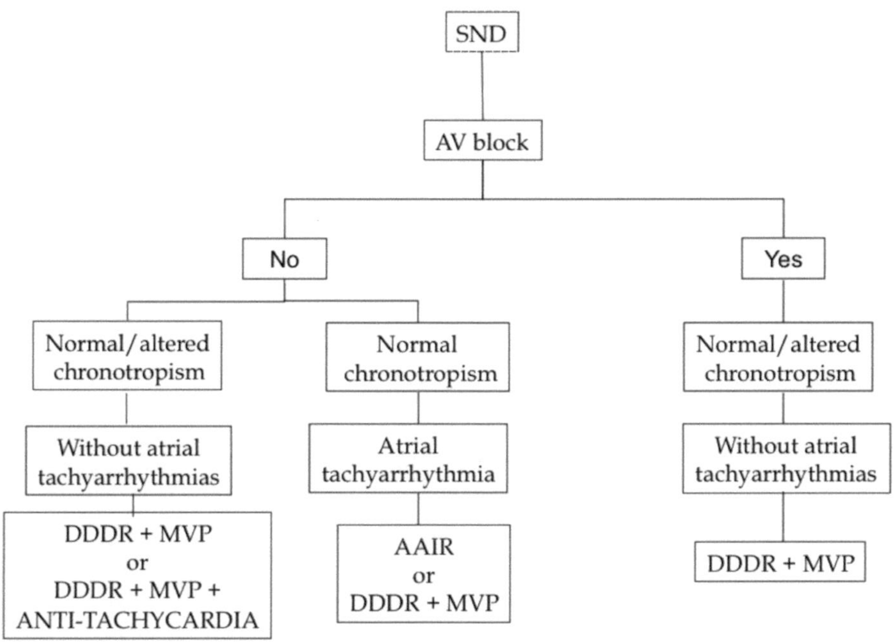

Fig. 1. Selecting the stimulation mode in SND.

4.3 Other indications

Apart from patients suffering from bradyarrhythmia (for example SND and AV block), other pacemaker indications deserve some specific comments about programming.

4.3.1 Neurocardiogenic syncope

Usually, patients do not have basal bradycardia and do not need permanent cardiac stimulation. Pacemaker only stimulates if patient develop bradycardia or asystole as part of a cardioinhibitory response. Moreover, some current devices contain programmable drop rate response algorithms, which activates if sudden bradycardia develops.

4.3.2 Heart failure

Cardiac resynchronization therapy optimal response depends on assuring a constant cardiac stimulation. For this reason, programming an appropriate AV delay and confirming ventricular pacing events (by reviewing counters and histograms) is essential.

4.3.3 Tachyarrhythmias

In the rare cases treated with a pacemaker, algorithms that automatically detects arrhythmia and applies antitachycardia pacing (ATP) exists. ATP needs to be individualized according to the arrhythmia rate and response to therapy.

4.3.4 Hypertrophic cardiomyopathy (HCM)

As in patients with heart failure, LV outflow tract gradient reduction in HCM depends on a constant ventricular stimulation. Attention needs to be paid in programming an appropriate AV delay and confirm ventricular pacing.

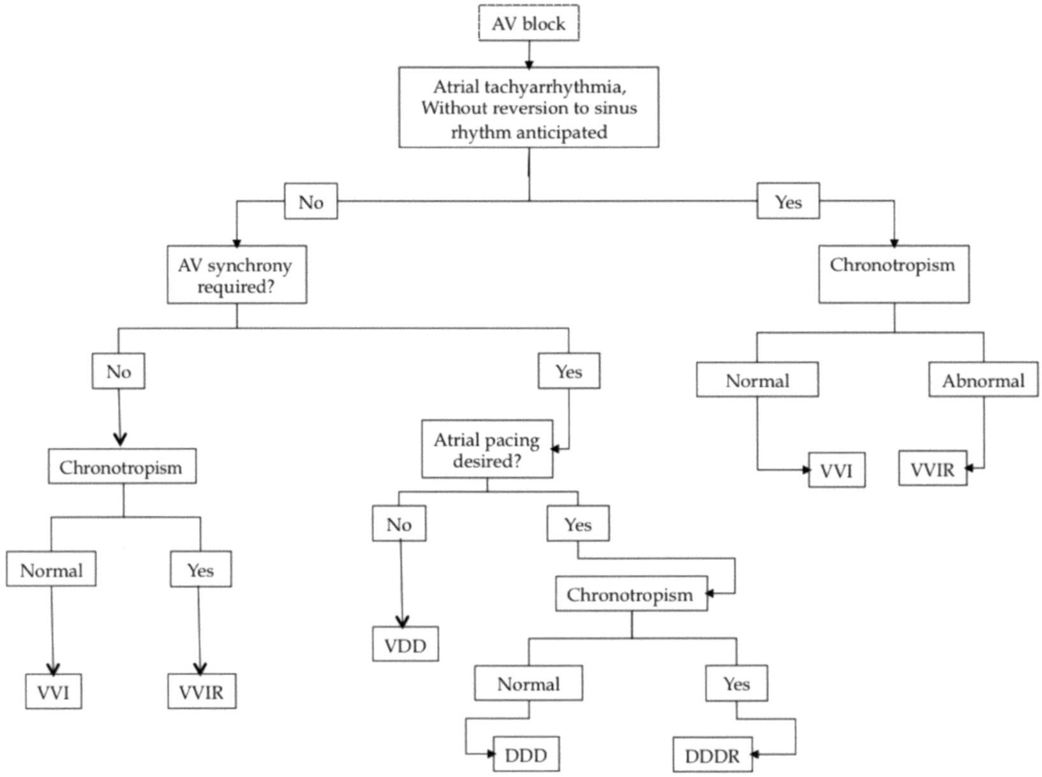

Fig. 2. Selecting the stimulation mode in AV block.

5. Device implantation techniques

A detailed description of the implantation techniques is beyond the scope of this chapter. We will approach some of the more important aspects to consider when a pacemaker is to be implanted.

5.1 Patient preparation

As in any invasive procedure, is mandatory to obtain written consent. A peripheral intravenous line must be placed, preferably in the arm of the planned implant side (of aid in case of requiring venography). Most of pacemaker implants are done in the left thoracic wall, mainly because of operator's choice and comfort. Conscious sedation is optional. Antibiotic prophylaxis is guaranteed and is determined by local antimicrobial guidelines, generally with coverage for G+ and staphylococcus. In the vast majority of cases, a single dose of a penicillin type antibiotic (for example a cephalosporin) can be used within 2 hours before operation. Antibiotics like vancomicyn and gentamicin are becoming more and more used, particularly in patients considered at high risk of infection.

Once in the operation room, implant area is prepared with antiseptic and delimited with sterile towels.[77,78]

5.2 Pocket formation

Three types of incisions are mostly used: deltopectoral, horizontal and oblique. By the time the incision site has been chosen, a local anesthetic is infiltrated at implantation area. In order to make the pacemaker pocket it should be decided if it will be subcutaneous or submuscular, depending on patient's characteristics (subcutaneous tissue thickness) and the pulse generator size. Subcutaneous pocket is easier to make and less painful, but it is imperative to reach the correct layer, the prepectoral fascia. The submuscular pocket requires a shallow incision in the pectoralis major, then blunt dissection up to pectoralis minor (intramuscular) or up to ribcage, beneath pectoralis minor (subpectoral). It is painful, but ordinarily can be performed under conscious sedation.

Pocket can be made before or after venous access, according to operator's preference.[77-79]

5.3 Venous access

Venous access is more frequently obtained by one of two techniques: dissection and vascular incision with direct vein visualization (commonly in the cephalic vein) and by venous puncture (usually directed to the subclavian vein). Cephalic vein dissection has lower pneumothorax and lead crush risk, however, more surgical skill is required and difficulties to introduce more than one lead can arise. Apart from the mentioned techniques, another venous access sites exists, for example, axillary, internal jugular or femoral veins. Nevertheless, although they can be used under certain circumstances, they are not of rutinary choice.[77-79]

5.4 Right ventricular lead placement

Lead placement is facilitated by positioning fluoroscopy in the right anterior oblique (RAO) projection, which helps to define the apex of the RV. The stylet is manually curved in a moderate angle (this action is learned with the experience). With the curved stylet in place, the lead is advanced across the tricuspid valve and then out to the pulmonary artery. Retracting the stylet 1-2 cm usually facilitates passage to the pulmonary artery. Once in the pulmonary artery, the stylet is advanced again to the lead tip. Now, the electrode body is gently retracted up to the midpoint of the interventricular septum. The stylet is retracted 1-2 cm and the floppy lead tip drops into the RV apex. Because the stylet is retracted, the lead tip is supple, precluding perforation of the RV. Adjustment of the tip position can be made by retracting and advancing the electrode, and, if necessary, by changing the curved one for a straight stylet. Gently pulling the electrode is a reliable method to confirm that fixation of the lead has been achieved. This maneuver should not be performed in active fixation leads. Positioning an active fixation lead is similar, but once the lead tip is in the desired position, the helix fixation is released and the stylet removed.[77-79]

5.5 Atrial lead placement

Essentially, there are two techniques, depending on the type of lead selected. If a preformed, passive fixation mechanism, "J" curve lead is utilized, the straight stylet is used to straighten the preformed J. In this case, after the venous access, the lead is advanced to the mid right atrium, and then, the stylet is withdrawn several centimeters while the lead tip gains its J configuration. The lead body is then slowly advanced to push it into the right atrial appendage, which is confirmed by fluoroscopy (in the antero-posterior projection, the tip of the lead will move medial to lateral with each atrial contraction).

When a straight, active fixation lead is selected, then a preformed J stylet is used to take the lead tip to the desired position. Once in there, helix fixation is released and the J stylet removed.[77-79]

5.6 Measuring pacing and sensing thresholds

Every time each lead is positioned and suture-fixed, pacing and sensing thresholds are measured to determine its correct performance.

Table 8 summarizes the acceptable thresholds for the atrial, RV and coronary sinus (CS) leads. Once thresholds are measured, leads are screwed into pacemaker generator and pocket is sutured.[77-79]

	Atrial lead	**RV lead**	**CS (LV) lead**
Voltage threshold	<1.0 V (0.5 ms)	<1.0 V (0.5 ms)	<3.0 V (0.5 ms)
P/R amplitude	≥2.0 mV	≥4.0 mV	≥5.0 mV
Impedance	200-1000 ohm	200-1000 ohm	300-1000 ohm

Table 8. Acceptable pacing and sensing thresholds.

5.7 Procedure related complications

The more frequent procedure related complications are mentioned in Table 9.[80,81]

Eberhardt and colleagues reported the main factors related to procedural complications. They underwent a retrospective analysis of 1884 patients who received a pacemaker. The global complication rate was 4.5%. Complication occurrence was increased by age, reduced LV function, and RV dilatation. Dual-chamber system implantation led to a higher complication rate (6.3%) than implantation of single-chamber (2.6%) or VDD pacemakers (3.2%). These differences were encountered only among operators with a low or medium level of experience.[81]

Moreover, a recent study, with a very large cohort, reported that implant related infections are relatively rare (192 cases/236,888 pacemaker-years, which counts for an incidence rate of 4.82 cases/1000 pacemaker-years) after first implantation. Independent factors associated with an increased risk of infection were a greater number of surgical procedures (including replacements), male sex, younger age, implantation during the earliest part of the study period, and absence of antibiotics.[82]

Pocket complications	Lead complications
Pocket hematoma Infection Erosion Migration of generator Twiddler´s syndrome Generator extrusion	Dislodgement Infection Vein thrombosis Air embolization Diaphragmatic stimulation CS dissection/perforation Myocardial perforation/tamponade

Table 9. Pacemaker implant complications

6. Clinical follow up for patients with pacemaker

Follow up office visits after a pacemaker implant, varies according to each center, but in general, may be performed twice in the first 6 months and then once every 6-12 months. More commonly, patients come to pacemaker checking several times during the first year, and then once or twice a year after that. As elective replacement is approaching, visits should be more frequent. The technician and/or nurse is a very valuable allied in this setting, because they carry out the majority of pacemaker checks at the outpatient consult.[83]

6.1 Main programming parameters

A normal follow-up visit to the outpatient pacemaker clinic may take a few minutes if patient is asymptomatic, there are no activated alarms and main parameters are normal. However, as technology advances, device complexity is arising and today we have multiple programmable parameters. The knowledge of theses parameters and its programmability enables the clinician in the follow-up problem solving process.[84,85]

Table 10 summarizes the main programming parameters and its possible applications.

7. Cost-benefit in pacemakers

Any measure oriented to optimize battery longevity will positively impact cost-efectiveness. Such measures may consist in improving pulse generator and leads technology or in optimizing pacemaker programming (above all, output voltage, pulse width and AV delay). In fact, reprogramming pulse generator may extend the estimated longevity by 4.25 years at a low cost, according to a report of Crossley et al.[86] It is expected that software algorithms, like automatic capture verification, help in increasing battery duration.

Obviously, dual-chamber systems are more expensive. However, considering aspects like quality of life is important in the evaluation of costs. Rinfret et al performed a cost-effectiveness analysis of pacemakers in SND and concluded that dual-chamber pacing increases quality-adjusted life expectancy at a cost that is generally considered acceptable.[87]

Parameter	Programmability	Application
Rate	Increase	Optimize cardiac output. After AV node RF ablation.
	Decrease	Minimize RV pacing. Adjust rate below angina threshold.
Voltage	Increase	Adapt to higher pacing threshold.
	Decrease	Enhance battery longevity. Reduce extracardiac stimulation (phrenic nerve, pectoral muscle).
Sensitivity	Increase	Correction of undersensing of P/R waves.
	Decrease	Correction of oversensing (T wave, myopotentials).
Refractory period	Increase	Atrial: minimize sensing of V far-field potentials. RV: minimize sensing of A far-field potentials (crosstalk).
	Decrease	Detection of early premature ventricular beats.
Hysteresis		Minimize RV pacing.
Detection/stimulation polarity	Conversion to unipolar mode	Optimize signal sensing. To obtain a more secure stimulation.
	Conversion to bipolar mode	Minimize electromagnetic or myopotential interference. Elimination of extracardiac anodal stimulation.
AV interval	Increase or decrease to optimize LV function	Increase: minimize RV pacing. Decrease: adaptative shortening according to heart rate (more physiologic). Optimize AV synchrony in HF.
PVARP	Increase	Prevent sensing of retrograde P waves, treatment of PMT.
PVARP extension after a PVC	On/off	Prevent sensing of retrograde P waves after a PVC
Post-atrial ventricular blanking period	Increase	Prevent crosstalk
Ventricular safety pacing	On/off	Assurance of ventricular stimulation in the presence of crosstalk

Abbreviations: AV= atrioventricular; RF= radiofrequency; RV= right ventricle; V= ventricular; LV= left ventricle; HF= heart failure; PVARP= post ventricular atrial refractory period; PMT= pacemaker mediated tachycardia; VPC= premature ventricular contraction.

Table 10. Main programming parameters and its applications.

8. Future perspectives on cardiac stimulation

There are many areas under investigation and others that need to be covered. The following is a selection of these areas.

Pacemakers availability. Above all in developing countries, further efforts needs to be done to extend pacemaker access to all eligible population.

Pacemakers technology. Improvements in hardware, software, battery and leads technology, will permit to obtain better clinical results as well as improved device performance and duration.

Pacemaker indications. Clinical applications of cardiac stimulation are under extensive research. Aspects like biventricular or LV pacing in patients with normal systolic function or in congenital heart disease needs to be determined.

Remote monitoring. This technology seems to represent a cost-effective tool to maintain an efficient and secure follow-up evaluation as a part of a well organized program. It is necessary to develop guidelines to norm its use.[7]

9. Conclusion

Permanent pacing is a therapy that can be lifesaving, established indications for main clinical syndromes and other specific conditions should be evaluated to offer the patient the best possible treatment. Once implanted determining the optimal stimulation mode is crucial, as it is to keep in mind all the possible complications inherent to the procedure. Clinical follow-up is as important as the implantation technique, to assure the patient the best quality of life possible.

10. References

[1] Ferrer, I. (1968). The sick sinus syndrome in atrial disease. *JAMA,* Vol. 206, pp. 645-652.

[2] James, TN. (2003). Structure and function of the sinus node, AV node and His bundle of the human heart: part II-structure. *Prog Cardiovasc Dis*, Vol. 45, pp. 327-360.

[3] Boyett, MR. (2003). Sophisticated architecture is required for the sinoatrial node to perform its normal pacemaker function. *J Cardiovasc Electrophysiol,* Vol. 14, pp. 104-106.

[4] Sweeney, M.O. (2006). Sinus node dysfunction, In: *Cardiac Electrophysiology,* Douglas P. Zipes and José Jalife, pp. 879-83, Elsevier Inc, New York, USA.

[5] Dreifus, LS. (1983). Bradyarrhythmias: clinical significance and management. *J Am Coll Cardiol,* Vol. 1, pp. 327-338.

[6] Menozzi, C. (1998). The natural course of untreated sick sinus syndrome and identification of variables predictive of infavorable outcome. *Am J Cardiol,* Vol.82, pp. 1205-1209.

[7] Epstein, AE. (2008). ACC/AHA/HRS 2008 Guidelines for Device-Based Therapy of Cardiac Rhythm Abnormalities: A Report of the American College of Cardiology / American Heart Association Task Force on Practice Guidelines (Writing Committee to Revise the ACC/AHA/NASPE 2002 Guideline Update for Implantation of Cardiac Pacemakers and Antiarrhythmia Devices): Developed in Collaboration With the American Association for Thoracic Surgery and Society of Thoracic Surgeons. *Circulation,* Vol. 117, pp. e350-e408.

[8] Rosenqvist, M. (1989). Atrial pacing and the risk for AV block: Is there a time for change in attitude? *Pacing Clin Electrophysiol*, Vol. 12, pp. 97-101.

[9] Mangrum, JM. (2000). The evaluation and Management of bradycardia. *N Engl J Med*, Vol. 342, pp. 703-709.

[10] Kusumoto, FM. (1996). Cardiac pacing. *N Engl J Med*, Vol. 334, pp. 89-98.

[11] Krahn, AD. (2001). Randomized assessment of syncope trial. *Circulation*, Vol. 104, pp. 46-51.

[12] Conti, CR. (1989). ACC/AHA Task force report. Guidelines for clinical intracardiac electrophysiologic studies. *J Am Coll Cardiol*, Vol. 14, pp. 1827-1842.

[13] Sra, JS. (1993). Comparison of cardiac pacing with drug therapy in the treatment of neurocardiogenic (vasovagal) syncope with bradycardia or asystole. *N Engl J Med*, Vol. 328, pp. 1085–1090.

[14] Sugrue, DD. (1986). Symptomatic "isolated" carotid sinus hypersensitivity: natural history and results of treatment with anticholinergic drugs or pacemaker. *J Am Coll Cardiol*, Vol. 7, pp. 158-162.

[15] Dreifus, LS. (1983). Bradyarrhythmias: clinical significance and management. *J Am Coll Cardiol*, Vol. 1, pp. 327–338.

[16] Donmoyer, TL. (1967). Experience with implantable pacemakers using myocardial electrodes in the management of heart block. *Ann Thorac Surg*, Vol. 3, pp. 218-227.

[17] Edhag, O. (1976). Prognosis of patients with complete heart block or arrhythmic syncope who were not treated with artificial pacemakers. A long-term follow-up study of 101 patients. *Acta Med Scand*, Vol. 200, pp. 457-463.

[18] Mymin, D. (1986). The natural history of primary first-degree atrioventricular heart block. *N Engl J Med*, Vol. 315, pp. 1183–1187.

[19] Walsh, EP. (2007). Arrhythmias in adult patients with congenital heart disease. *Circulation*, Vol. 115, pp. 534-545.

[20] Dorostkar, PC. (2005). Asystole and severe bradycardia in preterm infants. *Biol Neonate*, Vol. 88, pp. 299–305.

[21] Fisch, GR. (1980). Bundle branch block and sudden death. *Prog Cardiovasc Dis*, Vol. 23, pp. 187–224.

[22] McAnulty, JH. (1982). Natural history of "high-risk" bundle-branch block: final report of a prospective study. *N Engl J Med*, Vol. 307, pp. 137–143.

[23] Englund, A. (1995). Diagnostic value of programmed ventricular stimulation in patients with bifascicular block: a prospective study of patients with and without syncope. *J Am Coll Cardiol*, Vol. 26, pp. 1508–1515.

[24] Twidale, N. (1988). Clinical implications of electrophysiology study findings in patients with chronic bifascicular block and syncope. *Aust N Z J Med*, Vol. 18, pp. 841–847.

[25] Goldberg, RJ. (1992). Prognosis of acute myocardial infarction complicated by complete heart block (the Worcester Heart Attack Study). *Am J Cardiol*, Vol. 69, pp. 1135–1141.

[26] Col, JJ. (1972). The incidence and mortality of intraventricular conduction defects in acute myocardial infarction. *Am J Cardiol*, Vol. 29, pp. 344–350.

[27] Petrina, M. (2006). The 12-lead electrocardiogram as a predictive tool of mortality after acute myocardial infarction: current status in an era of revascularization and reperfusion. *Am Heart J*, Vol. 152, pp. 11–18.

[28] Chen-Scarabelli, C. (2004). Neurocardiogenic syncope. *BMJ*, Vol. 329, pp. 336-34.

[29] Kurbaan A. (2000). "Malignant" neurocardiogenic syncope. *Indian Pacing and Electrophysiology Journal*. Vol. 12, pp. 11-18.

[30] Connolly, SJ. (1999). The North American Vasovagal Pacemaker Study (VPS): a randomized trial of permanent cardiac pacing for the prevention of vasovagal syncope. *J Am Coll Cardiol*, Vol. 33, pp. 16–20.

[31] Sutton, R. (2000). Dual-chamber pacing in the treatment of neurally mediated tilt positive cardioinhibitory syncope: pacemaker versus no therapy: a multicenter randomized study. *Circulation*, Vol. 102, pp. 294–299.

[32] Ammirati, F. (2001). Permanent cardiac pacing vs. medical treatment for the prevention of recurrent vasovagal syncope: a multicenter, randomized, controlled trial. *Circulation*. Vol. 104, pp. 52–57.

[33] Connolly, SJ. (2003). Pacemaker therapy for prevention of syncope in patients with recurrent severe vasovagal syncope: Second Vasovagal Pacemaker Study (VPS II). *JAMA*, Vol. 289, pp. 2224–2229.

[34] Giada, F. (2003). The vasovagal syncope and pacing trial (SYMPACE): a randomized placebo-controlled study of permanent pacing for treatment of recurrent vasovagal syncope. *Pacing Clin Electrophysiol*, Vol. 26, pp. 1016-1020.

[35] Sutton, K. (2003). Has cardiac pacing a role in vasovagal syncope? *J Intervent Cardiovasc Electrophysiol*, Vol. 9, pp. 145–149.

[36] Fitzpatrick, A. (1991). Dual-chamber pacing aborts vasovagal syncope induced b head-up 60 degree tilt. *PACE*, Vol. 14, pp. 13-19.

[37] Samoil, D. (1993). Comparison of single and dual-chamber pacing techniques in prevention of upright tilt-induced vasovagal syncope. *Eur J Cardiac Pacing Electrophysiol*, Vol. 3, pp. 36-41.

[38] Peterson, M. (1994). Permanent pacing for cardioinhibitory malignant vasovagal syndrome. *Br Heart J*, Vol. 71, pp. 274-281.

[39] Benditt, D. (1997). Clinical experience with Thera DR rate-drop response pacing algorithm in carotid sinus syndrome and vasovagal syncope. The International Rate-Drop Investigators Group. *Pacing Clinic Electrophysiol*, Vol. 20,pp. 832-839.

[40] Sheldon, R. (1998). Effect of dual-chamber pacing with automatic rate-drop sensing on recurrent neurally medicated syncope. *Am J Cardiol*, Vol. 81, pp. 158-162.

[41] Grubb, BP. (1991). Differentiation of convulsive syncope and epilepsy with head-up tilt testing. *Ann Intern Med*, Vol. 115, pp. 871–876.

[42] Ammirati, F. (1998). DDD pacing with rate drop response function versus DDI with rate hysteresis pacing for cardioinhibitory vasovagal syncope. *Pacing Clin Electrophysiol*, Vol. 21, pp. 2178-2191.

[43] McLeod, K. (1999). Cardiac pacing for severe childhood neurally mediated syncope with reflex anoxic seizures. *Heart*, Vol. 82, pp. 721-725.

[44] Kurbaan, A. (1999). Is there an optimal pacing intervention rate for vasovagal syncope? *PACE*, Vol. 22, pp. 707-710.

[45] Giada, F.(2001). Efficacy of a patient-activated drug delivery system using phenylephrine as active drug in aborting tilt-induced syncope. *Pacing Clin Electrophysiol*, Vol. 24, pp. 573-575.

[46] Brignole, M. (2001). Task Force on Syncope, European Society of Cardiology. Guidelines on management, diagnosis and treatment of syncope. *European Heart Journal*, Vol. 22, pp. 1256-1306.

[47] Lazarus, A. (2002). Long-term follow-up of arrhythmias in patients with myotonic dystrophy treated by pacing: a multicenter diagnostic pacemaker study. *J Am Coll Cardiol*, Vol. 40, pp. 1645–1652).

[48] Clements, SD. (1976). Myotonia dystrophica: ventricular arrhythmias, intraventricular conduction abnormalities, atrioventricular block and Stokes-Adams attacks successfully treated with permanent transvenous pacemaker. *Am J Cardiol*, Vol. 37, pp. 933-935.

[49] Viskin, S. (2000). Prevention of ventricular arrhythmias in the congenital long QT syndrome. *Curr Cardiol Rep*, Vol. 2, pp. 492-497.

[50] Viskin, S. (2000). Cardiac pacing in the long QT syndrome: review of available data and practical recommendations. *J Cardiovasc Electrophysiol*, Vol. 11, pp. 593-600.

[51] Kron, J. (1990). The automatic implantable cardioverter-defibrillator in young patients. *J Am Coll Cardiol*, Vol. 16, pp. 896-902.

[52] Nishimura, RA. (1996). Effect of dual-chamber pacing on systolic and diastolic function in patients with hypertrophic cardiomyopathy: acute Doppler echocardiographic and catheterization hemodynamic study. *J Am Coll Cardiol*, Vol. 27, pp. 421-430.

[53] Nishimura, RA. (1997). Dual-chamber pacing for obstructive hypertrophic obstructive cardiomyopathy: a randomized, double-blind, crossover study. *J Am Coll Cardiol*, Vol. 29, pp. 435-441.

[54] Fananapazir, L. (1994). Long-term results of dual-chamber (DDD) pacing in obstructive hypertrophic cardiomyopathy: evidence for progressive symptomatic and hemodynamic improvement and reduction of left ventricular hypertrophy. *Circulation*, Vol. 90, pp. 2731-2742.

[55] Komsuoglu, Baki. (2006). Effect of Biventricular pacing on left ventricular outflow tract pressure gradient in a patient with hypertrophic cardiomyopathy and normal interventricular conduction. *J Cardiovasc Electrophysiol*, Vol. 17, pp. 207-209.

[56] Betocchi, S. (1996). Effects of dual chamber pacing in hypertrophic cardiomyopathy on left ventricular outflow tract obstruction and diastolic function. *Am J Cardiol*, Vol. 77, pp. 498–502.

[57] Jeanrenaud, X. (1992). Effects of dual-chamber pacing in hypertrophic obstructive cardiomyopathy. *Lancet*, Vol. 339, pp. 1318–1323.

[58] Slade, AK. (1996). DDD pacing in hypertrophic cardiomyopathy: a multicentre clinical experience. *Heart*, Vol. 75, pp. 44–49.

[59] Kappenberger, L. (1997). The PIC Study Group. Pacing in hypertrophic obstructive cardiomyopathy.A randomized crossover study. *Eur Heart J*, Vol. 18, pp. 1249–1256.

[60] Maron, BJ. (1999). Assessment of dual-chamber pacing as a treatment for drug-refractory symptomatic patients with obstructive hypertrophic cardiomyopathy: cardiomyopathy: A randomized double-blind, crossover study (MPATHY). *Circulation*, Vol. 99, pp. 2927-2933.

[61] Linde, C. (1997). Does pacemaker implantation have a placebo-effect? Results from the PIC study group. *J Am Coll Cardiol*, Vol. 29, Suppl A:74A.

[62] Lakkis, NM. (1998). Echocardiography-guided ethanol septal reduction for hypertrophic obstructive cardiomyopathy. *Circulation*, Vol. 98, pp. 1750-1755.

[63] Kappenberger, L. (1999). Clinical progress after randomized on/off pacemaker treatment for hypertrophic obstructive cardiomyopathy. Pacing in Cardiomyopathy (PIC) Study Group. *Europace*, Vol.1, pp. 77-84.

[64] Linde, C. (1999). Placebo effect of pacemaker implantation in obstructive hypertrophic cardiomyopathy. Pacing in Cardiomyopathy. *Am J Cardiol*, Vol. 83, pp. 903-907.
[65] Gadler, F. (1999). Significant improvement of quality of life following atrioventricular synchronous pacing in patients with hypertrophic obstructive cardiomyopathy. Data from 1 year of follow-up. PIC Study group. Pacing in Cardiomyopathy. *Eur Heart J*, Vol. 20, pp. 1044-1050.
[66] Frananapazir, L. (1995). Long-term results of dual chamber (DDD) pacing in pediatric patients with obstructive hypertrophic cardiomyopathy. *Circulation*, Vol. 92, Suppl 1, pp. 121-126.
[67] Moss, M. (1996). A US experiment on young children ignites painful database. *The Wall Street Journal*, Vol. 134, pp. A-1 to A-10.
[68] Yufu, K. (2004). Improved hypertrophic obstructive cardiomyopathy by left ventricular apex epicardial pacing. *Intern Med*, Vol. 43, pp. 295-299.
[69] Nielsen, JC. (2003). A randomized comparison of atrial and dual-chamber pacing in 177 consecutive patients with sick sinus syndrome: echocardiographic and clinical outcome. *J Am Coll Cardiol*, Vol. 42, pp. 614–623.
[70] Andersen, HR. (1994). Prospective randomized trial of atrial versus ventricular pacing in sick-sinus syndrome. *Lancet*, Vol. 344, pp. 1523–1528.
[71] Andersen, HR. (1997). Long-term follow-up of patients from a randomized trial of atrial versus ventricular pacing for sick-sinus syndrome. *Lancet*, Vol. 350, pp. 1210–1216.
[72] Sweeney, MO. (2003). Adverse effect of ventricular pacing on heart failure and atrial fibrillation among patients with normal baseline QRS duration in a clinical trial of pacemaker therapy for sinus node dysfunction. *Circulation*, Vol. 107, pp. 2932–2937.
[73] Wilkoff, BL. (2002). Dual-chamber or ventricular backup pacing in patients with an implantable defibrillator. The Dual Chamber and VVI Implantable Defibrillator (DAVID) Trial. *JAMA*, Vol. 288, pp. 3115–3123.
[74] Healey, JS. (2006). Cardiovascular outcomes with atrial-based pacing compared with ventricular pacing: meta-analysis of randomized trials, using individual patient data. *Circulation*, Vol. 114, pp. 11–17.
[75] Sweeney, MO. (2007). The Search AV Extension and Managed Ventricular Pacing for Promoting Atrioventricular Conduction (SAVE-PACE) trial. *N Engl J Med*, Vol. 357, pp. 1000-1008.
[76] Lamas, GA. (2002). Ventricular pacing or dual-chamber pacing for sinus-node dysfunction. *N Engl J Med*, Vol. 346, pp. 1854–1862.
[77] Kim, R. (2009). Permanent pacemaker implantation technique: part I. *Heart*, Vol. 95, pp. 259.
[78] Hayes, DL. (2008). Implantation and extraction techniques. In: *Cardiac pacing, defibrillation and resynchronization. A clinical approach. Second Edition*, Hayes DL, Friedman PA. pp: 144-201. Wiley-Blackwell, ISBN-13:978-1-4051-6748-2, New York, USA.
[79] Bellot, PH. (2008). Device implantation (Pacing Lead Implant techniques). In: *Cardiac pacing for the clinician. Second Edition*, Kusumoto FM, Goldschlager NF, pp 107-256. Springer Science+Business Media, ISBN-13:978-0-387-72762-2, New York, USA.
[80] Hayes, DL. (2008). Implantation-related complications. In: *Cardiac pacing, defibrillation and resynchronization. A clinical approach. Second Edition*. Hayes DL, Friedman PA, pp: 144-201. Wiley-Blackwell, ISBN-13:978-1-4051-6748-2, New York, USA.

[81] Eberhardt, F. (2005). Long term complications in single and dual chamber pacing are influenced by surgical experience and patient morbidity. *Heart*, Vol. 91, pp. 500-506.
[82] Johansen, JB. (2011). Infection after pacemaker implantation: infection rates and risk factors associated with infection in a population-based cohort study of 46299 consecutive patients. *Eur Heart J*, Vol. 32, pp. 991-998.
[83] Van Eck, JW. (2008). Routine follow-up after pacemaker implantation: frequency, pacemaker programming and professionals in charge. *Europace*, Vol. 10, pp. 832–837.
[84] Barold, SS. (2004). Overview of cardiac pacemakers. In: *Cardiac pacemakers step by step. First Edition,* pp: 291-328, Futura-Blackwell Publishing. ISBN 1-4051-1647-1, New York, USA.
[85] Hayes, DL. (2008). Programming. In: *Cardiac pacing, defibrillation and resynchronization. A clinical approach. Second Edition.* Hayes DL, Friedman PA, pp: 301-379. Wiley-Blackwell. ISBN-13:978-1-4051-6748-2, New York, USA.
[86] Crossley, GH. (1996). Reprogramming pacemakers enhances longevity and is cost-effective. *Circulation,* Vol. 94(9 Suppl):II245-7.
[87] Rinfret, S. (2005). Cost-effectiveness of dual-chamber pacing compared with ventricular pacing for sinus node dysfunction. *Circulation,* Vol. 111, pp. 165–172.

4

Permanent Cardiac Pacing in Adults with High Grade Atriovetricular Block and Preserved Left Ventricular Function: Optimal Mode and Site of Pacing

Ouali Sana
Sahloul Hospital University, Sousse
Tunisia

1. Introduction

Cardiac pacing is the only effective treatment for patients with sick sinus syndrome and atrioventricular conduction disorders. In permanently paced patients, cardiac performance and exercise capacity depend on 3 main parameters: the quality of chronotropic function, atrioventricular synchrony, and the ventricular activation sequence.

Dual chamber pacing is believed to have an advantage over single chamber ventricular pacing in that it resembles cardiac physiology more closely by maintaining atrioventricular (AV) synchrony and dominance of the sinus node, which in turn may reduce cardiovascular morbidity and mortality thus contributing to patient survival and quality of life.

However, the prospective studies designed with the objective of analyzing the impact of maintaining AV synchrony on mortality were disappointing. The PASE (Lamas et al, 1998), CTOPP (Connolly et al, 2000), MOST (Lamas et al, 2002) and UKPACE (Toff et al, 2005) studies demonstrated only secondary benefits, such as the decrease in the incidence of atrial fibrillation and improved quality of life, but without any effect on mortality. It has been proposed that the probable deleterious effects of right ventricular stimulation leading to dyssynchrony can annul the benefits obtained with the atrioventricular synchronism. At the same time, there is increasing evidence that conventional pacing from the right ventricular apex was associated with dyssynchronous activation of the left ventricle, resulting in impaired haemodynamic function (Leclercq et al,1995;Wilkoff et al,2002; Schmidt et al, 2007; Tops et al, 2006; Tops et al, 2007).

The detrimental effects of ventricular apical pacing on left ventricular (LV) haemodynamics were demonstrated as early as 1925 by Wiggers (Wiggers, 1925). However, it was not until recently that it became abundantly clear that the time has come to seek alternative ways to minimize or avert the adverse clinical outcomes resulting from the asynchronous contraction pattern that RVA stimulation induces (Wilkoff et al, 2002; Tops et al, 2007, Sweeney et al,2003).

In this Chapter, we attempt to discuss in patients with high grade atrioventricular block and preserved LV function, 1) the optimal mode of pacing (VVI(R)= single chamber, ventricular pacing in the inhibited mode vs DDD=dual chamber pacing and sensing, both triggered and inhibited mode) particularly in elderly patients, 2) the effectiveness and safety of alternative

RV pacing, 3) to compare the effects of alternative RV pacing to RVA pacing on electric and mechanic LV synchrony, systolic and diastolic LV function and outcomes.

2. Pacing mode selection

The pacemaker prescription has the greatest impact on procedural time and complexity, follow-up, patient outcome, and cost: the choice among single-chamber ventricular pacing, and dual-chamber pacing. In 2008, revision of the "ACC/AHA/NASPE Guidelines for Implantation of Cardiac Pacemakers and Antiarrhythmia Devices" have updated the previous versions published in 1984, 1991, 1998, and 2002 (Epstein et al ,2008). These guidelines have included sections on selection of pacemakers in patients with atrioventricular block (Figure 1).

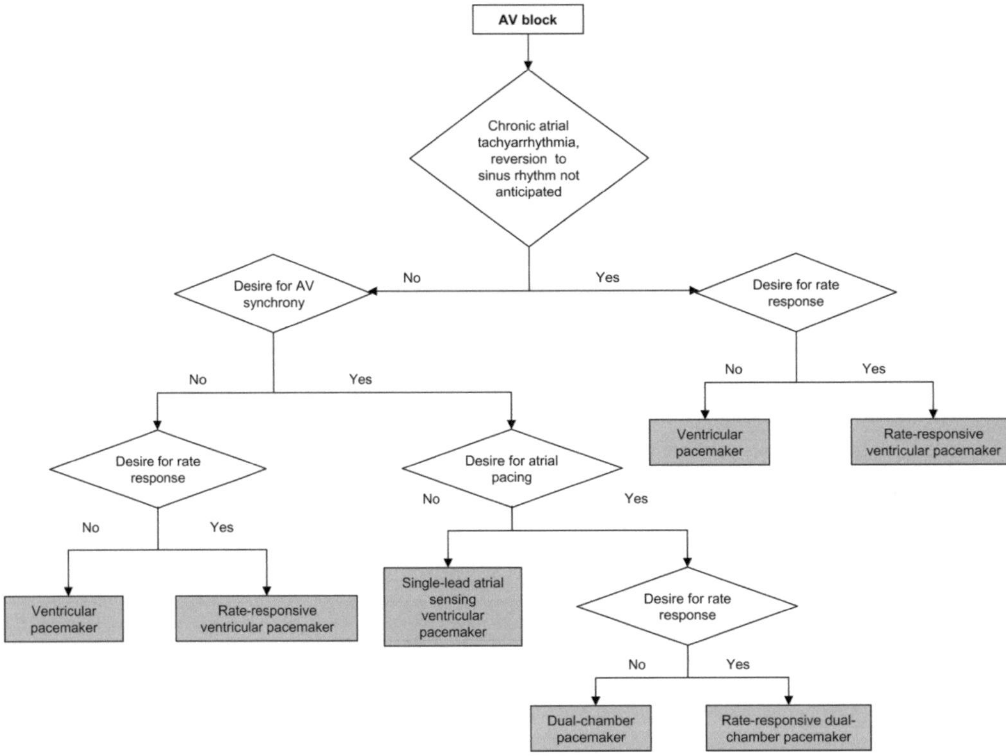

Fig. 1. Selection of Pacemaker Systems for Patients With Atrioventricular Block. Decisions are illustrated by diamonds. Shaded boxes indicate type of pacemaker. AV indicates atrioventricular. (Epstein et al,2008).

As with all clinical practice guidelines, the 2008 recommendations have focused on treatment of an average patient with a specific disorder and may be modified by patient comorbidities, limitation of life expectancy because of coexisting diseases, and other situations that only the primary treating physician may evaluate appropriately.

Augmented life expectancy and increasing health care expenditures have led to questions concerning the routine use of electrotherapy in elderly patients. More than 80% of pacemaker recipients are aged > 65 years. So the selection of the pacing system has important clinical and economic implication. Despite the results of randomized trial (Lamas,1998; Connolly, 2000; Toff, 2005), the use of dual chamber systems, continues to provoke debate particularly in elderly. The several randomized clinical trials such as PASE (Lamas et al,1998), CTOPP (Connolly et al, 2000), MOST (Lamas et al, 2002), and UKPACE (Toff et al, 2005) demonstrated that DDD pacing (dual chamber pacing and sensing, both triggered and inhibited mode), is not superior to VVI (R) pacing (single chamber, ventricular pacing in the inhibited mode with or without rate responsive) in the prevention of death and stroke in patients with conduction disease.

UKPACE (Toff et al, 2005) is a prospective multicenter,randomized, parallel-group trial comparing the clinical benefits of ventricular pacing and dual-chamber pacing in elderly patients with AV block. In this population, the pacing mode does not influence the rate of death from all causes during the first 5 years or the incidence of cardiovascular events during the first 3 years after implantation of a PM. These findings have questioned the justification for implantation of DDD (R) pacing mainly in elderly patients. Unfortunately, a subgroup analysis (Jahangir, 2003) based on pacemaker dependency has not been presented for either the MOST or UKPACE.

Several previous studies have compared dual chamber pacemaker (DDD) and rate-responsive ventricular pacemaker VVIR pacing in elderly patients, and they showed an improvement in symptom scores and objective exercise performances (Jordaens et al,1988; Hargreaves et al,1995; Channon et al,1994). Most studies have demonstrated that the haemodynamic benefits of DDD pacing during maximal exercise result largely from the increase in heart rate rather than from atrioventricular synchrony (Kritensson et al, 1985; Faerestrand & Ohm,1985; Buckingham et al, 1992; Fananapazir,1985). Rate responsive ventricular demand (VVIR) pacing may therefore represent an alternative to DDD pacing in the elderly.

In a recent study published by our institution, we (Ouali et al, 2010) have demonstrated in elderly population (over 70 years) with dual chamber pacemakers inserted for complete AV block, significant benefit from DDD pacing compared with VVIR pacing. There were improvements in HR-QOL questionnaire (SF36), NYHA functional class and echocardiographic parameters. On the contrary, the 6 min walking distance was similar in the two groups.

In this study, 36,6 % of patients deteriorated in NYHA functional class during VVI R pacing (from NYHA class 2,1 ± 0,6 to NYHA class 2,5±0,5), a rate which is consistent with previously published results from studies of a similar design (Naegeli et al, 2007; Rediker et al, 1988; Heldman et al, 1990). Hargreaves et al (Hargreaves et al, 1995) demonstrated that in their elderly population (over 75 years), both total and pacemaker syndrome symptom scores were significantly lower during DDD mode compared with VVI and VVIR modes. However, both exercise performance and the perceived level of exercise (Borg scores) during DDD and VVIR modes were similar. In the opposite, Oldroyed et al (Oldroyed et al,1991) have not identified significant differences between pacing mode (VVIR, and DDD) in patients with complete AV block, in symptoms scores for dyspnea, fatigue, exercise time and maximal oxygen consumption. However, resting plasma concentrations of atrial natriuretic peptide were raised in complete heart block and were restored to normal by DDD pacing but not by VVIR pacing ((Oldroyed et al,1991).

Frielingsdorf et al (Frielingsdorf et al, 1995) have showed that in patients with normal left ventricular function, may profit most from preserved AV synchrony (VDD = ventricular pacing with atrial tracking vs VVIR) as shown by the higher maximum uptake on exercise

and conclude that rate responsive single chamber pacemakers largely enable the same work capacity as dual chamber pacemakers in patients with high degree AV block.
Elderly patients are assumed to have a more sedentary lifestyle, and consequently to have less need for physiological pacing. On the other hand, haemodynamic studies have shown that the atrial contribution to ventricular systolic function becomes more important with advancing age (Kuo et al, 1987; Miller et al, 1986). Hoïijer et al (Hoïijer et al, 2002) showed improved cardiac function and quality of life following upgrade to dual chamber pacing after long-term ventricular stimulation in 19 patients (age: 75,5 ± 7,3 years) with AV block or sinus node disease. Left ventricular systolic function was significantly superior in the DDDR mode (mean aortic velocity time integral; P<0,001) and left atrial diameter was significantly smaller in the DDDR mode than in VVIR mode (P=0,01). The plasma level of brain natriuretic peptide was significantly lower in DDDR pacing (p=0,002)
Considering ventricular systolic function, Ouali et al (Ouali et al, 2010) have demonstrated decreased LV-EF and myocardial systolic velocities assessed by Tissue Doppler Imaging following VVI pacing, results which are in agreement with those of previous studies in which non physiologic pacing was found to affect the LV contractile efficiency negatively (Naegeli et al,2007; Höijer et al, 2002).
Naegeli et al (Naegeli et al,2007) showed that patients experience a highly significant, two to three fold increase of BNP and NT-proBNP levels during VVI(R) pacing compared with synchronized atrioventricular pacing which was reversible after restoring AV synchrony. So the authors (Naegeli et al,2007) suggested that the loss of atrioventricular synchrony, while on VVI(R) pacing is directly responsible for increased levels of natriuretic peptides, most likely as a result of increased atrial and ventricular stretch and pressure (Levin et al, 1998). These subtle improvement in haemodynamic performance detected by natriuretic peptides in AV pacing was associated with a mild but significant increase in left ventricular ejection (p=0,036). These mild changes in left ventricular function may not be clinically relevant, but need to be interpreted with regard to the short periods in these different studies.
The subjective response to VVI(R) pacing is highly dependent on whether there had been previous exposure to dual chamber pacing. Since having a pacemaker implanted, whether it be VVI(R) or DDD(R), results in a great improvement in quality of life compared to having an untreated AV block or sinus node disease. All paced patients are likely to feel considerably better, making it difficult to ascertain which group improved the most.
DDD pacing preserves AV synchrony, but disturbs inter and intra-ventricular synchrony resulting from RV pacing like VVI. Echocardiographic data have demonstrated inter and intra-ventricular dyssynchrony as assessed by interventricular delay and the aortic pre ejection period (152,6±23,1ms vs 151,4 ± 25,3 ms) in the two pacing modes (ouali et al, 2010). The hemodynamic deleterious effect via RV apical pacing could be exaggerated in elderly patients, in whom reduced ventricular compliance is frequently present (Connolly et al, 2000).
Even elderly, patients with complete heart block and sinus rhythm, DDD pacing is associated with improved quality of life and systolic ventricular function compared with VVI pacing. In active elderly patients with complete heart block, efforts should be made to maintain AV synchrony and VVI (R) pacing should not be used instead of DDD pacing.

3. Pacing site selection

Modern pacemakers currently provide pacing modes and algorithms minimizing unnecessary ventricular pacing, but in patients with atrioventricular conduction system disease in whom a high percentage of ventricular stimulation is mandatory, there is no way to exclude it. Especially for these patients, the need for identification of more 'physiological' pacing sites has become more and more compelling. Right Ventricular Apical permanent pacing could have negative hemodynamic effects. Initially, attention was directed to RV outflow tract/septum pacing and His/para-Hisian pacing in patients with LV dysfunction (Mera et al, 1999; Schwaab et al, 1999; Buckingham et al, 1997; Buckingham et al, 1998; de Cock et al, 1998) and latter in preserved LV function patients (Giudici et al, 1997; Karpawich & Mital, 1997; Kolettis et al, 2000; Bourke et al, 2002; Tse et al, 2002; Occhetta et al, 2006; Victor et al, 2006; Yu et al, 2007; Kypta et al, 2008; Flevari et al, 2009; Ng et al, 2009; Dabrowska-Kugacka et al, 2009; Takemoto et al, 2009; Tse et al, 2009; Gong et al, 2009; Rosso et al, 2010; Verma et al , 2010;106:806-9; Leong et al, 2010; Cano et al,. 2010; Yoshikawa et al, 2010) while subsequently biventricular stimulation began to emerge as an appealing alternative proposal (Yu et al, 2009; Simantirakis et al, 2009; Doshi et al, 2005). Despite attempts to corroborate the theoretical superiority of alternative RV pacing sites, such as septal and His/para-Hisian pacing, the reported outcomes remain conflicting and their efficacy equivocal.

3.1 His/ ParaHissian pacing

Direct His Bundle Pacing (DHBP) was documented as reliable and effective for preventing the desynchronization and negative effects of right ventricular apical pacing. It is, however, a complex method that requires longer average implant times, cannot be carried out on all patients and presents high pacing thresholds (Deshmukh et al, 2000; Deshmukh et al, 2004, Zanon et al, 2006). On the contrary, the parahisian pacing, with simpler feasibility and reliability criteria, seems to guarantee an early invasion of the His-Purkinje conduction system, with a physiological ventricular activation, very similar to the one that can be obtained with direct His bundle pacing (Occhetta et al, 2006).

The parameters that allow for the direct pacing of the His bundle were defined(Deshmukh et al, 2004):

1. the morphology and the duration of the native QRS and the paced QRS must be identical on the 12 standard ECG derivations
2. the HV interval on the original rhythm and the spike-QRS distance in the paced signal must be equal (with a tolerance margin of 10 ms)
3. the pacing threshold must be high (> 2V), since it must capture a specific non-muscular conduction tissue;
4. the pacing lead should be positioned with the distal pole (screw in) at the same level as one of the two electrodes of a mapping catheter on the His bundle (x-ray in both right and left anterior oblique projections)

The criteria for the realization of parahisian pacing are (Deshmukh et al, 2004):

the distal pole of the catheter (screw-in) must be positioned as much as possible next to the mapping dipole of the electrophysiological catheter of reference (within 1 cm in the right and left oblique projections)

1. the duration of the paced QRS can be larger than the spontaneous QRS, but the duration must be at least 50 ms shorter than the QRS obtained with the RVA pacing and, in any case, not more than 120-130 ms.
2. the electrical axis of the paced QRS must be concordant with the electrical axis of the spontaneous QRS;

3. the interval between the spike and start of paced QRS is less than the HV time of the original rhythm;
4. the pacing threshold must be less than 1 V, since the muscular portion of the interventricular septum is paced.

Indication of His or para-His bundle pacing is limited to patients without significant distal conduction abnormalities particularly after ablation of the AV node for chronic atrial fibrillation (Deshmukh et al, 2004, Occhetta et al, 2006).

In these selected patients, His or para-His bundle pacing might be optimal (Zanon et al, 2008; Occhetta et al, 2006) but its feasibility is limited by the technical difficulties (Occhetta et al, 2006; Deshmuck et al, 2000; Deshmuck et al, 2004). His bundle pacing in patients has been shown to result in better hemodynamic performance (Deshmukh et al, 2004) and more uniform distribution of perfusion when compared with RV pacing (Deshmuck et al, 2000). Inversely, Padeletti et al (Padeletti et al; 2007) have demonstrated that acute His bundle pacing did not improve LV function compared with alternate site RV pacing (RVA, RVS and free wall portions of the RVOT) and may be inferior to LV pacing.

3.2 RV septal pacing

3.2.1 Technical aspect of lead implantation for alternative RV pacing site

To attain the septal position, the pacing site was usually determined on a topological rather than functional basis (Giudici & Karpawich, 1999). Different parameters were used variably. In old literature, all authors have used fluoroscopic images, defined as a leftward orientation of the lead confirmed by LAO projection, and considered as the standard approach in the daily practice for a septal site access. Many papers do not define the LAO angle, whereas the Mond papers use 40° (Medi & Mond, 2009). Indeed from experience, it is very hard to manipulate leads with fluoroscopy at 40° either from the left or right sided approach. However, electrocardiographic criteria such as negative deflection of lead I and positive initial R-waves of the paced ventricular complex in leads II and III (Schwaab et al, 2001; McGavigan et al,2006; Lieberman et al, 2004; Balt et al, 2010) or the narrowest paced QRS complex available during the mapping of the interventricular septum (Tse et al, 2002; Tse et al, 2009a; Tse et al, 2009b; Schwaab et al, 2001), were not used uniformly.

Tse et al (Tse et al; 2002) and Mera et al (Mera et al, 1999) have postulated that the paced QRS duration is a practical indicator for determining the optimal RV pacing site. However, Schwab et al (Schwaab et al, 2001) have found the detailed mapping of the RV with precise measurements of QRS duration has been found to be impractical.

This lack of uniform definitions of where the alternate RV sites actually lie and the inadequacy of tools to consistently reach these locations and verify correct placement may account for the variability in lead positioning within the RVS and may have contributed to the mixed results regarding the long-term hemodynamic benefits of RVS pacing (Lieberman et al, 2004; Balt et al, 2010; Iaizzo et al, 2004).

In a recent study, Balt et al (Balt et al, 2010) have concluded that in 143 patients in whom lead implantation in the RVOT was performed, a septal position was achieved in only one-third of patients. The paced QRS complexes resulting from different stimulation sites within the RVOT (anterior, septal, and free wall) were found to differ significantly, but a considerable overlap of QRS patterns was demonstrated, and the authors, could not define clear cut-off point or devise flow-charts to match ECG and pacing site. Differences in ventricular conduction and electrical activation were proposed to explain this overlap (Balt et al, 2010).

Using anatomical reconstruction of the RV in 31 patients to validate pacing sites, Burri et al (Burri et al, 2011) have analyzed and compared 12-lead ECGs wile pacing from a para-Hissian position, from the mid-septum, and from the anterior free wall. The authors (Burri et al, 2011) have concluded that a negative QRS complex in lead I is an inaccurate criterion for validating septal pacing. A negative QRS or the presence of q-wave in lead I tended to be more frequent with anterior than with mid-septal pacing (9/31 vs 3/31, P=0.2 and 8/31 vs 1/31, P= 1, respectively).

In the daily practice, the standard approach of septal site is based generally on only fluoroscopic images during the implantation procedure.

Several studies have demonstrated the feasibility, and the safety of alternative pacing sites (Rosso et al, 2010; Vlay et al, 2006; Medi & Mond, 2009, Schwaab et al, 2001). With active fixation technology, lead placement and stability in the RVS are no longer a problem. Moreover, recently commercially approved stylets (Models 4140, 4150; St. Jude Medical, Sylmar,CA, USA) are available for septal positioning of ventricular leads, which resembles the manually shaped stylet described by the senior author in previous publications (Kypta et al, 2008; Rosso et al, 2010; McGavigan et al, 2006).

In a large study, including 460 patients, Vlay et al. (Vlay et al, 2006) reported on a 9 year experience of right ventricular outflow tract pacing, an excellent success rate and stable lead measurements over time, without an increased risk for acute or chronic complications compared with RVA pacing. There was a reported overall implantation success rate of 84%, with improving success as experience was obtained. Rosso et al (Rosso et al, 2010) have also confirmed that conventional active-fixation pacing leads can be successfully and safely deployed onto the RV septum either in the RVOT or mid RV locations using a purposely-shaped stylet guided only by fluoroscopic views. In this study, it has been quicker to deploy the RVOT lead than the mid-RV lead. Acute electrical parameters for the RV leads at implant were satisfactory, regardless of their positioning at the RVOT or mid-RV septum. The primary success rates of ventricular pacing lead positioning in mid RV septal and RVOT locations were respectively 88.2% and 100% of patients undergoing PM implantation.

In a recent manuscript, Mond (Mond, 2010) have described the implant tools and techniques required for consistent and successful placement of pacing leads onto the RV septum. The PA or approximately 10° RAO projection is recommended. Rather than using the commercial product, the stylet for septal lead placement can be hand prepared at the time of implant. The 40° LAO projection should be performed to confirm septal positioning after the screw deployment. There is at least a 90% success in septal positioning using these techniques with a 97% success rate for the RVOT (Medi & Mond, 2009) with an excellent long-term (1 year) electrical stability in 92 patients undergoing pacemaker implantation for bradycardia indication.

3.2 Electric and mechanic LV synchrony

Since 1925, Wiggers (Wiggers, 1925) have postulated that the longer the distance from the artificial stimulation site to the entry of the His-Purkinje system the weaker the beats that occur. This was supported by the electrophysiological maps obtained in dogs by Lister et al (Lister et al, 1964).

In experimental studies, RVS pacing using a screw-in electrode was shown to produce a synchronous LV electrical activation via stimulation of the genuine intraventricular conduction system deep in the septum, and to prevent the development of adverse cellular changes (Laske et al, 2006; Karpawich & Mital, 1991).

Inversely, in other animal studies (Mills et al, 2009; Peschar et al, 2003), it was demonstrated in canine hearts with normal ventricular conduction that LV function is maintained at SR level when pacing the LV apex or the LV endocardial surface of the interventricular septum (Mills et al, 2009; Peschar et al, 2003) and that electric desynchronization pacing was significantly greater in RV apical and RV septal than LV apical and LV septal pacing (Mills et al, 2009; Wyman et al, 2002). It was also demonstrated by using tagged magnetic resonance imaging that RV apex and RV septal pacing increased significantly mechanical dyssynchrony, discoordination (MRI tagging) and blood flow redistribution (microspheres) and reduced LV contractility, relaxation, and myocardial efficiency (stroke work/myocardial oxygen consumption). In contrast, LV apical and LV septal pacing did not significantly alter these parameters as compared with the values during intrinsic conduction. At 16 weeks, acute intrasubject comparison showed that single-site LV apical and LV septal pacing generally resulted in similar or better contractility, relaxation, and efficiency as compared with acute biventricular pacing (Mills et al, 2009).

In the animal study described by Mills et al (Mills et al, 2009), the lead was implanted in the RV midseptum, based solely on position and not optimizing the QRS complex. Surprisingly, none of the parameters investigated in this study (electric mapping, hemodynamic, regional strains, efficiency) showed a significant difference between RV apical and RV septal pacing. Similarly, no apparent benefit of RV septal pacing over RV apical pacing was observed in a human clinical study of LV pressure-volume loops that also used purely anatomic lead positioning (Lieberman et al, 2006). In the same way, a recent comparison of chronic RV apex and RV septal pacing, based entirely on lead position, showed that RV septal pacing was associated with more impaired circumferential strain and worse LV dyssynchrony than apical pacing (Ng et al, 2009).

In contrast, it has been shown that the RV pacing site, which leads to the best LV function, is not predicted by anatomical position or by QRS duration (Peschar et al, 2003). The hemodynamic superiority of LV apex and LV septum pacing may be explained by a relatively physiological sequence of electrical activation when pacing from these sites (Mills et al, 2009; Peschar et al, 2003).

Some investigators have proposed the idea of a hemodynamic "sweet spot," where each patient has a particular optimal pacing site (Karpawich & Mital, 1997; Tse et al, 2002; Tse et al, 2009 b). The ideal ventricular pacing site should resemble the normal activation and synchronicity of ventricular activation observed with an undamaged conduction system. A pacing site that is in closer proximity with the proximal portion of His bundle at the RV septum should lead to a narrower QRS which in turn might reflect a lesser degree of activation delay compared with RVA pacing (Mera et al, 199; Schwaab et al, 1999; Tse et al, 2002) and less dyssynchrony, as demonstrated by multiple echocardiographic techniques (Tse et, 2002; Flevari et al, 2009; Takemoto et al, 2009; Gong et al, 2009; Leong et al, 2010; Cano et al, 2010).

Pacing on the right ventricular (RV) septum, at high (septal RVOT pacing) (Giudici et al, 1997; Kolettis et al, 2000; Bourke et al, 2002; Tse et al, 2002; Dabrowska-Kugacka et al, 2009; Gong et al, 2009; Leong et al, 2010; Yoshikawa et al, 2010), mid (Yu et al, 2007; Cano et al, 2010; Muto et al, 2007) or lower (Flevari et al, 2009) septal pacing position has been introduced as a potentially favorable alternative to RVA pacing to preserve a more physiologic ventricular activation.

Previous investigations of alternative pacing sites have yielded inconsistent results (Mera et al, 1999; Giudici et al, 1997; Bourke et al, 2002; Victor et al, 2006; Kypta et al, 2008;

Dabrowska-Kugacka et al, 2009; Tse et al Europace 2009; Victor et al, 1999) which may be attributable, in part, to the fact that the pacing site was determined on a topological rather than functional basis (Giudici & Karpawich, 1999).

Many previous studies (Schwaab et al, 1999; Victor et al, 2006; Yu et al, 2007; Ng et al, 2009; Takemoto et al, 2009; Tse et al, Europace 2009, Gong et al, 2009; Leong et al, 2010; Schwaab et al, 2001), have showed that septal pacing induced shorter paced QRS duration than RVA pacing did. These results indicated that RVS pacing resulted in better electric synchrony compared with RVA pacing. However, the duration of the QRS complex was not found to be significantly shorter when pacing from the mid-septum compared with the anterior free wall (Lister et al, 1964).

In 120 consecutive patients with standard pacing indications, Schwab et al (Schwab et al, 2001) have tested the feasibility of RV septal lead implantation technique guided by surface ECG and the degree to which this technique reduces paced QRS duration compared to RV apical stimulation when passive-fixation leads are used. Pace-mapping of the septum was performed until QRS was minimal. QRS could be reduced by 5-55 ms in 83 (69%) of 120 patients. In 22 (18%) patients, QRS was identical with apical and septal pacing, and in 15 (13%) patients, QRS was 5-20 ms (delta QRS) longer despite septal stimulation. Average QRS was significantly shorter during septal pacing compared with apical pacing (151 ± 20 vs 162 ± 23 ms, $P < 0.001$). There was a tendency towards greatest QRS reduction when the high septum was stimulated (22±11 ms reduction) as compared with mid- (18±11 ms) or apical parts of the RV septum (16 ± 10 ms). QRS reduction was most likely if apical QRS width was > 170 ms ($P = 0.0002$), and there was an inverse correlation between apical QRS and delta QRS ($r = 0.53, P < 10^{-7}$).

In the Rosso study (Rosso et al, 2010), two pacing leads were simultaneously and temporarily positioned at the RVOT septum and mid-RV septum in order to determine which pacing site was associated with a narrower QRS. The mean QRS duration in the RVOT septum was similar to the mid- RV septum. The QRS was narrower when pacing from the mid-septal RV in nine patients, whereas it was shorter while pacing the RVOT in three patients . In the remaining patients, there was no difference in QRS duration.

Many recent studies have compared the mechanic synchrony between septal pacing and RVA pacing (Schwaab et al, 1999; Yu et al, 2007; Flevari et al, 2009; Ng et al, 2009; Takemoto et al, 2009; Leong et al, 2010; Cano et al, 2010; Yoshikawa et al, 2010) and have showed a more inter and intraventricular synchrony with septal pacing than apical pacing immediately after implantation and at midterm (after 6 to 12 months of follow-up), excepted for the study of Ng et al (Ng et al, 2009).

Moreover, patients in the RVAP group had significantly more inter and intraventricular dyssynchrony than did the controls, and patients in the RVSP group had comparable values to those obtained from the control group (Flevari et al, 2009; Verma et al, 2010; Cano et al, 2010).

In contrast; Takemoto et al (Takemoto et al, 2009) have revealed that, RVS pacing caused a significant increase in the interventricular mechanical delay (IVMD) compared with AAI pacing, which indicates that the onset of the LV activation is delayed even during RVS pacing. These authors explained that, such an increase in interventricular dyssynchrony may be a result of the initial impulse propagation through a slow muscular conduction region. The increase in the time to peak systolic velocity dispersion among the 12 LV segments (Tsys) during RVS pacing compared with AAI pacing, may also be attributable to the initial delay of the impulse propagation.

Authors measured dyssynchrony by different indices (Flevari et al, 2009; Takemoto et al, 2009; Gong et al, 2009; Leong et al, 2010; Yoshikawa et al, 2010) and available parameters quantifying intraventricular dyssynchrony could not contain all information of dyssynchrony. A positive and statistically significant correlation was found between the paced QRS duration and global dyssynchrony (Victor et al, 2006; Flevari et al 2009; Takemoto et al, 2009; Muto et al, 2007).
However, it has been shown in experimental studies that RV pacing sites maintaining an optimal LV function, are not correlated with the narrowest paced QRS complexes (Peschar et al, 2003). In addition, the correlation between QRS duration and the degree of electromechanical LV dyssynchrony has been disputed (Ng et al, 2009; Bordachar et al, 2003; Tournoux et al, 2007; Bleeker et al, 2004). Using tissue Doppler-derived basal septal-to-lateral wall delay, Bleeker et al (Bleeker et al, 2004) demonstrated a lack of relation between QRS duration and mechanical LV dyssynchrony. In the same way Ng et al (Ng et al, 2009), have concluded that correlations between QRS duration and tissue Doppler-derived systolic dyssynchrony and 2-dimensional speckle tracking-derived circumferential strain dyssynchrony indexes were weak, and there was no correlation with radial strain dyssynchrony (Ng et al, 2009).

3.3 Outcome

Results from acute and chronic studies are summarized in table 1 and show mixed results with a tendency toward better hemodynamic outcome when pacing at these alternative sites (Giudici et al, 1997; Kolettis et al, 2000; Tse et al, 2002; Yu et al, 2007; Flevari et al, 2009; Takemoto et al, 2009; Tse et al, 2009 a; Yoshikawa et al, 2010; Yu et al, 2009; de Cock et al, 2003).

Authors/ year of publication	Study design	N°	Pacing modes	Pacing sites	Septal approach	Conduction disturbances	Paced QRS with alternative RV pacing	Follow-up duration	less VA with RVS than RVAP	Results with alternative RV pacing
Giudici et al, 1997	Not randomized crossover	89	VVI	RVOT vs RVA	NA	14 SSS; 19 intrinsic AVB; 56 AVNA	NA	Acute results	NA	RVOT improves cardiac output
Karpawich & Mital, 1997	Not randomized Crossover	22	VVI/AAI	AAI vs RVA vs RVS	NA	Normal AV conduction	NA	Acute results	NA	RVS pacing, maintained comparable indices with intrinsic and atrial paced rhythms (LV dP/dt, Vmax, and Vpm, and LV end-diastolic pressure)
Kolettis et al, 2000	Randomized crossover	20	DDD	RVA vs RVOT vs AAI	Fluoroscop, ECG, narrowest QRS	Normal AV conduction	Shorter	Acute results	NA	PSP decreased from either site compared with AAI; RVOT is associated with more favorable diastolic function compared with RVA
Bourke et al, 2002	Not-randomized parallel	20	VVIR	10 RVOT vs 10 RVA	fluoroscopy	AVNA AF Narrow QRS	same	23 weeks	±	No major differences were identified in acute or chronic radionuclide parameters of ejection fraction
Tse et al, 2002	Randomized parallel	24	DDD	12 RVA vs 12 RVOT	fluoroscopy and ECG narrowest QRS	Complete AVB Sinus rhythm 75% Wide QRS	Shorter	18 months	+	Best myocardial perfusion and function
Occhetta et al, 2006	Randomized crossover	16°	VVIR	Parahissian / hissian vs RVA	ECG Pacing threshold	AVNA; chronic AF; narrow QRS	Shorter	6 months	+	The LVEF did not show any significant differences
Victor et al, 2007	Randomized crossover	28§	VVIR	RVA vs RVS	fluoroscopy narrowest QRS	AV node ablation chronic AF	shorter	3 months	NA	chronic RV septal pacing preserved LVEF in patients with baseline LVEF ≤ 45%. No effect in patients with preserved LVEF

Authors/ year of publication	Study design	N°	Pacing modes	Pacing sites	Septal approach	Conduction disturbances	Paced QRS with alternative RV pacing	Follow-up duration	less VA with RVS than RVAP	Results with alternative RV pacing
Yua et al, 2007	Randomized parallel	42	DDD	18 RVA vs 14 RV mid-septal vs 10 AAI	fluoroscopy narrowest QRS	Symptomatic bradycardia	shorter	72 h Acute results	+	better mechanical performance and preserved chronotropic response on myocardial contractility in comparison with apical pacing
Kypta et al , 2008	Randomized Parallel	98¥	DDD	53 RVS (RVOT or midseptal) vs 45 RVA	fluoroscopy and ECG	AV block 55% wide QRS	Shorter	18 months	NA	Changes of BNP levels, LVEF, and exercise capacity s were statistically not different
Flevari et al, 2009	Randomized Parallel	31	DDD	15 Apical vs 16 lower RVS	fluoroscopy ECG	First, 2nd and 3rd AVB 22,5% wide QRS	Shorter	12 months	+	increase in LVEF compared to RVAP
Ng et al , 2009	Not randomized parallel	34	DDD	17 RVS vs 17 RVA vs 22 controls	fluoroscopy	Complete or second AV B QRS duration : NA	Shorter	Median: 692 days	-	RV septal pacing group was associated with poorer long-term LV function
Dabrowska-Kugacka et al, 2009	Randomized parallel	122	DDD, VDD, VVIR	56 Septal RVOT vs 66 RVA	Fluoroscopy	AVB, SSS, AF QRS duration : NA	same	10 years	NA	The RVOT provides no additional benefit in terms of long-term survival over RVA pacing
Takemoto et al, 2009	Not randomized Parallel	55	DDD	40 RVS vs 15 RVA	Fluoroscopy narrowest QRS	AVB/SSS with narrow QRS	Shorter	4 years	+	RVS preserves long-term LV function.
Tse et al , 2009	Randomized Parallel	24	VVIR	12 RVS vs 12 RVA	fluoroscopy and ECG narrowest QRS	Permanent AF bradycardia Narrow QRS	Shorter	24 months	NA	the use of a VRR algorithm with RVS pacing, but not RVA pacing, improved exercise capacity and preserved LVEF
Gong et al, 2009	Randomized Parallel	96	DDD	48 RVOT vs 48 RVA	fluoroscopy and ECG narrowest QRS	AVB Mean QRS duration 97±9 ms	Shorter	12 months	+	no benefit over RVA pacing in aspect of preventing cardiac remodeling and preserving LV systolic function
Rosso et al, 2010	Not randomized crossover	15	VVI	RVOT septum vs mid RVS	fluoroscopy	5 AVB and 12 SSS Mean QRS duration: 0,97±0,23ms	same	Acute results	NA	no preferences in regard to acute lead performance or paced QRS duration with either position.
Verma et al, 2010	Randomized crossover	19*	AAI/ VVI	HRA vs RVS vs RVOT vs RVA vs sinus rhythm	Fluoroscopy and ECG	sinus rhythm Narrow QRS Normal AV conduction	NA	Acute results	+ (RVS vs RVA), ± (RVOT vs RVA)	the RV apex, demonstrated, with the RV outflow tract location, the least mechanically synchronous contraction during
Leong et al , 2010	Randomized parallel	58	DDD	32 RVOT vs 26 RVA	Fluoroscopy and ECG	32 AVB and 26 SSS QRS duration: NA	Shorter	29 ± 10 months	+	superior indices of LV structure and function compared with RVA-pacing, and less adverse LA remodeling.
Cano et al, 2010	Randomized Parallel	81	VVI DDD	28 RVA vs 32 mid RVS vs 21 control	Fluoroscopy ECG	59 AVB and 22 SSS QRS duration : NA	Shorter	12 months	+	No significant differences in terms of clinical outcomes or EF were found
Yoshikawa et al, 2010	Not randomized parallel	60	DDD	36 High RVS vs 24 RVA	Fluoroscopy	40 AVB and 20 SSS QRS duration : NA	shorter	Acute results	+	Left ventricular dyssynchrony was smaller in patients with high septal than apical pacing

AF: atrial fibrillation; AV : atrioventricular; AVNA: AV node ablation; AVB: atrioventricular block; DDD: dual chamber pacing; HRA: high right atrium ; NA: not available; PSP: Peak systolic pressure; RVS: right ventricle septum; RVOT: right ventricle outflow tract; RVA: right ventricle apex; SSS: sick sinus syndrome; VA: ventricular asynchrony; VRR : ventricular rate regularization; VVI: single chamber ventricular pacing; * the study population included only children; § LVEF ≤45% in 12 patients; ¥ LVEF <40% in 14% of patients; ° LVEF<40% in 1 patient.

Table 1. Results from studies comparing the alternative right ventricular pacing to RVA pacing in patients with preserved LVEF.

Data from the literature on the RVS vs RVA debate are still conflicting, which might be attributed to the inhomogeneity of the studies performed in different patient populations, differences in trial design (randomized vs not randomized, parallel vs cross-over), the small cohorts studied, the differing protocols used and the lack of accepted definitions of RV lead position, and verifying actual anatomic lead position.

The study patient populations previously published were heterogeneous and consisted of patients with an indication for permanent cardiac pacing because of atrioventricular block with normal or wide QRS duration, sick sinus syndrome or after AV node ablation for permanent atrial fibrillation. These conduction disturbances were not associated with a significant distal conduction abnormalities.

Of the 12 chronic studies (≥ 6 months), 6 demonstrated a significant benefit of RV septal over RV apical pacing (table 1). In 3 of these studies, RV septal pacing produced a shorter QRS duration (Tse et al, 2002; Takemoto et al, 2009; Tse et al, 2009a), whereas in the other positive studies, the septal access was based only on fluoroscopic images and ECG pattern.

Takemoto et al (Takemoto et al, 2009) have concluded that in patients undergoing dual-chamber pacemaker implantation with normal QRS duration (AVB and SND) and preserved LV function at baseline, RVS pacing guided by the paced QRS morphology preserves long-term LV function via minimizing LV dyssynchrony. After a long (~4 years) follow-up period, the LVEF decreased significantly in patients with RVA pacing but not in those with RVS pacing. In this study, paced QRS duration was significantly shorter during RVS than RVA pacing. Tsys dispersion among the 12 LV segments was significantly smaller during RVS than RVA pacing. There was a positive correlation between the paced QRS duration and Tsys dispersion ($R=0.65$, $P<0.0001$). The pacing-induced decrease in LVEF was positively correlated with the degree of Tsys dispersion ($R=0.42$, $P=0.008$).

More recently and in the same way, Leong et al (Leong et al, 2010) have showed in a similar population (AVB and SND and preserved LV function), a significant difference in LV ejection fraction, LV end-systolic volume , and LA volume favoring the RVOT-paced group over the RVA-paced patients after a mean follow up of 29 ± 10 months. RVA-pacing was associated with greater interventricular mechanical dyssynchrony and intra-LV dyssynchrony than RVOT-pacing.

In different studies, Tse et al (Tse et al, 2002; Tse et al, 2009 a; Tse et al, 2009 b) have demonstrated that RV septal pacing improves LV systolic and diastolic function and functional capacity in patients with preserved LV function in different conditions as high grade atrioventricular block (Tse et al, 2002), after AV ablation for atrial fibrillation (Tse et al, 2009 a) or after upgrading in case of previously permanent RV apical pacing (Tse et al, 2009 b). In one particular study (Tse et al, 2002), Tse et al have showed that after 18 months of follow-up in 24 patients with AV block, the group paced from the RVOT presented with fewer myocardial perfusion defects, fewer regional wall motion abnormalities, and an improved LV ejection fraction compared with the RVA-paced group. This finding was attributed to the fact that the detrimental effects of RVA pacing become evident after several months, especially in patients with preserved LV systolic function.

The RV septal pacing also resulted in shorter isovolumic relaxation than RV apical pacing (Yu et al, 2007), implicating better diastolic function that has been invasively demonstrated by Kolettis et al. (Kolettis et al, 2000) at the cardiac catheterization laboratory.

In fact despite the beneficial features of reducing electrical and mechanical dyssynchrony , different studies failed to demonstrate a positive effect on indices of LV structure and function and did not confirm the above mentioned clinical outcomes, at least during the 3-18 months after implantation (Bourke et al, 2002; Victor et al, 2006; Kypta et al, 2008; Dabrowska-Kugacka et al, 2009; Gong et al, 2009; Cano et al, 2010)

Kypta et al (Kypta et al, 2008) randomized 98 patients with atrioventricular block (AV-block) undergoing pacemaker implantation to positioning the ventricular lead in the high or mid septum (n =53) or in the apex (n = 45) of the right ventricle. The Changes of N-terminal pro-brain natriuetic peptide (BNP) levels, LVEF, and exercise capacity from baseline to 18 months were statistically not different between septal and apical stimulation. The clinical occurrence or deterioration of overt heart failure was similar in both treatment arms. Kypta et al (Kypta et al, 2008) concluded that septal stimulation site is not superior to conventional apical pacing in unselected patients undergoing pacemaker implantation for AVB.

Gong et al (Gong et al, 2009) demonstrated that RVOT pacing did not benefit over RVA pacing in the aspect of preventing cardiac remodeling and protecting LV systolic function after 12 months of pacing in patients with normal cardiac function although it caused more synchronous LV contraction compared with RVA pacing. Inversely Ng et al (Ng et al, 2009) have demonstrated that standard fluoroscopic and electrocardiographic implantation techniques for RVS pacing resulted in a heterogenous group of different pacing sites. They conducted a cross-sectional study in which they compared echocardiographic dyssynchrony and the LV function parameters between RVS (n = 17) or RVA (n = 17) pacing in complete or second AVB patients and a control group of non-paced patients (n = 22). They found that the RVS pacing patients had a lower LVEF, lower circumferential strain, and greater circumferential dyssynchrony despite achieving a narrower QRS complex. They concluded that these detrimental effects associated with RVS pacing might have resulted from the heterogeneity of the real pacing sites included under the umbrella of RVS pacing concept. These results are in accordance with other studies (Bourke et al, 2002; Dabrowska-Kugacka et al, 2009). Victor et al (Victor et al, 2006) found that in contrast to RVA pacing, RVS pacing preserved LVEF in patients with baseline LVEF ≤45%, but did not gain any advantage of LVEF in patients with baseline LVEF>45%. The absence of significant change in resting LV ejection fraction with both septal and apical pacing in patients with ejection fraction >45% is probably attributable to the time needed for pacing-induced ventricular remodeling in that population. Sweeney et al (Sweeney et al, 2003) showed that in patients with normal LV systolic function without myocardial infarction, the risk of heart failure after RVA pacing was low. So RVA pacing may do little harm to patients with normal LV systolic function and RVOT pacing may have no benefit over RVA pacing for these patients (Cano et al, 2010).

In patients with normal LV systolic function, ventricular synchrony may be of less importance and of more time needed for pacing-induced ventricular remodeling in that population. A longer follow-up, has indeed been able to unveil significant differences in LV volumes and systolic function. The similarity of chronic outcome between pacing in the outflow and the lower septum implies that these sites may be equally useful as more physiological RV pacing sites than the RVA, especially when RV pacing cannot be avoided (Flevari et al, 2009; Rosso et al, 2010).

The PACE study (Yu et al, 2009) showed that the mean left ventricular ejection fraction declined by almost 7 percentage points (from 61.5 ± 6.6 % to 54.8 ± 9.1 %) in the first year of RVA pacing in patients with a normal ejection fraction. Among nine patients in whom the LVEF decreased to less than 45% at 12 months, eight (89%) were in the right ventricular-

pacing group. The authors suggests that the ejection fraction could decrease rapidly in vulnerable patients and that these patients might benefit even more from biventricular pacing (Yu et al, 2009).
Nevertheless, the routine use of LV-based pacing for bradycardia in most patients without heart failure and preserved LVEF is impractical because of the longer procedure time, shorter battery life, higher cost and complications rates, such as lead dislodgement, and less reliability for long-term pacing.

4. Clinical implications and perspectives

This controversy is difficult or impossible to resolve by reviewing the old literature as the techniques for defining septal pacing, using fluoroscopic images in the left anterior oblique position and the tools to reliably direct leads onto the septum have only recently been described (Mond, 2010). the older methods of directing leads onto the septum using a simple curved stylet with torque are not reliable (Balt et al, 2010; McGavigan et al, 2006) and yet comfortably use the term "septal pacing" for many studies, where this was not convincingly demonstrated and the described methods of lead placement would make reliable septal positioning very unlikely. Of importance, there are trials currently underway that may answer the questions posed in this chapter (Kaye et al, 2009).
To address this issue, three randomized prospective multicenter clinical trials are in progress comparing the long-term effects of RV apical versus septal pacing on left ventricular (LV) function Kaye et al, 2009). The three trials are Optimize RV Selective Site Pacing Clinical Trial (Optimize RV), Right Ventricular Apical and High Septal Pacing to Preserve Left Ventricular Function (Protect Pace), and Right Ventricular Apical versus Septal Pacing (RASP). The RV septal lead is positioned in the mid-septum in Optimize RV, the high septum in Protect Pace, and the mid-septal inflow tract in RASP. Lead position is confirmed by fluoroscopy in two planes and adjudicated by a blinded panel. The combined trials will follow approximately 800 patients for up to 3 years. The primary outcome in each trial is LV ejection fraction evaluated by radionuclide ventriculography or echocardiography. Secondary outcomes include echo-based measurements of ventricular/atrial remodeling, 6-minute hall walk distance, brain natriuretic peptide levels, and clinical events (atrial tachyarrhythmias, heart failure, stroke, or death). These selective site ventricular pacing trials should provide evidence of the importance of RV pacing site in the long-term preservation of LV function in patients that require ventricular pacing and help to clarify the optimal RV pacing site.

5. Conclusion

There is actually sufficient evidence that patients with preexisting LV dysfunction and indication for standard "ventricular" pacing should preferentially be treated with resynchronization therapy (CRT) (de Teresa et al, 2007; Höijer et al, 2006). Although biventricular pacing therapy resynchronizes the ventricles of asynchronous hearts, the primary concern during ventricular pacing of otherwise normal hearts is to prevent mechanical desynchronization. It should be highlighted that not all patients develop LV dyssynchrony and newonset heart failure after RV pacing. Therefore, early predictive factors (Zhanget al, 2008; Siu et al,2008 ; Sagar et al, 2010), such as dyssynchrony at the time of implantation, paced QRS width, age, presence of atrial fibrillation, concomitant coronary artery disease, or compromised LVEF, or antibody status should be further evaluated, they may reveal the patients who are more prone to LV function deterioration and who are consequently better candidates for biventricular pacing. CRT use with milder degrees of LV dysfunction or even normal cardiac function as a means of maintaining cardiac mechanical synchrony is at this date, controversial. The time, cost, and experience required for LV lead placement and the high failure rates due to absent, unsuitable, or unattainable venous anatomy, coupled with eventual operative and postoperative complications, all argue that at the moment, CRT is not the option of choice in patients with conventional indications of pacing, particularly those with preserved LV function.

It is also recognized that the weight of evidence of harm from chronic RV apical pacing is great and that mechanical and safety benefits from RV septal lead positioning for pacing is sufficient in itself to recommend that we now leave the RV apex as a primary implant site (Mond & Vlay, 2010). A septal fixation of the ventricular pacing lead was not associated with increased short- or long-term complications when compared with conventional RVA pacing. In addition, implantation times and fluoroscopy times were shorter in the septal group (Kypta et al, 2008).Coupled to this are the potential physiologic benefits of LV performance that even unproven, cannot be ignored. Therefore, this stimulation site may becomes more and more the default position in different institution although different studies did not reveal a significant outcome benefit. Keeping in mind that there might be at least a subgroup of patients who could do better with septal pacing, the noninferiority of septal pacing could become an argument for a widespread use of this stimulation spot.

Disclosure: The authors designed the commercially available right ventricular septal stylet, but have no financial interest in the product.

6. References

Balt JC, van Hemel NM, Wellens HJ, & de Voogt WG.(2010). Radiological and electrocardiographic characterization of right ventricular outflow tract pacing. *Europace*, Vol.12, No.12, (December 2010), pp.1739-1744. PubMed PMID: 20876274

Bleeker GB, Schalij MJ, Molhoek SG, Verwey HF, Holman ER, Boersma E, Steendijk P, van der Wall EE & Bax JJ. (2004). Relationship between QRS duration and left ventricular dyssynchrony in patients with end-stage heart failure. *J Cardiovasc Electrophysiol*,Vol.15, No.5, (May 2004),pp. 544–549. PubMed PMID: 15149423

Bordachar P, Garrigue S, Lafitte S, Reuter S, Jaïs P, Haïssaguerre M & Clementy J.(2003). Interventricular and intra-left ventricular electromechanical delays in right ventricular paced patients with heart failure: implications for upgrading to biventricular stimulation. *Heart*, Vol.89, No.12 , (December 2003),pp.1401-1405. PubMed PMID: 14617545.

Bourke JP, Hawkins T, Keavey P, Tynan M, Jamieson S, Behulova R & Furniss SS. (2002). Evolution of ventricular function during permanent pacing from either right ventricular apex or outflow tract following AV-junctional ablation for atrial fibrillation. *Europace* ,Vol.4, No.3, (July 2002), pp. 219 - 228. PubMed PMID: 12134968.

Buckingham TA, Candinas R, Attenhofer C, Van Hoeven H, Hug R, Hess O, Jenni R & Amann FW. (1998). Systolic and diastolic function with alternate and combined site pacing in the right ventricle. *Pacing Clin Electrophysiol*, Vol.21, No.5, (May 1998), pp. 1077–84. PubMed PMID: 9604239.

Buckingham TA, Candinas R, Schläpfer J, Aebischer N, Jeanrenaud X, Landolt J & Kappenberger L.(1997). Acute hemodynamics effects of atrioventricular pacing at different sites in the right ventricle individually and simultaneously. *Pacing Clin Electrophysiol* , Vol.20, No.4, (April 1997), pp. 909–915. PubMed PMID: 9127395

Buckingham TA, Janosik DL & Pearson AC.(1992) .Pacemaker hemodynamics: Clinical implications. *Prog Cardiovasc Dis*, Vol.34, No.5, (March- April 1992), pp. 347–366. PubMed PMID: 1542730.

Burri H, Park CI, Zimmermann M, Gentil-Baron P, Stettler C, Sunthorn H, Domenichini G & Shah D.(2011). Utility of the surface electrocardiogram for confirming right ventricular septal pacing: validation using electroanatomical mapping. *Europace*, Vol.13, No.1, (January 2011), pp. 82-86. PubMed PMID: 20829188.

Cano O, Osca J, Sancho-Tello MJ, Sánchez JM, Ortiz V, Castro JE, Salvador A & Olagüe J. (2010). Comparison of effectiveness of right ventricular septal pacing versus right ventricular apical pacing. *Am J Cardiol*. Vol.105, No.10, (March 2010), pp .1426-32. PubMed PMID: 20451689.

Channon KM, Hargreaves MR, Cripps TR, Gardner M & Ormerod OJM.(1994). DDD vs VVI pacing in patients aged over 75 years with complete heart block: A double-blind crossover comparison. *Quart J Med*, Vol.87, No.4, (April, 1994), pp. 245–251. PubMed PMID: 8208915.

Connolly SJ, Kerr CR, Gent M, Roberts RS, Yusuf S, Gillis AM, Sami MH, Talajic M, Tang AS, Klein GJ, Lau C & Newman DM. (2000). Effects of physiologic pacing versus ventricular pacing on the risk of stroke and death due to cardiovascular causes: Canadian Trial of physiologic Pacing Investigators. N Eng J Med, Vol.342, No.19, (May 2000), pp. 1385–1391. PubMed PMID: 10805823.

Dabrowska-Kugacka A, Lewicka-Nowak E, Tybura S, Wilczek R, Staniewicz J, Zagozdzon P, Faran A, Kozłowski D, Raczak G & Swiatecka G. (2009). Survival analysis in patients with preserved left ventricular function and standard indications for permanent cardiac pacing randomized to right ventricular apical or septal outflow tract pacing. *Circ J*, Vol.73, No.10, (October 2009), pp. 1812-1819. PubMed PMID:19690393.

de Cock CC, Giudici MC & Twisk JW. (2003). Comparison of the haemodynamic effects of right ventricular outflow-tract pacing with right ventricular apex pacing: a quantitative review. *Europace*, Vol.3, No.3, (July 2003), pp. 275-8. PubMed PMID:12842643.

de Cock CC, Meyer A, Kamp O & Visser CA. (1998). Hemodynamic benefits of right ventricular outflow tract pacing: comparison with right ventricular apex pacing. *Pacing Clin Electrophysiol*, Vol.21, No.3, (March 1998), pp. 536–41. PubMed PMID: 9558684.

de Teresa E, Gómez-Doblas JJ, Lamas G, Alzueta J, Fernández-Lozano I, Cobo E, Navarro X, Navarro-López F & Stockburger M. (2007). Preventing ventricular dysfunction in pacemaker patients without advanced heart failure: rationale and design of the PREVENT-HF study. *Europace*, Vol.9, No.6, (June 2007), pp. 442-6. PubMed PMID:17460018.

Deshmukh P, Casavant DA, Romanyshyn M & Anderson K. (2000). Permanent, direct His-bundle pacing: A novel approach to cardiac pacing in patients with normal His-Purkinje activation. *Circulation*, Vol.101, No.8, (February 2000), pp. 869 - 877. PubMed PMID:10694526.

Deshmukh PM & Romanyshyn M. (2004). Direct His-bundle pacing: present and future. Pacing Clin Electrophysiol, Vol.27, No.6, (June 2004), pp.862-70. PubMed PMID: 15189517.

Doshi RN, Daoud EG, Fellows C, Turk K, Duran A, Hamdan MH, Pires LA; PAVE Study Group. (2005) Left ventricular-based cardiac stimulation post AV nodal ablation evaluation (the PAVE study). *J Cardiovasc Electrophysiol*, Vol.16, No.11, (December 2005), pp.1160-5. PubMed PMID: 16302897.

Epstein AE, DiMarco JP, Ellenbogen KA, Estes NA 3rd, Freedman RA, Gettes LS, Gillinov AM, Gregoratos G, Hammill SC, Hayes DL, Hlatky MA, Newby LK, Page RL, Schoenfeld MH, Silka MJ, Stevenson LW, Sweeney MO, Smith SC Jr, Jacobs AK, Adams CD, Anderson JL, Buller CE, Creager MA, Ettinger SM, Faxon DP, Halperin JL, Hiratzka LF, Hunt SA, Krumholz HM, Kushner FG, Lytle BW, Nishimura RA, Ornato JP,Page RL, Riegel B, Tarkington LG &Yancy CW; American College of Cardiology/American Heart Association Task Force on Practice Guidelines (Writing Committee to Revise the ACC/AHA/NASPE 2002 Guideline Update for Implantation of Cardiac Pacemakers and Antiarrhythmia Devices); American Association for Thoracic Surgery; Society of Thoracic Surgeons. (2008). ACC/AHA/HRS 2008 Guidelines for Device-Based Therapy of Cardiac Rhythm Abnormalities: a report of the American College of Cardiology/American Heart Association Task Force on Practice Guidelines (Writing Committee to Revise the ACC/AHA/NASPE 2002 Guideline Update for Implantation of Cardiac Pacemakers and Antiarrhythmia Devices): developed in collaboration with the American Association for Thoracic Surgery and Society of Thoracic Surgeons. *Circulation.*, Vol.117, No.21, (May 2008), pp.e350-408. PubMed PMID: 18483207.

Faerestrand S & Ohm OJ. (1985). A time-related study of the hemodynamic benefit of atrioventricular synchronous pacing evaluated by Doppler echocardiography. *Pacing Clin Electrophysiol*, Vol.8, No.6, (November 1985), pp. 838– 848. PubMed PMID: 2415937.

Fananapazir L, Rademaker M & Bennett DH.(1985). Reliability of the evoked response in determining the paced ventricular rate and performance of the QT or rate responsive (TX) pacemaker. Pacing Clin Electrophysiol 1985; 8: Vol.8, No.5, (September 1985), pp.701–714. PMID: 2414752.

Flevari P, Leftheriotis D, Fountoulaki K, Panou F, Rigopoulos AG, Paraskevaidis I & Kremastinos DT. (2009). Long-term nonoutflow septal versus apical right ventricular pacing: relation to left ventricular dyssynchrony. *Pacing Clin Electrophysiol*, Vol.32, No.3, (March 2009), pp. 354-362. PubMed PMID: 19272066.

Frielingsdorf J, Dur P, Gerberb AE, Vuilliomenet A & Bertel O. (1995). Physical work capacity with rate responsive ventricular pacing (VVIR) versus dual chamber pacing (DDD) in patients with normal and diminished left ventricular function. *Inter J Cardiol*, Vol.49, No.3, (May 1995), pp. 239–248. PubMed PMID: 7649670.

Giudici MC & Karpawich PP. (1999). Alternative site pacing: It's time to define terms. *Pacing Clin Electrophysiol*, Vol.22, No.4 Pt 1, (April 1999), pp 551-553. PubMed PMID: 10234707.

Giudici MC, Thornburg GA, Buck DL, Coyne EP, Walton MC, Paul DL & Sutton J. (1997). Comparison of right ventricular outflow tract and apical lead permanent pacing on cardiac output. *Am J Cardiol*, Vol.79, No.2, (January 1997), pp. 209–212. PubMed PMID: 9193029.

Gong X, Su Y, Pan W, Cui J, Liu S & Shu X. (2009). Is right ventricular outflow tract pacing superior to right ventricular apex pacing in patients with normal cardiac function? *Clin Cardiol*, Vol.32, No.12, (December 2009), pp 695-699. PubMed PMID: 20027661.

Hargreaves MR, Channon KM, Cripps TR, Gardner M & Ormerod OJM. (1995). Comparison of dual chamber and ventricular rate responsive pacing in patients over 75 with complete heart block. *Br Heart J*, Vol.74, No.4, (October 1995), pp.397–402. PubMed PMID: 7488454.

Heldman D, Mulvihill D, Nguyen H, Messenger JC, Rylaarsdam A, Evans K & Castellanet MJ. (1990). True incidence of pacemaker syndrome. *Pacing Clin Electrophysiol*, 1990; 13: Vol.13, No.12 Pt 2, (December 1990), pp.1742–1750. PubMed PMID: 1704534.

Höijer CJ, Brandt J, Willenheimer R, Juul-Moller S & Boström PA. (2002). Improved cardiac function and quality of life following upgrade to dual chamber pacing after long-term ventricular stimulation. Eur Heart J, Vol.23, No.6, (March 2002), pp.490–497. PubMed PMID: 11863352.

Höijer CJ, Meurling C & Brandt J. (2006). Upgrade to biventricular pacing in patients with conventional pacemakers and heart failure: a double-blind, randomized crossover study. *Europace*, Vol.8, No.1, (January 2006), pp.51-55. PubMed PMID: 16627409.

Iaizzo PA, Laske TG, Skadsberg NA, Vincent SA & Padeletti L. (2004) Right ventricular septal lead placement—Are you really on the anterior wall? (abstract). AHA Annual Meeting, New Orleans, LA, 2004.

Jahangir A, Shen WK & Minn R. (2003). Pacing in elderly patients. *Am Heart J*, Vol.146, No.5, (November 2003), pp. 750–753. PubMed PMID: 14597921.

Jordaens L, Backers G & Clement DL. Physiologic pacing in the elderly. Effects on exercise capacity and exercice induced arrhythmias. *Jpn Heart J*, Vol.29, No.1, (January 1988), pp. 35–44. PubMed PMID: 3398242.

Karpawich PP, Justice CD, Chang CH, Gause CY & Kuhns LR. (1991). Septal ventricular pacing in the immature canine heart: a new perspective. *Am Heart J*, 1991;121: Vol.121, No.3 Pt 1, (March 1991), pp. 827-833. PubMed PMID: 2000750.

Karpawich PP & Mital S. (1997). Comparative left ventricular function following atrial, septal, and apical single chamber heart pacing in the young. *Pacing Clin Electrophysiol*, Vol.20, No.8 Pt 1, (August 1997), pp. 1983–1988. PubMed PMID: 9272537.Kaye G, Stambler BS & Yee R. (2009). Search for the optimal right ventricular pacing site: design and implementation of three randomized multicenter clinical trials. *Pacing Clin Electrophysiol*, Vol.32, No.4, (April 2009), pp.426-433. PubMed PMID: 19335850.

Kolettis TM, Kyriakides ZS, Tsiapras D, Popor T, Paraskeraides IA & Kremastinos DT. (2000). Improved left ventricular relaxation during short-term right ventricular outflow tract compared to apical pacing. *Chest*, Vol.117, No.1, (January 2000), pp. 60–64. PubMed PMID: 10631200.

Kritensson BE, Arnman K, Ryden L.(1985). The haemodynamic importance of atrioventricular synchrony and rate increase at rest and during exercise. *Eur Heart J*, Vol.6, No.9, (September 1985), pp. 773–778. PubMed PMID: 4076212.

Kuo LC, Quinones MA, Rokey R, Sartori M, Abinander EG & Zoghbi WA. (1987). Quantification of atrial contribution to left ventricular filling by pulsed Doppler echocardiography and the effect of age in normal and diseased hearts. *Am J Cardiol*, Vol.56, No.12, (December 1987), pp.1174–1178. PubMed PMID: 2953229.

Kypta A, Steinwender C, Kammler J, Leisch F & Hofmann R. (2008). Long-term outcomes in patients with atrioventricular block undergoing septal ventricular lead implantation compared with standard apical pacing. *Europace*. Vol.10, No.5, (May 2008), pp. 574-579. PubMed PMID: 18403387.

Lamas GA, Lee KL, Sweeney MO, Silverman R, Leon A, Yee R , Marinchak RA, Flaker G, Schron E, Orav EJ, Hellkamp AS, Greer S, McAnulty J, Ellenbogen K, Ehlert F, Freedman RA, Estes NA 3rd, Greenspon A, Goldman L; Mode Selection Trial in Sinus-Node Dysfunction.(2002). Ventricular pacing or dual-chamber pacing for sinus-node dysfunction. N Eng J Med, Vol.346, No.24, (June 2002), pp. 1854–1862. PubMed PMID: 12063369.

Lamas GA, Orav EJ, Stambler BS, Ellenbogen KA, Sgarbossa EB, Huang SK, Marinchak RA, Estes NA 3rd, Mitchell GF, Lieberman EH, Mangione CM & Goldman L. (1998). Quality of life and clinical outcomes in elderly patients treated with ventricular pacing as compared with dual-chamber pacing. Pacemaker Selection in the Elderly Investigators. *N Engl J Med*, Vol.12, No.12, (April 1998), pp. 1097–1104. PubMed PMID: 9545357.

Laske TG, Skadsberg ND, Hill AJ, Klein GJ & Iaizzo PA. (2006). Excitation of the intrinsic conduction system through his and interventricular septal pacing. *Pacing Clin Electrophysiol*, Vol.29, No.4, (April 2006), pp. 397-405. PubMed PMID: 16650269.

Leclercq C, Gras D, Le Helloco A, Nicol L, Mabo P & Daubert C. (1995). Hemodynamic importance of preserving the normal sequence of ventricular activation in permanent cardiac pacing. *Am Heart J*, Vol.129, No.6, (June 1995), pp. 1133–1141. PubMed PMID:7754944.

Leong DP, Mitchell AM, Salna I, Brooks AG, Sharma G, Lim HS, Alasady M, Barlow M, Leitch J, Sanders P, & Young GD. (2010). Long-term mechanical consequences of permanent right ventricular pacing: effect of pacing site. *J Cardiovasc Electrophysiol*, Vol.21, No.10, (October 2010), pp. 1120-1126. PubMed PMID:20487122.

Levin ER, Gardner DG & Samson WK. (1998). Natriuretic peptides. *N Engl J Med*, Vol.339, No.5, (July 1998), pp .321–328. PubMed PMID: 9682046.

Lieberman R, Grenz D, Mond HG & Gammage MD. (2004). Selective site pacing: defining and reaching the selected site. *Pacing Clin Electrophysiol*, Vol.27, No.6, (June 2004), pp .883-886. PubMed PMID: 15189520.

Lieberman R, Padeletti L, Schreuder J, Jackson K, Michelucci A, Colella A, Eastman W, Valsecchi S & Hettrick DA. (2006). Ventricular pacing lead location alters systemic hemodynamics and left ventricular function in patients with and without reduced ejection fraction. *J Am Coll Cardiol*, Vol.48, No.8, (October 2006), pp .1634-1641. PubMed PMID: 17045900.

Lister JW, Klotz DH, Jomain SL, Stuckey JH & Hoffman BF. (1964). Effect of pacemaker site on cardiac output and ventricular activation in dogs with complete heart block, *Am J Cardiol*, Vol.14, (October 1964), pp. 494–503. PubMed PMID: 14215060.

McGavigan AD, Roberts-Thomson KC, Hillock RJ, Stevenson IH & Mond HG. (2006). Right ventricular outflow tract pacing: radiographic and electrocardiographic correlates of lead position. *Pacing Clin Electrophysiol*, Vol.29, No.10, (October 2006), pp. 1063-8.PubMed PMID: 17038137.

Medi C & Mond HG. (2009). Right ventricular outflow tract septal pacing: long-term follow-up of ventricular lead performance. Pacing Clin Electrophysiol, Vol.32, No.2, (February 2009), pp. 172-176. PubMed PMID: 19170905.

Mera F, DeLurgio DB, Patterson RE, Merlino JD, Wade ME & Leon AR. (1999) A comparison of ventricular function during high right ventricular septal and apical pacing after his-bundle ablation for refractory atrial fibrillation. *Pacing Clin Electrophysiol*, Vol.22, No.8, (August 1999), pp. 1234 –1239. PubMed PMID: 10461302.

Miller TR, Grossman SJ, Schectman KB, Biello DR, Ludbrook PA & Ehsani AA.(1986). Left ventricular filling and its association with age. *Am J Cardiol*, Vol.58, No.6, (September 1986), pp. 531–535. PubMed PMID: 3751916.

Mills RW, Cornelussen RN, Mulligan LJ, Strik M, Rademakers LM, Skadsberg ND, van Hunnik A, Kuiper M, Lampert A, Delhaas T & Prinzen FW. (2009). Left ventricular septal and left ventricular apical pacing chronically maintain cardiac contractile coordination, pump function and efficiency. *Circ Arrhythm Electrophysiol*, Vol.2, No.5, (October 2009), pp. 571–579. PubMed PMID: 19843926.

Mond HG & Vlay SC. (2010). Pacing the right ventricular septum: time to abandon apical pacing. *Pacing Clin Electrophysiol*, Vol.33, No.11, (November 2010), pp. 1293-7. PubMed PMID: 20723079.

Mond HG. (2010). The road to right ventricular septal pacing: techniques and tools. *Pacing Clin Electrophysiol*, Vol.33, No.7, (July 2010), pp 888-98. PubMed PMID: 20456643.

Muto C, Ottaviano L, Canciello M, Carreras G, Calvanese R, Ascione L, Iengo R,Accadia M, Celentano E & Tuccillo B. (2007). Effect of pacing the right ventricular mid-septum tract in patients with permanent atrial fibrillation and low ejection fraction. *J Cardiovasc Electrophysiol*, Vol.18, No.10, (September 2007), pp. 1032-1036. PubMed PMID: 17666060.

Naegeli B, Kurz DJ, Koller D, Straumann E, Furrer M, Maurer D, Minder E & Bertel O. (2007). Single-chamber ventricular pacing increases markers of left ventricular dysfunction compared with dual-chamber pacing. *Europace*, Vol.9, No.3, (February 2007), pp 194–199. PubMed PMID: 17272326.

Ng AC, Allman C, Vidaic J, Tie H, Hopkins AP & Leung DY. Long-term impact of right ventricular septal versus apical pacing on left ventricular synchrony and function in patients with second- or third-degree heart block. *Am J Cardiol*, Vol.103, No.8, (April 2009), pp. 1096-1101. PubMed PMID: 19361596.

Occhetta E, Bortnik M, Magnani A, Francalacci G, Piccinino C, Plebani L & Marino P. (2006). Prevention of ventricular desynchronization by permanent para- Hisian pacing after atrioventricular node ablation in chronic atrial fibrillation: a crossover, blinded, randomized study versus apical right ventricular pacing. *J Am Coll Cardiol*, 2006;47: Vol.47, No.10, (May 2006), pp. 1938–1945. PubMed PMID:16697308.

Oldroyd KG, Rae AP, Carter R, Wingate C & Cobbe SM.(1991). Double blind crossover comparison of the effects of dual chamber pacing (DDD) and ventricular rate-adaptive (VVIR) pacing on neuroendocrine variables, exercise performance, and symptoms in complete heart block. *Br Heart J*, Vol.65, No.4, (April 1991), pp. 188–193. PubMed PMID:1827588

Ouali S, Neffeti E, Ghoul K, Hammas S, Kacem S, Gribaa R, Remedi F & Boughzela E.(2010.) DDD versus VVIR pacing in patients, ages 70 and over, with complete heart block. *Pacing Clin Electrophysiol*, Vol.33, No.5, (May 2010), pp. 583-9. Epub 2009 Dec 10. PubMed PMID: 20015129.

Padeletti L, Lieberman R, Schreuder J, Michelucci A, Collella A, Pieragnoli P, Ricciardi G, Eastman W, Valsecchi S & Hettrick DA. (2007). Acute effects of His bundle pacing versus left ventricular and right ventricular pacing on left ventricular function. *Am J Cardiol*, Vol.100, No.10, (November 2007), pp. 1556-60. PubMed PMID: 17996519.

Peschar M, de Swart H, Michels KJ, Reneman RS & Prinzen FW. (2003). Left ventricular septal and apex pacing for optimal pump function in canine hearts. *J Am Coll Cardiol*, Vol.41, No.7, (April 2003), pp. 1218-26. PubMed PMID: 12679225.

Rediker DE, Eagle KA, Homma S, Gillam LD & Harthorne JW. (1988). Clinical and hemodynamic comparison of VVI versus DDD pacing in patients with DDD pacemakers. *Am J Cardiol*, Vol.61, No.4, (February 1988), pp.323–329. PubMed PMID: 3341209.

Rosso R, Medi C, Teh AW, Hung TT, Feldman A, Lee G & Mond HG.(2010). Right ventricular septal pacing: a comparative study of outflow tract and mid ventricular sites. *Pacing Clin Electrophysiol*, Vol.33, No.10, (October 2010), pp. 1169-1173. PubMed PMID: 20636311.

Sagar S, Shen WK, Asirvatham SJ, Cha YM, Espinosa RE, Friedman PA, Hodge DO, Munger TM, Porter CB, Rea RF, Hayes DL & Jahangir A. (2010). Effect of long-term right ventricular pacing in young adults with structurally normal heart. *Circulation*, Vol.121, No.15, (April 2010), pp.1698-705. PubMed PMID: 20368525.

Schmidt M, Bro¨msen J, Herholz C, Adler K, Neff F, Kopf C & Block M.(2007). Evidence of left ventricular dyssynchrony resulting from right ventricular pacing in patients with severely depressed left ventricular ejection fraction. *Europace*, Vol.9, No.1, (January 2007), pp. 34–40. PubMed PMID: 17224420.

Schwaab B, Fro¨ hlig G, Alexander C, Kindermann M, Hellwig N, Schwerdt H, Kirsch CM & Schieffer H. (1999). Influence of right ventricular stimulation site on left ventricular function in atrial synchronous ventricular pacing. *J Am Coll Cardiol*, Vol.33, No.2, (February 1999), pp. 317–23. PubMed PMID: 9973009.

Schwaab B, Kindermann M, Fröhlig G, Berg M, Kusch O & Schieffer H. (2001). Septal lead implantation for the reduction of paced QRS duration using passive-fixation leads. *Pacing Clin Electrophysiol*, Vol.24, No.1, (January 2001), pp. 28-33. PubMed PMID: 11227965.

Simantirakis EN, Arkolaki EG, Chrysostomakis SI & Vardas PE. (2009). Biventricular pacing in paced patients with normal hearts. *Europace*. Vol.11, No.suppl 5, (November 2009), pp. v77-81. PubMed PMID: 19861395.

Siu CW, Wang M, Zhang XH, Lau CP & Tse HF. (2008). Analysis of ventricular performance as a function of pacing site and mode. *Prog Cardiovasc Dis*, Vol.51, No.2, (September-October 2008), pp.171-182. PubMed PMID: 18774015.

Sweeney MO, Hellkamp AS, Ellenbogen KA, Greenspon AJ, Freedman RA, Lee KL & Lamas GA;. MOde Selection Trial Investigators. (2003). Adverse effect of ventricular pacing on heart failure and atrial fibrillation among patients with normal baseline QRS duration in a clinical trial of pacemaker therapy for sinus node dysfunction. *Circulation*, Vol.107, No.23, (June 2003), pp.2932–2937. PubMed PMID: 12782566.

Takemoto Y, Hasebe H, Osaka T, Yokoyama E, Kushiyama Y, Suzuki T, Kuroda Y, Ichikawa C, Kamiya K & Kodama I.(2009). Right ventricular septal pacing preserves long-term left ventricular function via minimizing pacing-induced left ventricular dyssynchrony in patients with normal baseline QRS duration. *Circ J*. Vol.73, No.10, (October 2009), pp. 1829-1835.PubMed PMID: 19690391.

Toff WD, Camm J & Skehan JD, for the United Kingdom Pacing and Cardiovascular Events (UKAPACE) Trial Investigators.(2005). Single chamber versus dual chamber pacing for high Grade atrioventricular block. *N Engl J Med*, Vol.353, No.2, (July 2005), pp.145–155. PubMed PMID:16014884.

Tops LF, Schalij MJ, Holman ER, van Erven L, van der Wall EE & Bax JJ. (2006). Right ventricular pacing can induce ventricular dyssynchrony in patients with atrial fibrillation after atrioventricular node ablation. *J Am Coll Cardiol*, Vol.48, No.8, (October 2006), pp.1642–1648. PubMed PMID: 17045901.

Tops LF, Suffoletto MS, Bleeker GB, Boersma E, van der Wall EE, Gorcsan J III, Schalij MJ & Bax JJ. (2007). Speckle-tracking radial strain reveals left ventricular dyssynchrony in patients with permanent right ventricular pacing. *J Am Coll Cardiol*, Vol.50, No.12, (September 2007), pp.1180–1188. PubMed PMID: 17045901.

Tournoux F, Donal E, Leclercq C, De Place C, Crocq C, Solnon A, Cohen-Solal A, Mabo P & Daubert JC.(2007). Concordance between mechanical and electrical dyssynchrony in heart failure patients: a function of the underlying cardiomyopathy? *J Cardiovasc Electrophysiol*, Vol.18, No.10, (September 2007), pp.1022-1027. PubMed PMID: 17666067.

Tse HF, Wong KK, Siu CW, Tang MO, Tsang V, Ho WY & Lau CP. (2009). Impacts of ventricular rate regularization pacing at right ventricular apical vs. septal sites on left ventricular function and exercise capacity in patients with permanent atrial fibrillation. *Europace*, Vol.11, No.5, (May 2009), pp.594-600. PubMed PMID: 19363054

Tse HF, Wong KK, Siu CW, Zhang XH, Ho WY & Lau CP. (2009). Upgrading pacemaker patients with right ventricular apical pacing to right ventricular septal pacing improves left ventricular performance and functional capacity. *J Cardiovasc Electrophysiol*, Vol.20, No.8, (August 2009), pp.901-905. PubMed PMID: 19490265.

Tse HF, Yu C, Wong KK, Tsang V, Leung YL, Ho WY & Lau CP. (2002). Functional abnormalities in patients with permanent right ventricular pacing: the effect of sites of electrical stimulation. *J Am Coll Cardiol*, Vol.40, No.8, (October 2002), pp. 1451–1418. PubMed PMID: 12392836.

Verma AJ, Lemler MS, Zeltser IJ & Scott WA. (2010). Relation of right ventricular pacing site to left ventricular mechanical synchrony. *Am J Cardiol.* Vol.106, No.6, (August 2010), pp. 806-809. PubMed PMID: 20816121.

Victor F, Leclerq C, Mabo P, Pavin D, Deviller A, de Place C, Pezard P,Victor J & Daubert C. (1999). Optimal right ventricular pacing site in chronically implanted patients. A prospective randomized crossover comparison of apical and outflow tract pacing. *J Am Coll Cardiol,* Vol.33, No.2, (February 1999), pp. 311-316. PubMed PMID: 9973008.

Victor F, Mabo P, Mansour H, Pavin D, Kabalu G, de Place C, Leclercq C & Daubert JC. (2006). A randomized comparison of permanent septal versus apical right ventricular pacing: short-term results. *J Cardiovasc Electrophysiol,* Vol.17, No.3, (March 2006), pp.238–242. PubMed PMID: 16643392.

Vlay SC. (2006) Right ventricular outflow tract pacing: practical and beneficial. A 9-year experience of 460 consecutive implants. *Pacing Clin Electrophysiol,* Vol.29, No.10, (October 2006), pp.1055–62. PubMed PMID: 17038136.

Wiggers C.J. (1925). The muscular reactions of the mammalian ventricles to artificial surface stimuli. Am J Physiol. Vol.73, (1925), pp. 346–378.

Wilkoff BL, Cook JR, Epstein AE, Greene HL, Hallstrom AP, Hsia H, Kutalek SP & Sharma A. Dual Chamber and VVI Implantable Defibrillator Trial Investigators. (2002). Dual chamber pacing or ventricular backup pacing in patients with an implantable defibrillator: the Dual Chamber and VVI Implantable Defibrillator (DAVID) Trial. *JAMA,* Vol.288, No.24, (December 2002), pp.3115–23. PubMed PMID: 12495391.

Wyman BT, Hunter WC, Prinzen FW, Faris OP & McVeigh ER. (2002). Effects of single- and biventricular pacing on temporal and spatial dynamics of ventricular contraction. *Am J Physiol Heart Circ Physiol,* Vol.282, No.1, (January 2002), pp.372–379. PubMed PMID: 11748084.

Yoshikawa H, Suzuki M, Tezuka N, Otsuka T & Sugi K. (2010). Differences in left ventricular dyssynchrony between high septal pacing and apical pacing in patients with normal left ventricular systolic function. *J Cardiol,* Vol.56, No.1, (July 2010), pp.44-50. PubMed PMID: 20350517.

Yu CC, Liu YB, Lin MS, Wang JY, Lin JL & Lin LC.(2007). Septal pacing preserving better left ventricular mechanical performance and contractile synchronism than apical pacing in patients implanted with an atrioventricular sequential dual chamber pacemaker. *Int J Cardiol,* Vol.118, No.1, (May 2007), pp.97–106. PubMed PMID: 16962674.

Yu CM, Chan JY, Zhang Q, Omar R, Yip GW, Hussin A, Fang F, Lam KH, Chan HC & Fung JW. (2009). Biventricular pacing in patients with bradycardia and normal ejection fraction. *N Engl J Med,* Vol.361, No.22, (November 2009), pp. 2123-2134. PubMed PMID: 19915220.

Zanon F, Bacchiega E, Rampin L, Aggio S, Baracca E, Pastore G, Marotta T,Corbucci G, Roncon L, Rubello D & Prinzen FW. (2008), Direct His bundle pacing preserves coronary perfusion compared with right ventricular apical pacing: a prospective, cross-over mid-term study. *Europace.* 2008;10, Vol.10, No.5, (May 2008), pp.580-7.PubMed PMID: 18407969.

Zanon F, Baracca E, Aggio S, Pastore G, Boaretto G, Cardano P, Marotta T, Rigatelli G, Galasso M, Carraro M & Zonzin P.(2006) A feasible approach for direct his-bundle pacing using a new steerable catheter to facilitate precise lead placement. *J Cardiovasc Electrophysiol,* Vol.17, No.1, (January 2006), pp. 29-33. PubMed PMID:16426396.

Zhang XH, Chen H, Siu CW, Yiu KH, Chan WS, Lee KL, Chan HW, Lee SW, Fu GS, Lau CP & Tse HF. (2008). New-onset heart failure after permanent right ventricular apical pacing in patients with acquired high-grade atrioventricular block and normal left ventricular function. *J Cardiovasc Electrophysiol,*Vol.19, No.2, (February, 2008), pp.136-41. PubMed PMID: 18005026.

5

Cardiac Resynchronization Therapy: Lead Positioning and Technical Advances

Karl Mischke[1] and Christian Knackstedt[2]
[1]*Department of Cardiology, RWTH Aachen University Hospital, Aachen,*
[2]*Department of Cardiology, Maastricht University Hospital, Maastricht,*
[1]*Germany*
[2]*The Netherlands*

1. Introduction

Cardiac resynchronization therapy (CRT) is a therapeutic option for heart failure patients with a severely reduced left ventricular ejection fraction and left bundle branch block (Cleland et al., 2001). Ventricular resynchronization is achieved by biventricular pacing, usually via electrodes in the right ventricular apex and a left ventricular (LV) electrode positioned in a coronary vein.
About one third of implanted patients do not respond to CRT (Derval et al., 2010). In order to reduce the percentage of non-responders, several strategies have been developed. They include optimization of patient selection, device programming as well as LV lead location. In cardiomyopathy with left bundle branch block, the lateral wall is the site of latest activation and should be the optimal location for LV pacing. Therefore, standard implantation sites for LV leads are lateral or posterolateral branches of the coronary sinus. Congruent to these pathophysiological findings, Butter et al. demonstrated a superiority of lateral wall pacing versus anterior wall pacing in CRT (Butter et al., 2001). However, a more detailed look at optimal pacing locations might be required to increase the effect of CRT and decrease non-responder rates.
Different imaging modalities have been used to both identify optimal pacing sites as well as to plan LV lead implantation.

2. Imaging for cardiac resynchronization therapy

Imaging for CRT is focused on imaging of the coronary venous (CS) system for CS lead implantation and on imaging techniques to asses the left ventricular function for patient selection, choose the optimal lead position and to evaluate the effect of CRT.
Contrast angiography is commonly used for imaging of the coronary venous system. To evaluate ventricular function including dyssynchrony, transthoracic echocardiography is commonly applied as it is widely availably and inexpensive. A lot of efforts have been done to improve patient selection by echoardiographic screening and there are hundreds of papers published on echocardiographic evaluation of mechanical dyssynchrony, including the use of tissue Doppler imaging, speckle tracking, three-dimensional and contrast

echocardiography. However, in the PROSPECT trial with almost 500 patients no single echocardiographic parameter could predict response with convincing sensitivity and specificity (Chung et al., 2008). Despite good results in single-center studies, echocardiography for assessment of dyssynchrony is limited by high intra- and inter-observer variability, measurement errors and in some patients low image quality. Alternatives to echocardiography include magnetic resonance imaging, computed tomography and nuclear imaging. Magnetic resonance imaging has the benefit of high spatial resolution, high reproducibility and information on viability. A high scar burden and pacing over a posterolateral scar are associated with poor response to CRT (Bleeker et al., 2006, White et al., 2006). Whereas magnetic resonance imaging is the gold standard to assess myocardial viability, computed tomography also provides information on scar burden and localization as well as left ventricular function and dyssynchrony. However, data on dyssynchrony measured by computed tomography are limited and there are no published data for the prediction of CRT response. In addition, computed tomography is associated with radiation exposure. Nuclear imaging with single photon computed tomography and positron emission tomography is also associated with radiation exposure. Nuclear imaging provides information on scar burden and scar localization, ventricular function and dyssynchrony. However, a major disadvantage of nuclear imaging is the low spatial resoluation.

2.1 Imaging of the coronary venous system

Left ventricular leads are usually implanted in a lateral or posterolateral branch of the coronary sinus. Contrast venography is a standard procedure performed either before or during implantation to identify suitable target veins. Table 1 displays imaging modalities for the coronary venous system.

	Advantages	**Disadvantages**	**Clinical relevance**
Retrograde contrast CS angiography	Good vessel visibility Can be performed during CRT implantation	invasive	standard procedure
Rotational CS angiography	3D imaging Can be performed during CRT implantation	invasive	limited experience
Computed tomography	Non-invasive	radiation exposure	limited experience
MRI	Non-invasive No radiation exposure	lower spatial resolution	limited experience
Venous phase CS angiography	Can be performed during standard coronary angiography	lower vessel visibility	limited experience

Table 1. Imaging modalities for the coronary venous system

Because a lot of patients with heart failure undergo a coronary angiogram, we compared retrograde occlusion venography with venous phase imaging of the coronary sinus in 24 patients (Mischke et al., 2007).

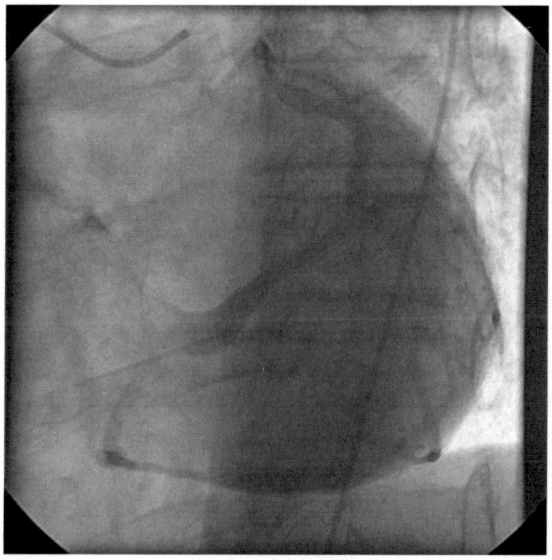

Fig. 1. Venous phase coronary sinus angiography (left anterior oblique projection).

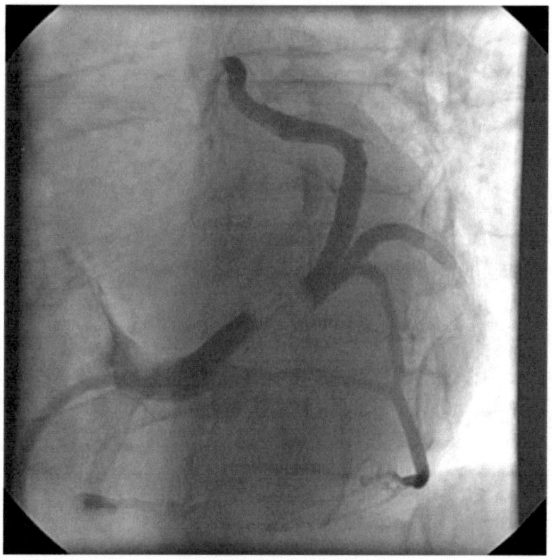

Fig. 2. Retrograde coronary sinus angiography (left anterior oblique projection).

Suitable target vessels for LV lead implantation were identified in all patients by both imaging modalities. Although visibility was superior in retrograde venography than in venous phase imaging, this technique might be an alternative to retrograde venography in patients undergoing a coronary angiogram. Venous phase angiography is time-saving and easy to perform. Figures 1 and 2 display a venous phase coronary sinus angiography and a retrograde occlusion venography.

Some of the standard C-arms used for fluoroscopy allow rotational angiography with a 3D image. In an animal model we compared rotational coronary sinus angiography to ECG-gated enhanced cardiac dual source computed tomography (Knackstedt et al., 2008a). We found no significant difference between these imaging modalities with respect to vessel diameters or vessel visibility. In contrast to computed tomography, rotational angiography images can be obtained within seconds in the catheter lab without a time lag between cardiac imaging and procedure. In addition, estimated radiation exposure and the amount of contrast medium were lower in rotational coronary sinus angiography.

We compared retrograde coronary sinus angiography with multi-slice computed tomography for visualization of the coronary venous system in 20 patients with congestive heart failure (Knackstedt et al., 2008b). Vessel visualization was better using retrograde coronary sinus angiography except for the middle cardiac vein and small veins, which were better seen with computed tomography. There was a trend that computed tomography detected more vessels. Overall, retrograde coronary sinus angiography offered a better display of target vessels commonly used for LV lead implantation.

Imaging of the coronary sinus via cardiac computed tomography correlates well with direct coronary sinus venography (Van de Verie et al., 2006). Imaging of the coronary venous anatomy by computed tomography is non-invasive and can help to plan coronary sinus lead implantation especially in patients with angulated coronary veins and in patients in whom a left marginal vein or a posterior vein is absent. It also provides information on the localization of the left phrenic nerve in relation to the target vein. However, it is associated with radiation and contrast agent exposure.

Magnetic resonance imaging of the coronary venous anatomy allows adequate assessment of localization, size and angulations of the veins (Ma et al., 2010; Nezafat et al., 2007). However, spatial resolution is inferior to computed tomography and magnetic resonance imaging cannot routinely be performed in patients with cardiac implants, e.g. patients scheduled for an upgrade from an implantable cardioverter defibrillator (ICD) to a CRT device.

2.2 Magnetic resonance imaging in CRT patients

Implanted devices like pacemakers and ICDs generally pose a contraindication to magnetic resonance imaging. However, magnetic resonance imaging might be performed with only small risks for the patient and device. In order to reduce the risks, careful patient selection, constant monitoring, specific absorption rate management and careful device programming before the scan have been used in the past. In a recent study Wilkoff et al. evaluated the safety of a pacemaker especially designed for safe magnetic resonance imaging (Wilkoff et al., 2011). Several modifications were used to improve the safety of magnetic resonance imaging, including modification of the leads to reduce lead tip heating, reduction of the amount of ferromagnetic materials, replacement of the reed switch by a Hall sensor, whose behaviour in a static magnetic field is predictable. In this prospective randomized study magnetic resonance imaging with a 1.5 T scanner could be performed without adverse events.

3. Left ventricular lead implantation

Cardiac resynchronization requires left ventricular pacing. The standard approach for left ventricular lead implantation is a transvenous implantation into a lateral or posterolateral tributary of the coronary sinus. Although dedicated instruments allow successful LV lead implantation in most patients, failure rates of 5-17% have been reported (Abraham et al., 2002; Al-Khadra et al., 2005; Purerfellner et al., 2000). In these patients, LV leads are usually implanted onto the LV epicardium through thoracotomy or thoracoscopy. In addition, there are several alternatives to standard LV lead implantation techniques, including endocardial LV lead implantation, LV lead implantation assisted by magnetic navigation and video-

assisted pericardioscopic epicardial LV lead implantation. As the access to LV regions is limited by the anatomy of the venous coronary system in standard procedures with transvenous CS lead implantation, some strategies aim at improved access to LV regions:
- Epicardial stimulation
- Endocardial LV stimulation
- Magnetic navigation for CS lead implantation
- Microcatheter LV stimulation

Table 2 lists advantages und risks of LV lead implantation techniques.

	Advantages	Disadvantages	Clinical relevance
Standard transvenous implantation into CS tributary	Low periprocedural risk	Limited access to LV regions Risk of dislocation Failure in 5-17%	Standard implantation procedure
Epicardial implantation via thoracotomy or thoracoscopy	Access to all LV regions	Surgical risks	First-line alternative to transvenous LV lead implantatoin
Endocardial LV lead implantation	Access to all LV regions Fast impulse propagation	Risk of thromboembolism	limited experience with patients
Magnetically navigated CS lead implantation	Possibly improved access to target vessels		Experimental/limited experience with patients
Video-assisted pericardioscopic epicardial implantation	Access to all LV regions		Experimental

Table 2. LV lead implantation techniques

3.1 Alternatives to right ventricular pacing

Whereas right ventricular apical pacing is the standard for patients requiring a pacemaker, this mode of stimulation is associated with electromechanical dyssynchrony and may contribute to worsening of the cardiac function (Tantengco et al., 2001). Because of the detrimental effects of right ventricular apical pacing several strategies have been suggested to avoid or reduce right ventricular apical pacing, including biventricular pacing either by de novo implantation of a CRT device or by upgrading an existing pacemaker, changes in programming to reduce the percentage of right ventricular pacing and alternative pacing sites. Careful patient selection and minimal ventricular pacing algorithms can substantially reduce the amount of right ventricular pacing and have been implemented into clinical practice (Tops et al., 2009). Several studies have demonstrated a hemodynamic and symptomatic benefit of upgrading right ventricular apical pacing to CRT as well as CRT in patient with indications for permanent pacing (Tops et al, 2009). However, so far it remains uncertain whether this will translate into a prognostic benefit. Alternative pacing sites have been suggested to avoid right ventricular apical pacing, including pacing the right ventricular outflow tract, septal pacing and direct His bundle pacing. A meta-analysis by de Cock (de Cock et al., 2003) showed a favorable hemodynamic effect, and a study by Venerio (Vanerio et al., 2008) demonstrated an improved survival in patients with right ventricular outflow tract pacing as compared to right ventricular apical pacing. However, most studies include rather small numbers of patients and are of short follow up, so more data are needed to evaluate the relevance of right ventricular outflow tract pacing for clinical routine. Septal pacing has been shown to decrease ventricular dyssynchrony compared to right ventricular apical pacing (Yu et al., 2007) but there was no difference in left ventricular ejection fraction in a prospective study by Kypta (Kypta et al., 2008). Direct His-bundle pacing or para-Hisian pacing allows a more physiological impulse propagation than right ventricular apical pacing but is associated with difficulties in lead positioning and concerns about pacing thresholds (Tops et al., 2009).

Henz (Henz et al., 2009) demonstrated in a small animal study the feasibility of atrioventricular septal synchronous pacing with intramyocardial leads implanted deep within the atrioventricular septum; further animal studies are needed to evaluate this approach.

3.2 Optimized CS lead implantation

Already a decade ago Butter et al. demonstrated a hemodynamic superiority of pacing from a lateral vein compared to an anterior vein for CRT (Butter et al., 2001). The distance between stimulation site and the region of latest contraction may be crucial for hemodynamic benefit of CRT (Ypenburg et al., 2008). This is in line with findings from animal studies (Helm et al., 2007) and studies using echocardiographic parameters in patients (Becker et al., 2007a and 2007b).

We used computed tomography and MRI imaging prior to LV lead implantation in 20 patients with congestive heart failure (Knackstedt et al., 2010a). Computed tomography was used for imaging of the coronary venous system and MRI to detect the region of latest contraction. Computed tomography and MRI images were then over-imposed to determine a coronary side branch suitable for lead implantation that is closest to the region of latest contraction. There was a trend towards a shorter distance between the LV lead and the region of latest contraction in patients classified as responders.

Another approach is the use of myocardial deformation analysis assessed by circumferential strain analysis during echocardiography to determine the optimal site for CS lead implantation. In a study with 56 patients optimal LV lead position was defined as a lead position close to the segment with latest systolic strain prior to CRT (Becker et al., 2010). During follow up, patients with leads implanted in an "optimal position" experienced a significantly higher increase in left ventricular ejection fraction than patients with leads implanted at other sites.

In a smaller study Ducket et al. performed computed tomography and MRI to acquire 3D whole heart images. After segmentation, 3D anatomical models were overlaid over live fluoroscopy to guide LV lead implantation (Ducket et al., 2010).

3.3 Endocardial LV lead implantation

Endocardial lead implantation is associated with a high risk of systemic thromboembolism (van Gelder et al., 2000). However, endocardial LV lead implantation has several (potential) advantages to CS and epicardial LV leads: it allows access to all LV regions, endocardial ventricular layers offer faster impulse propagation than epicardial leyers and endocardial stimulation might result in improved hemodynamics. Van Deursen demonstrated in an

acute canine model a superior electrical resynchronization as well as +dP/dT(max) when endocardial biventricular stimulation was used instead of epicardial stimulation. In addition, whereas epicardial stimulation resulted in a transmural dispersion of repolarization, this was not observed in endocardial stimulation (van Deursen et al., 2009).
However, Spragg et al. compared the hemodynamic effects of endocardial pacing at sites directly transmural to the CS lead tip in a small study of patients and found no difference in hemodynamics (Spragg et al., 2010). In this study a superior hemodynamic result was seen in 8 of 11 patients when endocardial pacing was performed from extreme basal sites at positions adjacent to the mitral ring. In a study by Derval et al. (Derval et al., 2010) pacing at the best LV site in 35 patients with non-ischemic dilated cardiomyopathy was associated with twice the improvement in +dP/dT(max) compared to CS pacing.
In summary, the major benefit of endocardial left ventricular pacing seems to be the access to all LV regions, whereas endocardial stimulation per se seems to be only of minor relevance.
In a few patients with major surgical contraindications to epicardial LV leads have been implanted through a transseptal approach (Jaïs et al., 2000; Leclercq et al., 1999; van Gelder et al., 2007). However, this approach is technically challenging. In addition to the risk of thromboembolism due to leads in the LV cavity, the adjacency to the mitral valve carries the risk of mitral insufficiency as well as endocarditis in case of infectious complications. A transapical approach which has been described by Kassai et al. in a limited number of patients would avoid passage of the mitral valve (Kassai et al., 2008).

3.4 Magnetically navigated LV lead implantation

A tortuous course of the coronary venous tree and target veins with small diameters can sometimes be challenging for CS lead implantation. New wire and lead navigation systems might facilitate lead implantation. The Niobe System (Stereotaxis Inc., St. Louis, USA) allows remote magnet controlled navigation of catheters and guidewires. The magnetically navigation system consists of two permanent magnets creating a steerable magnetic field (figure 3). The magnetic guidewires include a small magnet at their tip and can be steered by changing the orientation of the outer magnets. The magnetic field vector is displayed on a monitor and can be changed from the control room or from a bedside touch-screen monitor with sterile covers (figure 4).
We studied 123 patients who were assigned to either conventional CS lead implantation or LV lead implantation using magnetic navigation (Mischke et al., 2009). Venography of the coronary venous system was performed to select a target vessel for lead implantation. Left ventricular lead placement was analyzed with regard to three endpoints: 1) engagement of the target vessel with the guidewire, 2) over-the-wire lead placement in the target vessel, and 3) final LV lead position. Guidewire access to the target vessel was achieved in all patients using magnetic navigation compared to 87% with the conventional approach ($p<0.05$). Implantation success rates, total procedure and fluoroscopy times did not differ significantly between groups. Gallagher et al. used the Niobe system for CRT implantation in 50 patients (Gallagher et al., 2007). In this study, vessels were engaged either by CS venography and the use of a magnetic guidewire or via a "bare wire" approach without venography or special CS delivery sheaths. For the "bare wire" approach, the guidewire was used to probe for a target vessel as a substitute for CS venography. This was associated with a reduction in procedure and fluoroscopy time compared to the use of CS sheaths and venography.

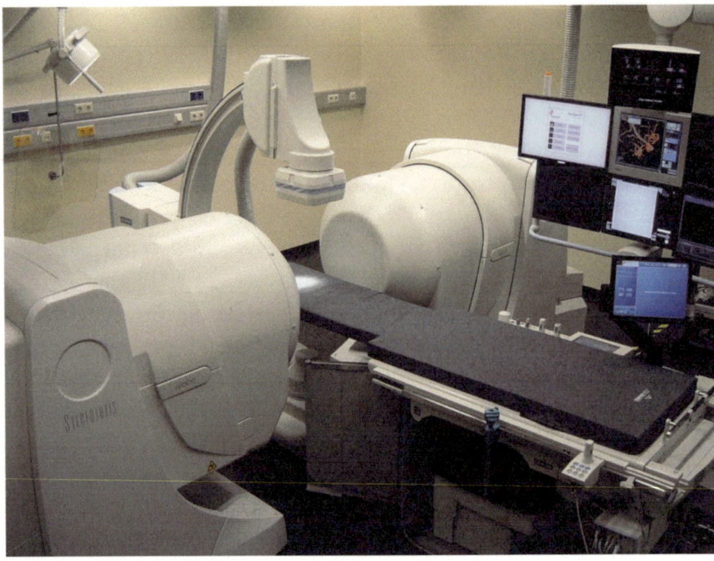

Fig. 3. Catheter suite with a magnetic navigation system (Niobe). Permanent magnets to both sides of the fluoroscopy table can be moved inside their casings to alter the magnetic field.

Magnetic navigation might be used as an additional tool for precise wire navigation and enable the operator to engage target vessels that are tortuous. In addition, technical advances in lead design might allow engagement of vessels which are now being considered inadequate due to morphology or size. We have recently demonstrated the feasibility of left ventricular stimulation via a miniaturized magnetized stimulation wire in an acute animal model (Knackstedt et al., 2010b). A conventional guide wire with a permanent magnet and a single stimulation electrode at its tip was coated with iridium oxide at the distal end and insulated except for the very tip. The stimulation wire was steered into side branches of the coronary sinus via magnetic navigation and successful left ventricular stimulation was performed via the wire.

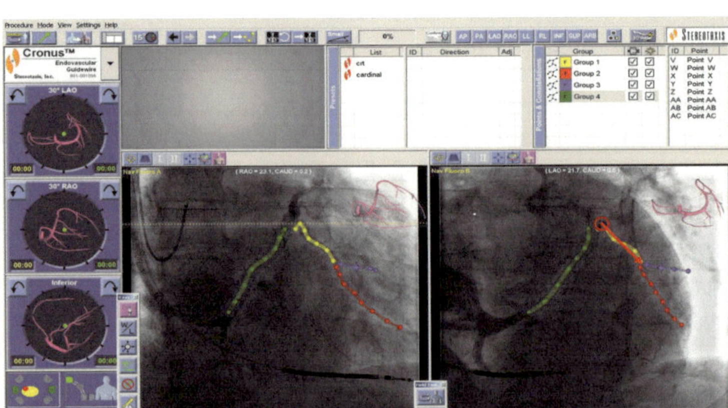

Fig. 4. Navigant screenshot. Two x-ray images have been transferred to the navigation software and tributaries of the CS have been marked with colors. The red arrow indicates the direction of the magnetic field vector.

3.5 Video-assisted pericardioscopic epicardial lead implantation

In an animal study we used flexible and rigid endoscopy for implantation of epicardial pacing leads via a subxiphoidal access (Hatam et al., 2010). Rigid endoscopy showed to be superior to flexible endoscopy with regard to stability and orientation within the pericardial space, and leads were successfully implanted onto all four cardiac chambers. This minimally invasive procedure allows access to all left ventricular regions. However, this technique requires a subxiphoidal access to the epicardial space and the endoscopy is associated with ventricular arrhythmias.

3.6 Leadless pacing

Pacing without pacemaker leads would decrease the risk of infection and might allow multisite pacing and thus decrease dyssynchrony. Ultrasound and magnetic field waves have been used to induce electrical stimulation via an intracardiac receiver electrode (Kapa et al., 2010; Lee et al., 2007). In an animal study Echt et al. (Echt et al., 2006) used burst ultrasound energy transmission through the chest to a receiver electrode mounted on a catheter that converted the ultrasound energy to electrical energy sufficient to pace the myocardium. Biventricular pacing was also possible in this acute animal study. Microscopic evaluation revealed no evidence of mechanical or thermal bioeffects. Lee et al. successfully tested this system in patients undergoing electrophysiological studies (Lee et al., 2006). The technology in this study is under development as a leadless implantable system for chronic use. Technical challenges include a high beat-to-beat variation in the receiver electrode output as well as inefficient energy conversion: less than 1% of the transmitted energy was used for cardiac pacing.

In an acute animal study Wieneke (Wieneke et al., 2009) demonstrated the feasibility of cardiac pacing via induction technology. The systems consisted of a transcutaneously implanted transmitter unit made of a ring-shaped copper coil and a receiver unit implanted in the right ventricular apex. The transmitter generated an alternating magnetic field of around 0.5 mT that was converted into a voltage pulse by the receiver in order to pace the ventricle. So far results have been published from one pig only, and no data on chronic pacing are availably.

A promising miniaturized leadless pacemaker is being developed by Medtronic (Minneapolis, USA): the small device can be deployed with a catheter from a venous access and implanted into the ventricular cavity. Up to now no animal or human data have been published about the device.

4. Electrical remodeling in CRT

In congestive heart failure (CHF), a complete left bundle branch block causes asynchronous ventricular contraction due to regional dispersion of ventricular depolarization, resulting in intra- and interventricular mechanical asynchrony. CRT reduces the heterogeneity of ventricular contraction by biventricular stimulation.

Especially patients with a very broad QRS-complex (> 150 msec) seem to profit most from CRT (Chung et al., 2008; Moss et al., 2009). Although QRS duration is not an optimal criterion for selecting patients amenable for CRT and some studies have failed to predict clinical and echocardiographic response to CRT, it remains an important criterion for dyssynchrony for the indication of CRT (Boriani et al., 2006; Gervais et al., 2009; Hawkins et al., 2006; Mollema et al., 2007).

In CRT, biventricular stimulation usually results in a narrowing of the stimulated QRS-complex and a reduction in left ventricular chamber size as well as improvement in ejection fraction. The extent of the QRS shortening induced by biventricular pacing seems to correlate with the structural remodeling (Boriani et al., 2006; Kronborg et al., 2010). However, about one third of patients fail to respond to CRT (Cleland et al., 2001; Chung et al., 2008; Lafitte et al., 2009). A lot of effort has been spent to both identify patients who are likely to benefit from CRT and to increase the benefit from CRT, e.g. by optimizing AV and VV delays (Strauss et al., 2010).

Although CRT has been shown to induce a structural remodeling resulting in reduction in left ventricular dimensions and improvement in ejection fraction, there is scarce and controversial data on a possible remodeling of the native conduction system (Dizon et al., 2004; Henrikson et al., 2007; Stockburger et al., 2008).

We studied the effect of CRT on the native conduction system in a small prospective study (Mischke et al., 2011). A CRT device was implanted in 38 patients with congestive heart failure (ejection fraction (EF): 26 ± 7%). 20 patients suffered from dilated cardiomyopathy and 18 from ischemic cardiomyopathy. Standard 12-lead ECGs with and without pacing as well as echocardiographies were obtained prior to implantation and after 6 and 12 months. Patients were classified as responders in case of an increase in EF ≥ 25% in combination with an increase in NYHA class ≥ 1. The EF increased to 36 ± 10% ($p<0.0001$) after 6 months and 40 ± 12% ($p<0.0001$) after 12 months of CRT. Intrinsic QRS duration decreased from 171 ± 18 ms before CRT to 164 ± 23 ms ($p=0.027$) after 6 months and 161 ± 25 ms ($p=0.002$) after 12 months of CRT (figure 5). 22 patients (58%) were classified as responders. Whereas a significant decrease in intrinsic QRS duration was observed in responders, only a slight decrease was seen in non-responders. However, two-factorial variance analyses did not show a significant influence of response or underlying heart disease (dilated or ischemic cardiomyopathy) on the change in QRS duration ($p=0.7$).

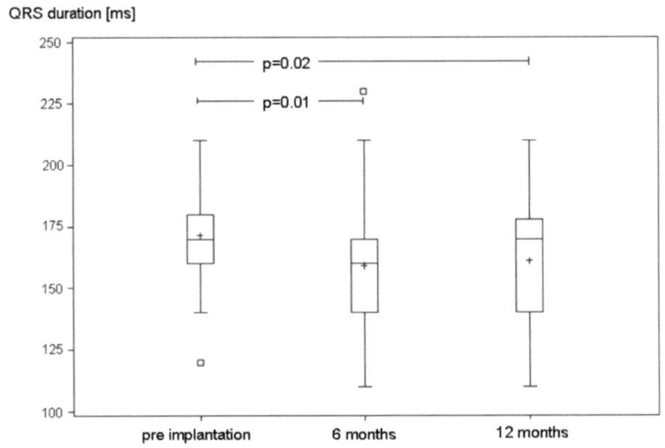

Fig. 5. Baseline and intrinsic QRS duration (from Mischke et al., 2011)

This was the first prospective study to demonstrate a decrease in intrinsic QRS duration in patients treated with CRT. Dizon et al. reported the first case of loss of bundle branch block in a patient 6 months after implantation of a CRT device (Dizon et al., 2004). However, data on intrinsic QRS duration is controversial. No change in intrinsic QRS duration was seen in the MUSTIC trial as well as in a study by Stockburger (Stockburger et al., 2008). Two studies displayed a trend towards a reduction in intrinsic QRS duration (Boriani et al., 2006; Vogt et al., 2000). Similar to our results, a retrospective study by Henrikson et al. showed a significant reduction in intrinsic QRS duration after 14 months of CRT in 25 patients (Henrikson et al., 2007). Experimental data suggest a subcellular redistribution of connexin43 and ion channel remodeling with a reduction in inward rectifier K+ current, delayed rectifier K^+ current and transient outward K^+ current) and abnormal Ca^{2+} homeostasis in left bundle branch block (Aiba et al., 2009; Spragg et al., 2005). CRT partially restored this ion channel remodeling and attenuated the regional heterogeneity of action potential duration. Although human data on intrinsic QRS duration in CRT is controversial, an impact on the conduction system by several factors including connexin redistribution and reduction in left ventricular dimensions is quite conceivable.

5. Conclusion

Cardiac resynchronization therapy is an effective treatment for patients with congestive heart failure and complete left bundle branch block. However, about one third of all patients who undergo CRT do not profit from it. Several strategies have been tried to reduce the percentage of non-responders, including optimized patient selection, device programming and optimized positioning of the left ventricular lead. However, due to high interpatient variability there seems to be no single best pacing site for all patients. Acute hemodynamic testing during implantation is time-consuming and good acute effects might not translate into a long-term clinical benefit.

None of these approaches has had a relevant impact on daily practice yet. In order to have the maximum benefit for our patients, we need to individualize the approach to CRT. Technical advances, like new lead designs and guiding catheters, are crucial for the further progress in CRT.

6. References

Abraham WT, Fisher WG, Smith AL, Delurgio DB, Leon AR, Loh E, Kocovic DZ, Packer M, Clavell AL, Hayes DL, Ellestad M, Trupp RJ, Underwood J, Pickering F, Truex C, McAtee P, Messenger J; MIRACLE Study Group. Multicenter InSync Randomized Clinical Evaluation. (2002). Cardiac resynchronization in chronic heart failure. *N Engl J Med*, Vol. 346, pp. 1845-1853.

Al-Khadra AS. (2005). Use of preshaped sheath to plan and facilitate cannulation of the coronary sinus for the implantation of cardiac resynchronization therapy devices: preshaped sheath for implantation of biventricular devices. *Pacing Clin Electrophysiol*, Vol. 28, pp. 489-492.

Aiba T, Hesketh GG, Barth AS Liu T, Daya S, Chakir K, Dimaano VL, Abraham TP, O'Rourke B, Akar FG, Kass DA, Tomaselli GF. (2009). Electrophysiological consequences of dyssynchronous heart failure and its restoration by resynchronization therapy. *Circulation*, Vol. 119, pp. 1220-1230

Becker M, Altiok E, Ocklenburg C, Krings R, Adams D, Lysansky M, Vogel B, Schauerte P, Knackstedt C, Hoffmann R. (2010). Analysis of LV lead position in cardiac resynchronization therapy using different imaging modalities. *JACC Cardiovasc Imaging*, Vol. 3, pp. 472-81

Becker M, Kramann R, Franke A, Breithardt OA, Heussen N, Knackstedt C, Stellbrink C, Schauerte P, Kelm M, Hoffmann R. (2007a). Impact of left ventricular lead position in cardiac resynchronization therapy on left ventricular remodelling. A circumferential strain analysis based on 2D echocardiography. *Eur Heart J*, Vol. 28, pp. 1211-20.

Becker M, Franke A, Breithardt OE, Kaminski T, Kramann R, Knackstedt C, Stellbrink C, Hanrath P, Schauerte P, Hoffmann R. (2007b). Impact of Left Ventricular Lead Position on the Efficacy of Cardiac Resynchronization Therapy. A Two-Dimensional Strain Echocardiography Study. *Heart*, Vol. 93, pp. 1197-203.

Bleeker GB, Kaandorp TA, Lamb HJ, Boersma E, Steendijk P, de Roos A, van der Wall EE, Schalij MJ, Bax JJ. (2006). Effect of posterolateral scar tissue on clinical and echocardiographic improvement after cardiac resynchronization therapy. *Circulation*, Vol. 113, pp. 969-76.

Boriani G, Biffi M, Martignani C, Ziacchi M, Saporito D, Grigioni F, Domenichini G, Valzania C, Diemberger I, Bertini M, Specchia S, Branzi A. (2006). Electrocardiographic remodeling during cardiac resynchronization therapy. *Int J Cardiol*, Vol. 108, pp. 165-170.

Butter C, Auricchio A, Stellbrink C, Fleck E, Ding J, Yu Y, Huvelle E, Spinelli J; Pacing Therapy for Chronic Heart Failure II Study Group. (2001). Effect of resynchronization therapy stimulation site on the systolic function of heart failure patients. *Circulation*, Vol. 104, No. 25, pp. 3026-9.

Chung ES, Leon AR, Tavazzi LJ, Sun JP, Nihoyannopoulos P, Merlino J, Abraham WT, Ghio S, Leclercq C, Bax JJ, Yu CM, Gorcsan J 3rd, St John Sutton M, De Sutter J, Murillo J. (2008). Results of the predictors of response to CRT (PROSPECT) trial. *Circulation* Vol. 117, pp. 2608–2616.

Cleland JG, Daubert JC, Erdmann E, Freemantle N, Gras D, Kappenberger L, Tavazzi L; Cardiac Resynchronization-Heart Failure (CARE-HF) Study Investigators. (2005). The effect of cardiac resynchronization on morbidity and mortality in heart failure. *N Engl J Med*, Vol. 352, pp. 1539-1549.

de Cock CC, Giudici MC, Twisk JW. (2003). Comparison of the haemodynamic effects of right ventricular outflow-tract pacing with right ventricular apex pacing: a quantitative review. *Europace*, Vol. 5, No. 3:275-8.

Derval N, Steendijk P, Gula LJ, Deplagne A, Laborderie J, Sacher F, Knecht S, Wright M, Nault I, Ploux S, Ritter P, Bordachar P, Lafitte S, Réant P, Klein GJ, Narayan SM, Garrigue S, Hocini M, Haissaguerre M, Clementy J, Jaïs P. (2010). Optimizing hemodynamics in heart failure patients by systematic screening of left ventricular pacing sites: the lateral left ventricular wall and the coronary sinus are rarely the best sites. *J Am Coll Cardiol*, Vol. 55, pp. 566 –75.

Dizon J, Horn E, Neglia J Medina N, Garan H (2004) Loss of Left Bundle Branch Block following Biventricular Pacing Therapy for Heart Failure: Evidence for Electrical remodeling? *JICE*, Vol. 10, pp. 47-50.

Duckett SG, Ginks MR, Knowles BR, Ma Y, Shetty A, Bostock J, Cooklin M, Gill JS, Carr-White GS, Razavi R, Schaeffter T, Rhode KS, Rinaldi CA. (2010) Advanced Image Fusion to Overlay Coronary Sinus Anatomy with Real-Time Fluoroscopy to Facilitate Left Ventricular Lead Implantation in CRT. *Pacing Clin Electrophysiol* doi: 10.1111/j.1540-8159.2010.02940.x. [Epub ahead of print]

Echt DS, Cowan MW, Riley RE, Brisken AF. (2006). Feasibility and safety of a novel technology for pacing without leads. *Heart Rhythm*, Vol. 3, No. 10 pp.1202-6

Hatam N, Amerini AL, Steiner F, Lazeroms M, Mischke K, Schauerte P, Autschbach R, Spillner J. (2010). Video-assisted pericardioscopic surgery: refinement of a new technique for implanting epimyocardial pacemaker leads. *Eur J Cardiothorac Surg* [Epub ahead of print]

Henz BD, Friedman PA, Bruce CJ, Okumura Y, Johnson SB, Danielsen A, Packer DL, Asirvatham SJ. (2009). Synchronous ventricular pacing without crossing the tricuspid valve or entering the coronary sinus--preliminary results. *J Cardiovasc Electrophysiol*, Vol. 20, No. 12, pp.1391-7.

Gallagher P, Martin L, Angel L, Tomassoni G. (2007). Initial clinical experience with cardiac resynchronization therapy utilizing a magnetic navigation system. *J Cardiovasc Electrophysiol*, Vol. 18, pp.174-180.

Helm RH, Byrne M, Helm PA, Daya SK, Osman NF, Tunin R, Halperin HR, Berger RD, Kass DA, Lardo AC. (2007). Three-dimensional mapping of optimal left ventricular pacing site for cardiac resynchronization. *Circulation*, Vol. 115, pp. 953-61

Henrikson CA, Spragg DD, Cheng A, Capps M, Devaughn K, Marine JE, Calkins H, Tomaselli GF, Berger RD. (2007). Evidence for electrical Remodeling of the Native Conduction System with Cardiac Resynchronization Therapy. *Pacing Clin Electrophysiol* Vol. 30, pp. 591-595.

Jaïs P, Takahashi A, Garrigue S, Yamane T, Hocini M, Shah DC, Barold SS, Deisenhofer I, Haïssaguerre M, Clémenty J. (2000). Mid-term follow-up of endocardial biventricular pacing. *Pacing Clin Electrophysiol*, Vol. 23, pp. 1744–7.

Kapa S, Bruce CJ, Friedman PA, Asirvatham SJ. (2010). Advances in cardiac pacing: beyond the transvenous right ventricular apical lead. *Cardiovasc Ther*, Vol. 28, No. 6, pp. 369-79.

Kassai I, Foldesi C, Szekely A, Szili-Torok T. (2008). New method for cardiac resynchronization therapy: transapical endocardial lead implantation for left ventricular free wall pacing. *Europace*, Vol. 10, No. 7, pp. 882-3.

Knackstedt C, Mühlenbruch G, Mischke K, Bruners P, Schimpf T, Frechen D, Schummers G, Mahnken AH, Günther RW, Kelm M, Schauerte P. (2008a). Imaging of the Coronary Venous System: Validation of Three-Dimensional Rotational Venous Angiography Against Dual-Source Computed Tomography. *Cardiovasc Intervent Radiol*,Vol. 31, No. 6, pp. 1150-8

Knackstedt C, Mühlenbruch G, Mischke K, Schimpf T, Spüntrup E, Günther RW, Sanli B, Kelm M, Schauerte P, Mahnken AH. (2008b). Imaging of the coronary venous system in patients with congestive heart failure: comparison of 16 slice MSCT and retrograde coronary sinus venography: Comparative imaging of coronary venous system. *Int J Cardiovasc Imaging*, Vol. 24, No. 8, pp. 783-91

Knackstedt C, Mühlenbruch G, Mischke K, Schummers G, Becker M, Kühl H, Franke A, Schmid M, Spuentrup E, Mahnken A, Lang RM, Kelm M, Günther R, Schauerte P. (2010a). Registration of Coronary Venous Anatomy the Site of Latest Mechanical Contraction. *Acta Cardiol*, Vol. 65, pp. 161-70

Knackstedt C, Schimpf T, Napp A, Wessling B, Rothe C, Mischke K, Schnakenberg U, Schauerte P. (2010b). Super-Selective Electrical Stimulation of the Left Ventricle via a Miniaturized Magnetized Stimulation Wire -Proof of Concept Study-. *Biomed Tech (Berl)*, Vol. 55, pp.285-90.

Kronborg, MB, Nielsen JC, Mortensen PT. (2010). Electrocardiographic patterns and long-term clinical outcome in cardiac resynchronization therapy. *Europace*, Vol. 12, pp. 216-222.

Kypta A, Steinwender C, Kammler J, Leisch F, Hofmann R. (2008). Long-term outcomes in patients with atrioventricular block undergoing septal ventricular lead implantation compared with standard apical pacing. *Europace*, Vol. 10, No. 5, pp. 574-9.

Lafitte S, Reant P, Zaroui A, Donal E, Mignot A, Bougted H, Belghiti H, Bordachar P, Deplagne A, Chabaneix J, Franceschi F, Deharo JC, Dos Santos P, Clementy J, Roudaut R, Leclercq C, Habib G. (2009). Validation of an echocardiographic multiparametric strategy to increase responders patients after cardiac resynchronization: a multicentre study. *Eur Heart J*, Vol. 30, pp. 2880-2887.

Leclercq F, Hager FX, Macia JC, Mariottini CJ, Pasquié JL, Grolleau R. (1999). Left ventricular lead insertion using a modified transseptal catheterization technique: a totally endocardial approach for permanent biventricular pacing in end-stage heart failure. *Pacing Clin Electrophysiol*, Vol. 22, pp. 1570 –5.

Lee KL, Lau CP, Tse HF, Echt DS, Heaven D, Smith W, Hood M. (2007). First human demonstration of cardiac stimulation with transcutaneous ultrasound energy delivery: implications for wireless pacing with implantable devices. *J Am Coll Cardiol*, Vol. 50, No. 9, pp. 877-83

Ma H, Tang Q, Yang Q, Bi X, Lu H, Ge L, Lin K, Xu D, Du X, Lu J, An J, Jin L, Jerecic R. Li K, Li D. (2010). Contrast-enhance whole heart coronary MRA at 3.0T for the evaluation of cardiac venous anatomy. *In J Cardiovasc Imaging*, in press

Mischke K, Knackstedt C, Fache K, Reith S, Rana O, Saygili E, Gemein C, Becker M, Marx N, Schauerte P. (2011). Electrical remodelling in cardiac resynchronization therapy: decrease in intrinsic QRS duration. *Acta Cardiol*, in press

Mischke K, Knackstedt C, Schmid M, Hatam N, Becker M, Spillner J, Fache K, Kelm M, Schauerte P. (2009). Initial experience with remote magnetic navigation for left ventricular lead placement. *Acta Cardiol*, Vol. 64, No. 4, pp. 467-475

Mischke K, Knackstedt C, Mühlenbruch G, Schimpf T, Neef N, Zarse M, Plisiene J, Stanzel S, Eickholt C, Spüntrup E, Frechen D, Hanrath P, Kelm M, Schauerte P. (2007). Imaging of the coronary venous system: retrograde coronary sinus angiography versus venous phase coronary angiograms. *Int J Cardiol*, Vol. 119, No. 3, pp.339-43

Moss AJ, Hall WJ, Cannom DS, Klein H, Brown MW, Daubert JP, Estes NA 3rd, Foster E, Greenberg H, Higgins SL, Pfeffer MA, Solomon SD, Wilber D, Zareba W; MADIT-CRT Trial Investigators. (2009). Cardiac-resynchronization therapy for the prevention of heart-failure events. *N Engl J Med*, Vol.. 361, pp.1329-1338.

Nezafat R, Han Y, Peters DC, Herzka DA, Wylie JV, Goddu B, Kissinger KK, Yeon SB, Zimetbaum PJ, Manning WJ. (2007). Coronary magnetic resonance vein imaging: imaging contrast, sequence, and timing. *Magn Reson Med*, Vol. 58, pp. 1196-206

Purerfellner H, Nesser HJ, Winter S, Schwierz T, Hornell H, Maertens S. (2000). Transvenous left ventricular lead implantation with the EASYTRAK lead system: the European experience. *Am J Cardiol*, Vol. 86, pp. 157K-164K.

Spragg DD, Akar FG, Helm RH, Tunin RS, Tomaselli GF, Kass DA. (2005). Abnormal conduction and repolarization in late-activated myocardium of dyssynchronously contracting hearts. *Cardiovasc Res*, Vol. 67, pp. 77-86.

Spragg DD, Dong J, Fetics BJ, Helm R, Marine JE, Cheng A, Henrikson CA, Kass DA, Berger RD. (2010). Optimal left ventricular endocardial pacing sites for cardiac resynchronization therapy in patients with ischemic cardiomyopathy. *J Am Coll Cardiol*, Vol. 56, No. 10, pp. 774-81.

Stockburger M, Nitardy A, Fateh-Moghadam S, Krebs A, Celebi O, Karhausen T, Dietz R. (2008). Electrical remodeling and cardiac dimensions in patients treated by cardiac resynchronization and heart failure controls. *Pacing Clin Electrophysiol*, Vol. 31, pp. 70-77.

Strauss M, Becker T, Kleemann T, Dyck N, Birkenhauer F, Seidl K. (2010). Impact of moderate exercise workload on predicted optimal AV and VV delays determined by an intracardiac electrogram-based method for optimizing cardiac resynchronization therapy. *Clin Res Cardiol*, Vol. 99, pp. 735-41.

Tantengco MV, Thomas RL, Karpawich PP. (2001) Left ventricular dysfunction after long-term right ventricular apical pacing in the young. *J Am Coll Cardiol*, Vol. 37, No. 8, pp. 2093-100.

Tops LF, Schalij MJ, Bax JJ. (2009). The effects of right ventricular apical pacing on ventricular function and dyssynchrony implications for therapy. *J Am Coll Cardiol*, Vol. 54, No. 9, pp. 764-76.

Van de Verie NR, Schuij JD, De Sutter J, Devos D, Bleeker GB, de Roos A, van der Wall ÄEE, Schalij MG, Bax JJ. (2006). Non-invasive visualization of the cardiac venous system in coronary artery disease patients using 64-slice computed tomography. *J Am Coll Cardiol*, Vol. 48, pp. 1832-8.

van Deursen C, van Geldorp IE, Rademakers LM, van Hunnik A, Kuiper M, Klersy C, Auricchio A, Prinzen FW. (2009). Left ventricular endocardial pacing improves resynchronization therapy in canine left bundle-branch hearts. *Circ Arrhythm Electrophysiol*, Vol. 2, pp. 580 -7.

Vanerio G, Vidal JL, Fernández Banizi P, Banina Aguerre D, Viana P, Tejada J. (2008). Medium- and long-term survival after pacemaker implant: Improved survival with right ventricular outflow tract pacing. *J Interv Card Electrophysiol*, Vol. 21, No. 3, pp.195-201.

van Gelder BM, Scheffer MG, Meijer A, Bracke FA. (2007). Transseptal endocardial left ventricular pacing: an alternative technique for coronary sinus lead placement in cardiac resynchronization therapy. *Heart Rhythm*, Vol. Vol. 4, pp. 454–60.

van Gelder BM, Bracke FA, Oto A, Yildirir A, Haas PC, Seger JJ, Stainback RF, Botman KJ, Meijer A. (2000). Diagnosis and management of inadvertently placed pacing and ICD leads in the left ventricle: a multicenter experience and review of the literature. *Pacing Clin Electrophysiol*, Vol. 23, No. 5, pp. 877-83.

Vogt J, Krahnefeld O, Lamp B, Hansky B, Kirkels H, Minami K, Körfer R, Horstkotte D, Kloss M, Auricchio A. (2000). Pacing Therapies in Congestive Heart Failure Study Group. Electrocardiographic remodeling in patients paced for heart failure. *Am J Cardiol*, Vol. 86, pp. 152K-156K.

Wieneke H, Konorza T, Erbel R, Kisker E. (2009). Leadless pacing of the heart using induction technology: a feasibility study. *Pacing Clin Electrophysiol*, Vol. 32, No. 2, pp. 177-83.

White JA, Yee R, Yuan X, Krahn A, Skanes A, Parker M, Klein G, Drangova M. (2006). Delayed enhancement magnetic resonance imaging predicts response to cardiac resynchronization therapy in patients with intraventricular dyssynchrony. *J Am Coll Cardiol*, Vol. 48, pp. 1953-60.

Ypenburg C, van Bommel RJ, Delgado V, Mollema SA, Bleeker GB, Boersma E, Schalij MJ, Bax JJ. (2008). Optimal left ventricular lead position predicts reverse remodeling and survival after cardiac resynchronization therapy. *J Am Coll Cardiol*, Vol. 52, pp. 1402-9.

Yu CC, Liu YB, Lin MS, Wang JY, Lin JL, Lin LC. (2007). Septal pacing preserving better left ventricular mechanical performance and contractile synchronism than apical pacing in patients implanted with an atrioventricular sequential dual chamber pacemaker. *Int J Cardiol*, Vol. 118, No. 1, pp. 97-106.

6

Implantable Loop Recorder in Clinical Practice

Dominique Babuty, Bertrand Pierre, Nicolas Clémenty, Bénédicte Lallemand, Olivier Marie and Laurent Fauchier
François Rabelais University / Hospital Trousseau Tours
France

1. Introduction

Implantable Loop Recorder (ILR) or Insertable Cardiac Monitor (ICM) is a tool developed in the 1990's which allows permanent monitoring of cardiac rhythm during a period exceeding one year. The major interest of this new tool is to establish a closed correlation between symptoms and heart rhythm. The first application of ICM was the diagnosis of recurrent syncope. Syncope is a common disorder which may recur and impair the survival and the quality of life of the patients. The objective of the investigation of syncope is to diagnose the cardiac aetiology because the mortality in this case is high. About half of the patients implanted with an ICM complains of a new syncope and about 50% of these patients had documented cardiac rhythm disturbances. The most frequent is a sinus bradycardia or sinus arrest but these results depend on the age of patients, resting ECG abnormalities and structural cardiac disease. A classification of the mechanisms of recurrent syncopes has been defined with the results of the ISSUE study separating the syncope due to primary cardiac arrhythmia from neurally-mediated syncope and from unknown syncope. The analysis of the presyncopal phase on the ICM restored ECG allows physicians to adapt the treatment (antiarrhythmic (with 2 h) agents or pacemaker) and optimize the programming of the pacemaker when necessary. It is recommended to implant the ICM early in the syncope patients with a normal physical examination, normal ECG and without structural heart disease and negative tilt testing. In the presence of cardiac disease, it is recommended to implant the ICM after performing an electrophysiological study and tilt testing. In syncope patients with depressed left ventricular ejection fraction, the implantation of an automatic implantable cardiac defibrillator is preferable. Early application of an ICM reduces the cost of the investigation of the patients suffering from syncope, especially when the electrophysiological study is avoided. The indications of the ICM tend to be extended to new syncope populations such as pediatric patients, the epileptic population and older patients suffering from unexplained falls. New algorithms are developed by the manufacturers which allow a good analysis of electrical atrial activity and open new applications of the ICM in the managements of patients treated for atrial arrhythmias.

2. Syncopes and unexplained recurrent syncopes

Syncope is a common disorder with an annual incidence of 1.3-2.7 episodes/1000 per year. Recurrent syncopes are also frequent, accounting for 3% of emergency visits and 1% of hospital admissions in the US. The diagnosis of cardiac syncope remains the principal objective in these patients because the mortality rates exceed 30% in this subgroup of patients (Kapoor et al., 1983; Soteriades et al., 2002). However, their diagnosis is often difficult, leading to repetitive hospitalizations and clinical investigations. About 40% of diagnoses are established after the related history is considered and a meticulous physical examination and resting ECG recorded, but in 60% the diagnosis is probable or uncertain. The applications of the laboratory investigations are limited. The ambulatory ECG of 24 or 48 hours identified a rhythmic aetiology in 19% of cases; the electrophysiological study is only useful in patients with underlying structural cardiac disease or resting ECG abnormalities (Task force 2004; Strickberer et al., 2006). Tilt table testing is useful to provoke neurally-mediated syncope, but its specificity and sensitivity are still debated (Moya et al., 2001). Exercise stress testing is not recommended except in stress induced syncope. Neurological testings are also not recommended (Task force 2004; Moya et al., 2009). Since clear recommendations published in 2004 and 2009 about the diagnosis strategy of syncope a median of 13 performed tests per patient has been reported in a recent large prospective study before considering ICM implantation (Edvardsson et al., 2011).

After complete investigations, recurrent syncopes remain undiagnosed in about 20 - 30% (Krahn et al., 1999a; Brignole et al., 2005a; Vitale et al., 2010). The gold standard for the diagnosis of an arrhythmic event is the ECG recording during a syncopal episode which can be obtained by a prolonged ECG recording. The first developed method was the external loop recorder but patient compliance is low and the duration is limited to a few weeks. About 20 % of the patients failed to activate their loop recorder properly, resulting in an undiagnosed test (Sivakumaran et al., 2003). The second method is the implantable loop recorder which now allows for a monitoring of cardiac rhythm over three years. This method of investigation for recurrent syncope is recommended by the Task force (Task force, 2004; Moya et al., 2009). A recent study estimated that ICM should be implanted in two thirds of the patients suffering from unexplained recurrent syncopes (Vitale et al., 2010) but only 18 % of these patients were implanted. Although the ICM has been recognized as a useful tool in the diagnosis of recurrent syncopes in the latest guidelines for the management of recurrent syncope it is always underutilized.

3. Methods

3.1 Principle

We describe for example the first device manufactured for the market. It is a small (62x19x8 mm) titanium box of 9 cm^3 in volume and weighing 17 g. The ICM is a single-lead ECG recording device with an initial battery life of 14 months (Reveal® 9525, 9526 Medtronic USA, Minneapolis) and which is now 36 months (Reveal® DX 9528 Medtronic USA, Minneapolis). The two sensing bipoles are separated by a distance of 37 mm. For the most recent device the bipolar electrocardiogram signal is stored in a circular memory of 49.5 minutes. After spontaneous symptoms, the memory is frozen with a patient assistant: 6.5 minutes of the preceding ECG signal are stored and 1 minute after activation. Three spontaneous episodes can be stored. The rhythmic events can be automatically stored in accordance with the alert programmed limits (27 episodes – 0.5 minutes pre and 0.5 minutes post-activation). The ECG can be retrieved by a standard programmer (Medtronic 2090, Medtronic USA, Minneapolis) (figure 1). New detection algorithms proved their efficiency to detect the presence of atrial arrhythmias (Reveal® XT, Medtronic USA, Minneapolis)

(Hindricks et al., 2010) and will participate in the extension of the indications of the ICM implantation to patients suffering from palpitations, atrial fibrillation etc...
Others devices (Paruchuri et al., 2011) are in development by others manufacturers (Confirm ILR, St Jude Medical and Sleuth ILR, Transoma Medical, Arden Hills, MN).

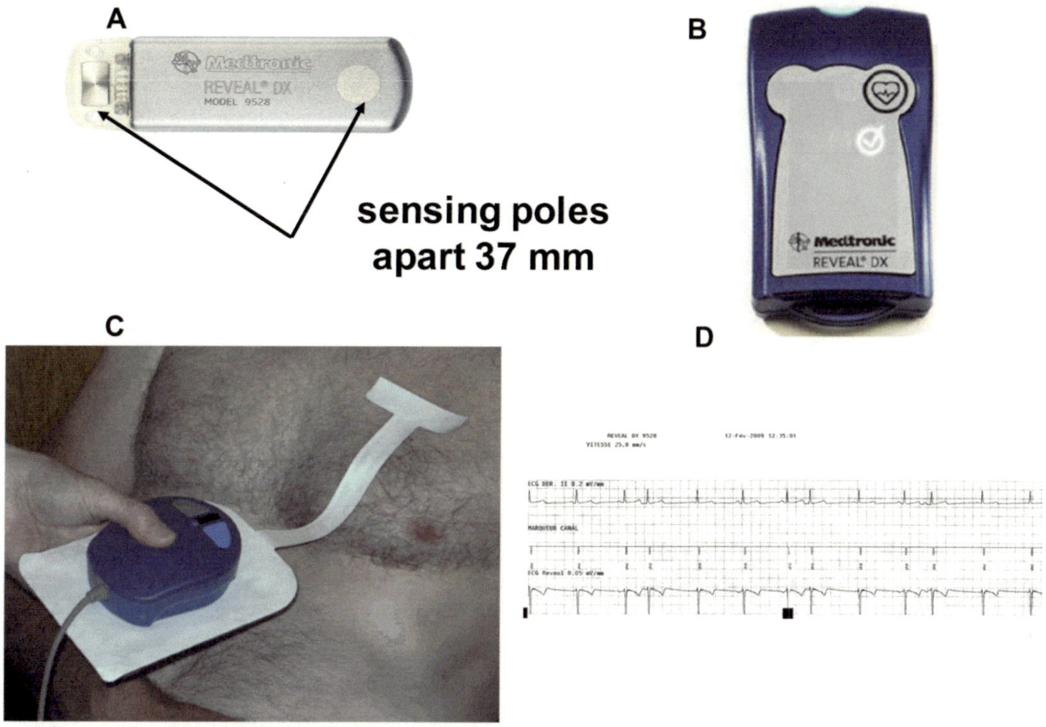

Fig. 1. A. Insertable cardiac monitor. B Reveal patient assistant in the pocket of the patient. C. Reveal Vector Check helps the physician to define the optimal implantation site based on the signal detection. D. Example of ECG recording with the Reveal Vector Check.

3.2 Implantation technique and positions (anterior chest or left axillary)

The ICM is easily inserted in the left chest using a local anesthetic with thorough asepsis in an operating room. A pocket is fashioned and the device is inserted with the electrodes towards the skin. The best implantation site is vertically to the right or left of the sternum between the fourth and the fifth intercostal spaces (Zellerhoff et al., 2000) (figure 2). With the latest version (Reveal DX) we can use the Reveal Vector Check to confirm the optimal implantation site based on signal detection. Sometimes an unusual site can be chosen, such left axillary implantation (figure 2). Miracapillo et al implanted 10 patients with an ICM in axillary position with success. The high R-wave amplitude obtained in this position was higher than with the standard position. The quality of the ECG recorder was always excellent and always allowed easy diagnosis interpretation (Miracapillo et al., 2010). This site of implantation might be very useful in younger patients for aesthetic reasons but also in obese patients to improve the amplitude of the R-wave recorded.

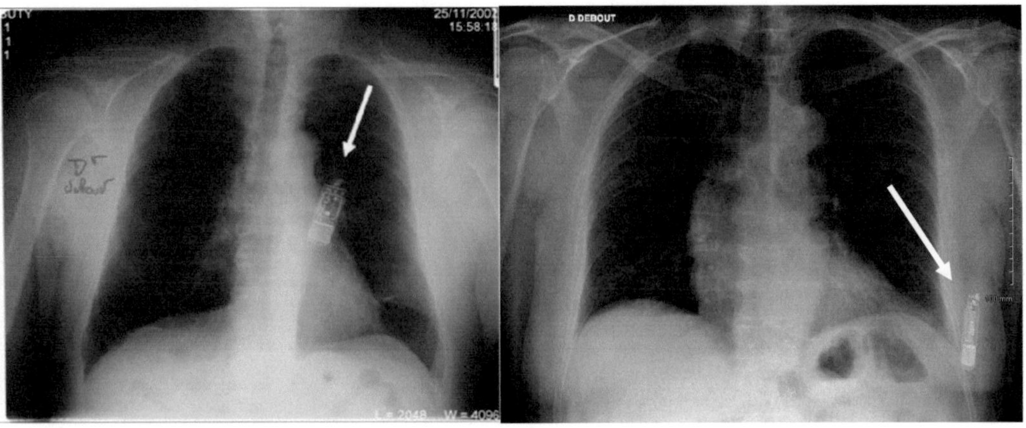

Fig. 2 Left. Anteroposterior chest radiography displays Reveal in a usual site. Right. Chest radiography shows Reveal inserted in a left axillary site in a young girl.

3.3 Program parameters and control

After implantation, the ICM is programmed. In the latest version of ICM, sensing and detection are automatically programmed (dynamic sensing threshold). Physicians can optimize the sensing of R-waves by adjusting the sensitivity parameters. Automatic ECG memory storage of episodes is activated by the physician (fast ventricular tachycardia, ventricular tachycardia, asystole, bradycardia) and the upper limits are defined. We can customize the detection criteria for each type of episode. Activation by the patient after syncope is possible with the Patient Assistant.

3.4 Follow up

Regular interrogation of the device is adviced to detect symptomatic or non-symptomatic arrhythmias or paroxysmal bradycardia. However for the past months it has been possible to control the ICM by telecardiology. This technology has several advantages, the control is permanent, the patient remains at home and the alerts are chosen by the cardiologist depending upon the clinical characteristics of the patient.

3.5 False positive recording or limits of the method

Five to 30 % of patients failed to appropriately activate the device after syncope. That was a problem with the first generation of the device which has disappeared with the newer generations of the device. The second and third generations have the ability to record an event either automatically or by manual activation. The effectiveness of the automatic activation has been evaluated by Ermis et al. in 50 patients. The auto-activation mode was found to be more efficient in documenting arrhythmia episodes than the manual activation mode (48% arrhythmia versus 6%) (Ermis et al., 2003). One limit of the ICM is related to the transient loss of signal which generates a false flat baseline tracing (figure 3). A false ventricular pause can also be recorded with the latest generation of ICM characterized by an autodetection sensing of the QRS. The change in the R wave amplitude leads to their undersensing. Conversely, the oversensing of myopotential noises can lead to the detection of false ventricular tachycardia or fibrillation (Figure 4). The second limit of the ICM is the lack of contemporary recording of blood pressure values. Neurally-mediated syncopes are not always associated with bradycardia, but exclusive vasodepressor response is possible. These kinds of syncope cannot be diagnosed with the ICM nor the syncope linked to the modification or adjustment to the upright position. The exact nature of the syncope remains unknown in these conditions.

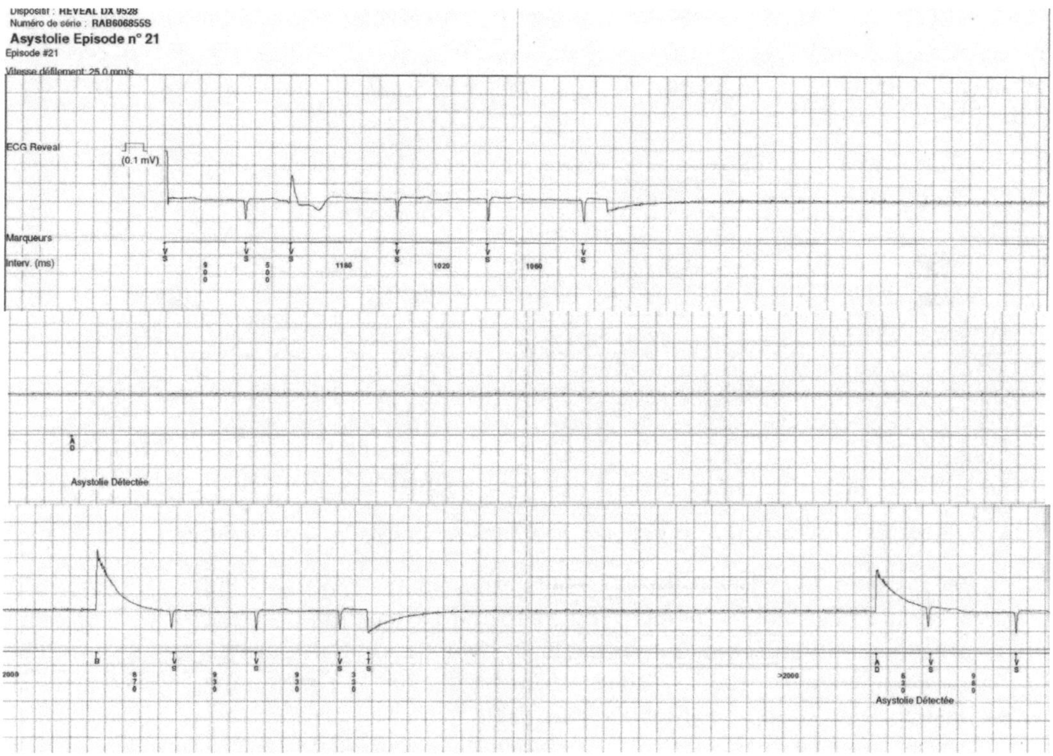

Fig. 3. Transient loss of signal which generates a false flat baseline tracing indicated as asystole in absence of presyncope or syncope.

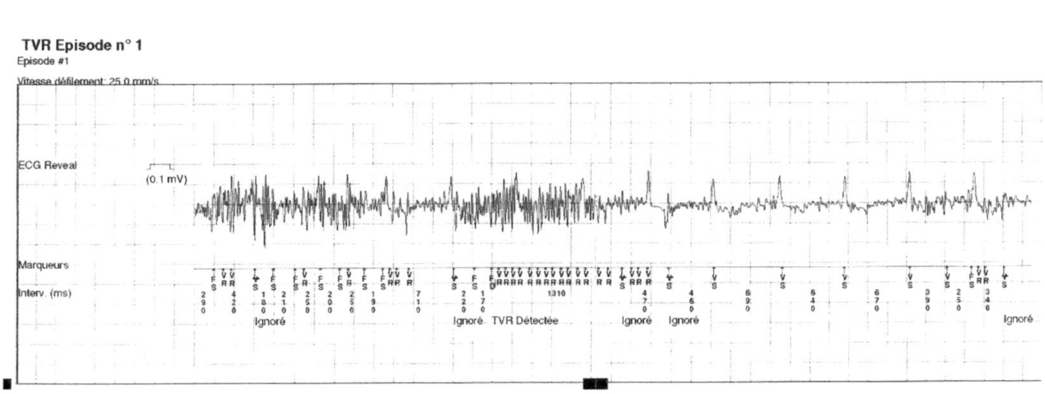

Fig. 4. Paroxysmal oversensing of R waves confounded to myopotentiels (Reveal® 9528). Fast ventricular tachycardia is the diagnosis retained by the device.

4. ICM implanted for recurrent syncopes

4.1 Results

Initially, the implantation of the ICM was limited to patients with recurrent syncopes and thorough negative investigations including an electrophysiological study. After the implantation of the ICM about 50% of the patients complained of a new syncope (Krahn et al., 1999a; Nierop et al., 2000; Lombardi et al., 2005; Pierre et al., 2008; Entem et al., 2009). The syncope is correlated to a rhythmic event in about 50% of cases (Table 1). These results are confirmed in the largest registry published in 2011 (PICTURE registry): 38 % of recruited patients complained of a recurrent syncope whose 59 % have a cardiac aetiology (Edvardsson et al., 2011).

Authors	Patients n	Syncope recurrence n (%)	Rhythmic event n (%)
Krahn 1999a	85	58 (68.2)	21(42)
Nierop 2000	35	14 (40)	8 (57)
Seidll 2000	133	83 (62)	32 (39)
Chettaoui 2002	32	15 (46.8)	10 (71)
Pierre 2008	95	43 (45.2)	27 (62.8)
Entem 2009	140	54 (38.5)	33 (64.5)
Edvardsson 2011	650	218 (38)	128 (59)

Table 1. Frequency of recurrent syncope and rhythmic events in ICM patients

The most frequent recorded event is a sinus arrest or bradycardia (figure 5); a complete atrio-ventricular block is less frequent (figure 6) and tachycardia is rare (figures 7, 8). Sinus bradycardia or sinus arrest account for the majority of the rhythmic events, and the duration of the events is widely variable (Table 2) (Chenet al., 2008). The ventricular pause can be severe, lasting up to 70 seconds (Babuty et al., 2001).

Authors	Syncope	Rhythmic event	Bradycardia	AVB	SupraVT	VT	others
Krahn 1999a	58	21	18	?	3		
Nierop 2000	14	14	4	?	4		
Seidl 2000	83	32	22	?	6	3	1
Krahn 2001	30	11	10		1		3
Chettaoui 2002	15	21	2	?	5	3	
Brignole 2005b	22	17	3	14			
Pierre 2008	43	27	16	5	2	4	
Entem 2009	51	33	18	9	2	4	

Table 2. Arrhythmic events documented by ICM

However these results depend upon the patient's age: in older patients arrhythmic events are more frequent (3.1 higher probability of an arrhythmia) (Brignole et al., 2005a). In patients older than 65 years of age, complete atrio-ventricular block accounts for 53% of arrhythmia events.

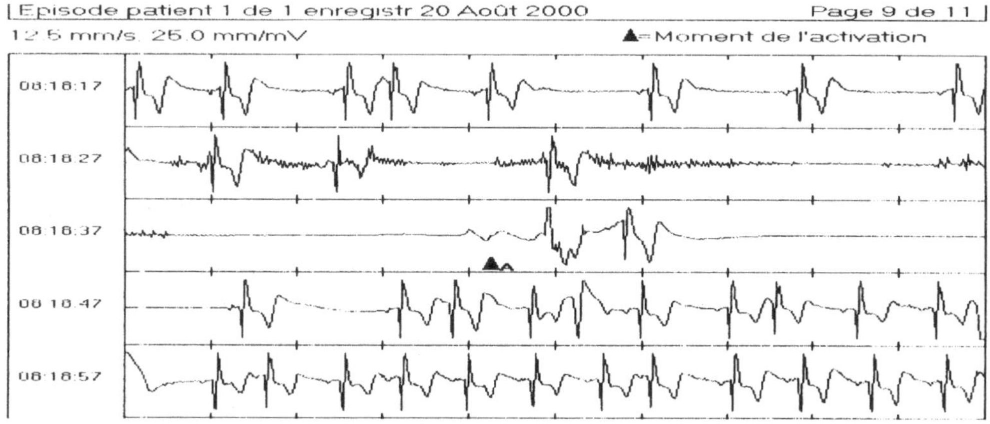

Fig. 5. Symptomatic sinus arrest during 9 seconds

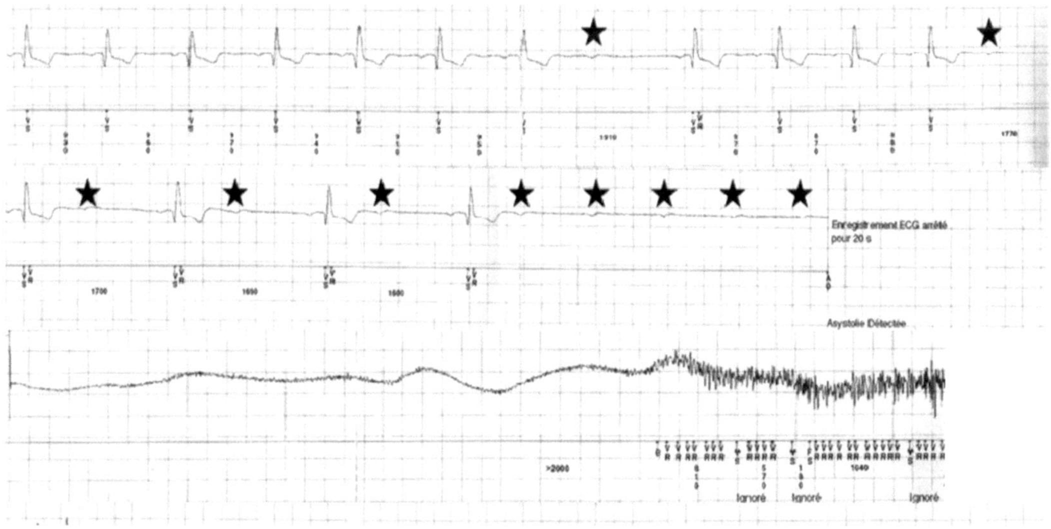

Fig. 6. Reveal's auto-activation captured a ventricular pause due to complete atrioventricular block. P waves are indicated by black stars.

The timeframe for recurrent symptoms shows that most events occur shortly after the implantation of the ICM: 31% within 30 days, 50% within 2 months, 78% within 6 months and 93% within one year (Assar et al., 2003).

Syncope is more likely to be associated with an arrhythmia than presyncope. Krahn et al reported a higher incidence of arrhythmic events in the group of patients suffering from syncope (64%) than in the group suffering from presyncope (25%) (Krahn et al., 1999a, 2001a).

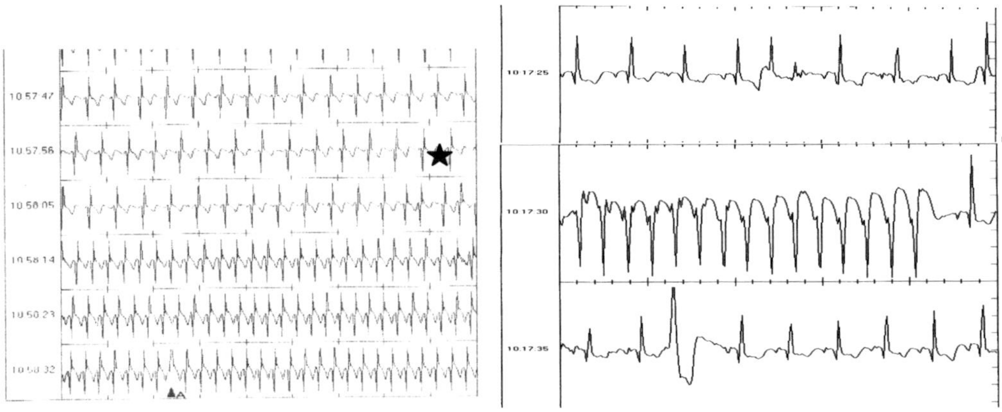

Fig. 7. Left. Symptomatic paroxysmal supraventricular tachycardia (black star). The electrophysiological demonstrated the atrioventricular nodal reentrant tachycardia. Right. Presyncope due to fast irregular tachycardia with wide QRS recorded in a patient without structural heart disease. During the electrophysiological study a right functional bundle branch block was induced by rapid atrial pacing. Atrial fibrillation was the final diagnosis and the patient was successfully treated with an antiarhythmic drug.

The International Study on Syncope of Uncertain Etiology (ISSUE) proposed a classification of spontaneous syncope documented by an implantable loop recorder (Brignole et al., 2005b) dependent on the mechanism of syncope (Table 3). The advantage of this classification is that of separating the syncope due to primary cardiac arrhythmia (Type 1C, type 4 B, 4C, 4D) from neurally-mediated syncope (type 1A, 1B, type 2) and from unknown syncope (type 3). However this classification probably overestimated the number of neurally-mediated syncope because some sick sinus syndrome patients are included in type 2.

Arrhythmia	Mechanism
Type 1 Asystole (pause ≥ 3 seconds) Type 1A Sinus arrest initiated by progressive bradycardia or tachycardia Type 1B Sinus bradycardia and AV block Type 1C AV block sudden with concomitant increase in sinus rate	Neurally-mediated syncope Neurally-mediated syncope Primary cardiac arrhythmia
Type 2 Bradycardia Type 2A decrease of heart rate > 30 % Type 2B Heart rate < 40 for 10 seconds	Neurally mediated syncope
Type 3 No or slight rhythm variations	Unknown
Type 4 Tachycardia increase in heart rate > 30 % or > 120 /min Type 4A progressive sinus tachycardia Type 4B atrial fibrillation Type 4C supraventricular tachycardia Type 4D ventricular tachycardia	Inadaptation to the upright position Primary cardiac arrhythmia Primary cardiac arrhythmia Primary cardiac arrhythmia

Table 3. The ISSUE classification of ECG-documented spontaneous syncope

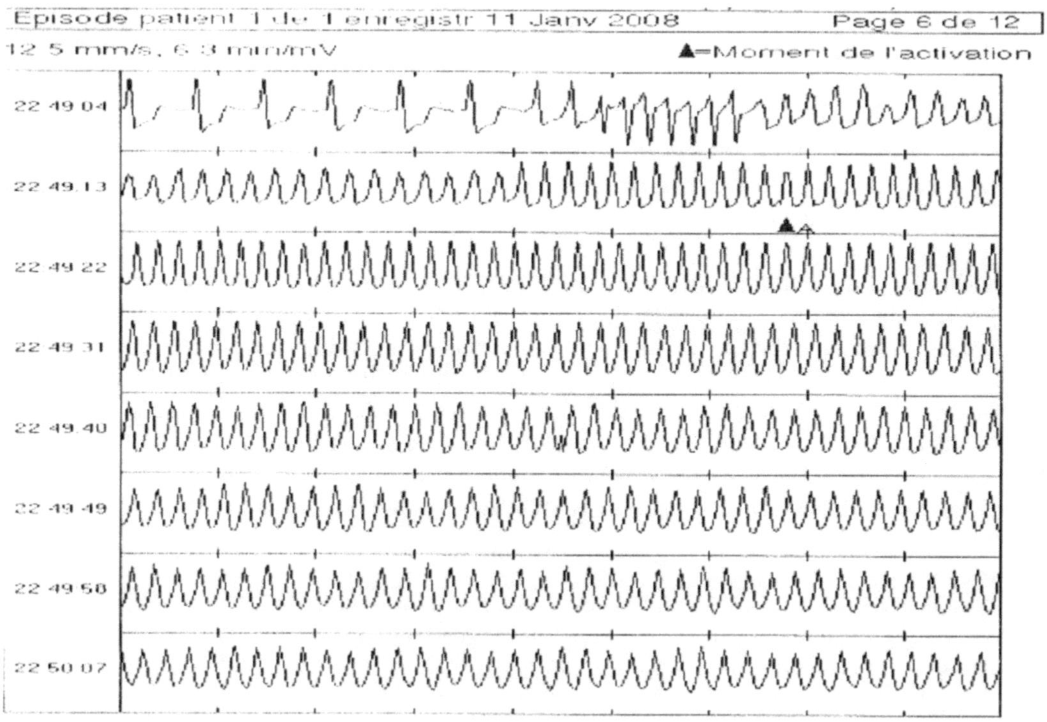

Fig. 8. Syncope due to fast ventricular tachycardia. Note the change of the QRS morphology at the beginning of the tachycardia.

4.2 Influence of resting ECG and structural heart disease on results of ICM recordings

One generally analyzes with caution the patients suffering from syncope in the presence of abnormalities on resting ECG or in the presence of structural heart disease. The Task force defined some electrocardiographic conduction abnormalities suggesting an arrhythmic syncope: bifascicular block, QRS duration ≥ 0.12 s, Mobitz I atrio-ventricular block, sinus bradycardia <50/min, or sinus pause ≥ 3s, non-sustained ventricular tachycardia, Pre-excited QRS complexes and T wave abnormalities suggesting a primary electrical disease (Moya et al., 2009). However, some of these abnormalities are frequent and may not justify the implantation of a definitive pacemaker (Epstein et al., 2008) in the absence of infrahissian conduction disturbance or inducible arrhythmias recorded during the electrophysiological study. We recently reported in populations with a normal infrahissian conduction time that arrhythmic events were not more frequent in syncope patients with cardiac conduction abnormalities on resting ECG (Pierre et al., 2008) than in patients without them (27.5% versus 28.7%). Paroxysmal complete atrio-ventricular block remains rare in this selected population (13.7% versus 1.5%). That was explained by the high frequency of symptomatic sinus arrest in the group of patients without cardiac conduction abnormalities on resting ECG and the very low frequency of complete atrio-ventricular block in bifascicular block defined by right bundle branch block and left axis deviation (Nierop et al., 2000; Brignole et al., 2001; Pierre et al., 2008).

However caution should be exercised in the presence of right bundle branch block associated with right axis deviation. In this case, the frequency of complete paroxysmal atrio-ventricular block is high (36%) (Brignole et al., 2001). At the present time, patients with recurrent syncopes and right bundle branch block and right axis deviation are usually implanted with a permanent pace maker without prior implantation of the ICM (Epstein et al., 2008).

In the risk of stratification at the initial evaluation of syncope, the presence of cardiovascular disease and /or history of congestive heart failure are considered as major risk factors accounting for 3 points in EGSYS score and 1 point in OESIL score and these parameters are recognized as a predictive factor for cardiac arrhythmia in the latest guidelines for the diagnosis and the management of syncope (Task Force 2004; Moya et al., 2009). However, this conclusion cannot be applied to patients having recurrent syncopes and having undergone profound clinical cardiac investigation, especially when electrophysiological studies were unremarkable (Table 4). Several studies with the ICM demonstrated that cardiac arrhythmia was not correlated to the presence of structural heart disease (Mason et al., 2003; Solano et al., 2004; Pierre et al., 2008; Pezawas et al., 2008) in patients with recurrent syncopes. An arrhythmic event was documented more frequently in patients without structural heart disease than in patients with structural heart disease (33.7 % versus 9.5 %) (Pierre et al., 2008).This significant difference was not observed in other studies (Mason et al., 2003; Pezawas et al., 2008). The aetiology of arrhythmia is controversial with regard to the presence or absence of structural heart disease: Solana et al reported a greater prevalence of primary cardiac arrhythmia (atrioventricular block and ventricular arrhythmia) in patients with structural heart disease than in patients without structural heart disease (sinus arrest primarily) (Solano et al., 2004). In contrast Pierre et al (Pierre et al., 2008) observed only one AV block and no ventricular arrhythmia in structural heart disease patients.

However, we must specify that in these studies, most patients with structural heart disease have normal or limited alteration of left ventricular ejection fraction (Menozzi et al., 2002). We should be cautious in patients with severe depressed left ventricular ejection fraction. In this population, the implantation of an automatic implantable defibrillator has to be discussed because the probability of severe ventricular arrhythmia is high (Epstein et al., 2008).

Authors	Cardiac disease Documented arrhythmia (%)	Without Cardiac disease Documented arrhythmia (%)
Mason 2003	31	29
Solano 2004	52	28
Pierre 2008	9.5	33.7
Pezawas 2008	45	51

Table 4. Documented arrhythmia in patients with or without structural heart disease

4.3 Interest of ICM in patients without structural heart disease and normal ECG

Moya was the first author to report the results of ICM in patients suffering from recurrent syncopes with a normal physical examination and normal ECG without structural heart disease. These syncopes evoke a neuro-mediated mechanism. In this study (ISSUE), the rate of recurrence was high (34%) and the major arrhythmic event documented in the ICM was prolonged asystole (> 3 secondes) regardless of the results of the tilt-testing (Moya et al.,

2001). Typically, a progressive sinus bradycardia precedes a ventricular asystole due to sinus arrest. Most of the asystolic pauses were very long at the time of the syncope (from 15 ± 6 to 17 ± 9 seconds). These findings suggested that the syncope was neurally-mediated with a strong cardioinhibitory reflex. Deharo et al observed no correlation between the heart rhythm recorded by the ICM during a spontaneous vasovagal syncope and the heart rhythm recorded during the tilt testing or the ATP test (Deharo et al., 2006). ICM appears to better define the therapeutic strategy in these patients in accordance with heart rhythm contemporary to the syncope. The implantation of a definitive pacemaker in the group of patients with severe bradycardia proved its efficiency in preventing the recurrence of syncopes (only 0.05 episodes per patient per year) (Brignole et al., 2006). A multicenter prospective, double-blind randomized placebo-controlled study (ISSUE 3) is underway to assess the effectiveness of pacemaker therapy for syncopal asystolic pause (ISSUE 3, 2007).

4.4 Value of asymptomatic arrhythmias in unexplained syncope

The major interest of the ICM is to establish a closed correlation between symptoms and ECG. However long-term monitoring of patients with unexplained syncope with the ICM demonstrated frequent severe arrhythmic events (Krahn et al., 2004). Severe asymptomatic arrhythmia was documented in 15% of patients in Krahn's study: sinus bradycardia, atrioventricular block, supraventricular tachycardia and ventricular tachycardia. Specific treatment resulted in the resolution of syncope. Asymptomatic arrhythmias are often clinically relevant, especially in syncope patients leading to pacemaker implantation in the case of bradycardia or ICD in case of ventricular tachycardia (Epstein et al., 2008). The guidelines of 2009 (Moya et al., 2009) retained the following diagnosis criteria in the absence of a clear correlation between symptoms and ECG monitoring: ECG monitoring is diagnostic when periods of Mobitz II or III degree AV block or ventricular pause > 3 s or rapid prolonged paroxysmal supraventricular tachycardia or ventricular tachycardia are detected. Caution should be considered with the possible exception of young trained persons, during sleep, medical patients, or rate-controlled atrial fibrillation.

4.5 ICM in diagnosis and management of syncope: Theory and practice

The first reports on ICM demonstrated the superiority of the ICM in terms of diagnosis over the conventional diagnostic testing. In the RAST trial including 60 recurrent syncope patients, a diagnosis was obtained in 43% of the patients randomized to ICM compared to 20% in the patients undergoing conventional diagnostic testing (Krahn et al., 2001). The Eastbourne Syncope Assessment Study recruited 201 patients randomized in the conventional investigation group (n=98) and ICM group (n=103). The superiority of the ICM in terms of diagnosis was evident: 42% versus 7% (hazard ratio for time to ECG diagnosis was 6.53). Moreover, the time to ECG directed therapy was quicker for the ICM group than for the conventional group (Farwell et al., 2006). The diagnosis performance of ICM depends on the duration of the follow-up and the segments of the patients. It varied from 27 to 50%. ICM is especially powerful in older patients: a diagnosis was made for every 1.7 patients selected for ICM implantation in Brignole's study (Brignole et al., 2005a).

In the recommendations published in 2004 and revisited in 2009, the ICM implantation is recommended in two kinds of situations: firstly the ICM implantation appears early in patients with recurrent syncope of uncertain origin without high risk criteria and a high likelihood of recurrence of syncope within battery longevity of the ICM (class IB). Secondly the ICM implantation is recommended in high risk patients in whom a comprehensive evaluation did not demonstrate a cause of syncope or lead to a specific treatment (class IB). Generally in patients with a normal physical examination, normal ECG and without familial history of sudden cardiac death and structural heart disease and negative tilt testing, the implantation of ICM must be considered early in the presence of recurrent syncope. Selective use of an electrophysiological study and tilt testing must be discussed before implanting the ICM (Garcia-Civera et al., 2003). In the presence of cardiac disease or high risk criteria suggesting arrhythmic syncope as defined in the 2009 guidelines, it is recommended to implant ICM after performing an electrophysiological study and tilt testing (Moya et al., 2009). Several studies previously discussed in this chapter demonstrated the benefit of a strategy based on a relatively straightforward initial clinical evaluation: the early implantation of an ICM and a therapy delivered in accordance with the arrhythmic event documented during an episode of recurrent syncope (Brignole et al., 2005a, Pierre et al., 2008). The analysis of the presyncopal phase on the ICM restored ECG allows physicians to adapt and optimize the programming of the pacemaker when necessary (Brignole et al., 2007).

Table 5 summarized the recommendations of the implantation of the ICM in unexplained recurrent syncope. Vitale et al reported in a multicenter study a discrepancy between clinical practice and standardized indications for the ICM in patients with unexplained syncope (Vitale et al., 2010) whereas no clinical characteristics distinguished the patients receiving the ICM or not. Only 18% of patients received an ICM whereas 69% of patients had appropriate criteria for implantation of an ICM. In this study the ICM strategy allowed 8.7 higher likelihood of ECG diagnosis. This study underlines the underutilization of ICM in the diagnosis of syncope.

Recommendations of ICM	Class	Level
Early phase of evaluation in patients with recurrent syncope of uncertain origin, absence of high risk criteria and high likelihood of recurrence within battery longevity of the device	I	B
High risk patients in whom a comprehensive evaluation did not demonstrate a cause of syncope or lead to a specific treatment	I	B
Should be considered to assess the contribution of bradycardia before embarking on cardiac pacing in patients with suspected or certain reflex syncope presenting with frequent or traumatic syncopal episodes	IIa	B

Table 5. Recommendations of Implantable Cardiac monitor in accordance to the 2009 guidelines (Moya et al.; 2009)

4.6 ICM in particular populations

4.6.1 ICM in children and young adults

As we have previously noted, in children the ICM implantation can be safety implanted in the left axillary region for aesthetic reasons. Only a few experiences with the ICM in a paediatric setting have been published. Two studies reported the results in children suffering from recurrent syncopes. Results similar to those of adults are obtained in children. A high degree of symptom-rhythm correlation was established. In the Sreeram study (Sreeram et al., 2008), 15/33 patients had documented arrhythmic events which required specific therapy. In Babikar's study of the 15 patients who experienced symptom recurrence, 8 (53%) had an arrhythmic event (polymorphic ventricular tachycardia n=1, supraventricular tachycardia n=5, sinus arrest n=1 and Mobitz II AV block =1) (Babikar et al., 2008). Al Dharhi et al reported 64% of diagnosis in 42 children implanted with ICM (Al Dharhi et al., 2009). Further studies are needed to confirm the benefit of ICM in the paediatric population and to confirm its tolerability.

4.6.2 ICM in older patients

Falls are a major health care concern in elderly patients. About 30 % of people over 65 years fall once. The falls can unmask recurrent syncopes (Kenny et al., 2001; Amstrong et al., 2003). Some overlap between syncopes and falls has been recognized in the elderly population. Several parameters explain this confusion between falls and syncope: the interrogation, the amnesia for loss of consciousness and the difficulty to investigate these patients. Moreover falls are often unwitnessed, rendering the diagnosis of fall more difficult. The ICM is a simple tool that can be used early in the diagnostic strategy. In a small study reported by Amstrong about half of patients who activated their Reveal documented cardiac arrhythmias (bradycardia and ventricular tachycardia) (Amstrong et al., 2003). In the SAFE PACE study, a strong correlation between non-accidental falls and cardio-inhibitory carotid sinus hypersensitivity has been established (Kenny et al., 2001). The bradycardia induces hypotension which favours the instability of old patients leading to falls without loss of consciousness. In the absence of positive carotid sinus massage, the ICM can document bradycardia preceding the fall. The consequence for these patients is of great interest because the implantation of a definitive pacemaker dramatically reduced the injurious events.

4.6.3 J wave syndromes and syncope

Brugada syndrome and early repolarization are primary electrical diseases responsible for sudden death by ventricular fibrillation. Implantation of an ICD in secondary prevention is a class I recommendation (Epstein et al., 2008), but in primary prevention its implantation is controversial because a high incidence of complications linked to the ICD was observed in this young population (Sacher et al., 2006). Brugada syndrome and early repolarization are two electrocardiographic criteria that must suggest a diagnosis of cardiac arrhythmia in patients complaining from syncope (Moya et al., 2009). Nevertheless, the mechanism of syncope may be heterogeneous in these subgroups of patients and the differential between benign and malignant forms of syncope is not always very easy. The implantation of the ICM has been proposed by some authors especially when the characteristics of syncope were not convincing or the primary implantation of an ICD is refused by the patient. In the early repolarization syndrome the implantation of an ICD is only indicated in patients with documented ventricular arrhythmias. ICM can be used in other symptomatic patients.

4.6.4 Epileptic patients, "convulsive syncope" and ICM

Two problems remain unexplained in the epileptic population: the overlap between convulsive syncope and epilepsy and the high frequency of sudden death. Convulsive syncope is defined as cerebral anoxic seizure activity secondary to transient global impairment of blood flow, often difficult to differentiate from epilepsy. Sudden death is higher in the epileptic population than in the general population and frequently syncopes remain unexplained in the epileptic population despite adequate doses of anticonvulsant drugs (Tomson et al., 2008). Several hypotheses have been evoked amongst them the cardiovascular cause. Cardiologic investigations in this population reported an alternative diagnosis in 40% of cases (Zaidi et al., 2000a). Two types of clinical events have been demonstrated in this population. The first is a cardiac event linked to seizure, the second is a primary cardiac event. ICM can be useful to diagnose a cardiac event in these selected patients. Twenty patients with refractory epilepsy received an ICM in order to record heart rhythm during seizure (Rugg-gunn et al., 2004). 377 episodes were analyzed and bradycardia and sinus arrest occurred in 8 recorded events (2.1%) but this represented four patients (21%). These bradycardia are linked to temporal seizure (ictal bradycardia). The mechanism may be parasympathetic activation. We recently reported that syncopal bradycardia could be the first manifestation of epilepsy (Dinan et al., 2008). Videotelemetry monitoring with electroencephalography is the gold standard for diagnosing this particular form of epilepsy. The implantation of a pacemaker has been proposed to prevent death and disability (Zaidi et al., 2000a). The second mechanism is a neurocardiogenic syncope. In some patients, the neurocardiogenic syncope can result in convulsive syncope which can be difficult to distinguish from epilepsy. Despite a careful clinical investigation and laboratory tests including head upright tilt table testing, sometimes it is uncertain to conclude on the nature of the syncope. In this situation IMC is a power tool to display the cardiac rhythm during convulsive episodes (Kanjwal et al., 2009). Frequently a prolonged asystole or paroxysmal atrio-ventricular block was reported. The neurally-mediated mechanism is suspected in these patients because a slowing of heart rhythm was recorded before the asystole episode. The second argument is the inefficacity of the anti epileptic drugs and the disappearance of seizure after implantation of a dual chamber pacemaker in these patients. It is important to diagnose the cardiac origin of a convulsive syncope in order to avoid a long term anticonvulsant treatment which is expensive, inefficient and can cause serious morbidity.

5. Cost-effectiveness of ICM in syncope patients

Syncope is a symptom with an extensive differential diagnosis which can be roughly divided into cardiac syncope, neurally-mediated syncope, orthostatic hypotension and vascular steal syndromes (Moya et al., 2009). Consequently there is no single diagnostic test and more often, many laboratory tests (24 hours ambulatory ECG, tilt testing, electrophysiological study and echocardiography) are done, but their sensitivity and specificity are low. These laboratory tests significantly add to the overall cost, but their contribution to the diagnostic yield is low. About 40 % of patients referred to the emergency department are hospitalized. Referred and hospitalized patients are known to generate a cost estimated between $3,000-25,000, a mean cost of $5400 per hospitalization in USA and €3506 in Italy (Moya et al.; 2009). The recording of the heart rhythm during the syncopal episode remains the only means to diagnosis an arrhythmic aetiology. Preliminary studies demonstrate the economic benefit of the ICM compared to the conventional strategy in reducing the cost of the diagnosis of syncope (Krahn et al.; 1999b; Zaidi et al.; 2000b; Ermis et al., 2003). The RAST study has the objective of comparing the cost of both strategies. In this study, the cost of a primary implantable loop recorder strategy is 26% less than that of conventional testing (Krahn et al., 2001b). Early application of ICM reduces the cost per patient ($1,878 versus 2,355 and per diagnosis $3,756 versus 5,045). In the EaSyAS study, the overall costs tended to be lower in the ICM group than in the conventional investigation group (Farwell et al., 2006).

6. Others applications of ICM - Diagnosis of atrial fibrillation

A new algorithm is proposed in the last version of ICM leading to a specific analysis of the atrial electrical activity and to improving the diagnosis of atrial fibrillation. This new device (Reveal® XT, Medtronic Inc, Minneapolis USA) has a good sensitivity (96.1%) and specificity (85.4%) for identifying patients with atrial fibrillation (Hindricks et al., 2010). Some teams already use these ICM after atrial fibrillation ablation in order to detect the recurrence of the arrhythmia. Such data offered a safer guide to continue or stop the anticoagulation and antiarrhythmic drugs (Pokushalov, et al., 2011). The application of this diagnosis method demonstrated in CARISMA study a high incidence of new-onset atrial fibrillation in patients recently hospitalized for myocardial infarction with left ventricular dysfunction (Jons, et al., 2011). The risk of major cardiovascular events in patients with new-onset atrial fibrillation longer than 30 seconds was increased (HR=2.04) suggesting to treat these atrial fibrillation episodes. The implantation of the old version of the ICM has been already proposed in other domains than syncope. About 50 % of strokes in young patients remain unexplained after non invasive investigations. One suspected diagnosis in this population is the occurrence of asymptomatic paroxysmal atrial fibrillation which can't be detected by the standard ECG or 24 hours ambulatory ECG. Some authors proposed to analyze the atrial vulnerability during an electrophysiological study but its specificity and sensibility are not defined in the prospective study. Dion et al tested the interest of the ICM (second generation Reveal Plus 9526) in young patients suffering from unexplained stroke. In this study the ICM did not display a high prevalence of atrial arrhythmias but the population was selected and the implantation was only performed three months after the stroke (Dion et al., 2010). Another limit of this study was the criteria to retain the diagnosis of atrial fibrillation which was an irregular tachycardia with narrow QRS complex. The application of the new algorithm to detect atrial arrhythmias in larger population of patients with unexplained stroke should be of great interest because the detection of symptomatic or not atrial fibrillation involves starting an oral anticoagulation. A new large randomized prospective study (CRYSTAL AF) is ongoing to evaluate the long term monitoring with the implantation of a subcutaneous cardiac monitor (Reveal XT) in patients with cryptogenic stroke (Sinha, AM.; 2010). Results are expected at the end of 2012. In the population of patients suffering from recurrent syncope or palpitations this new algorithm could also be useful to improve the diagnosis.

7. Conclusion

ICM or ILR is a new tool still underused in clinical practice. The longevity of the battery allows prolonged cardiac monitoring which is the most suitable investigation to correlate the symptom to an arrhythmic event. Recurrent syncope is the major indication of ICM implantation. Recurrent syncope may impair the survival and the quality of life of the patients, the capacity to work and the ability to drive. A long-term monitoring strategy with the ICM yields more diagnoses than with conventional testing. Early application of ICM is now recommended in patients with recurrent syncopes in order to diagnose the mechanism of the syncopes and to guide the effective therapy. New applications of the ICM are in development, especially in patients suffering from atrial fibrillation and in patients suffering from unexplained palpitations.

8. References

Al Dharhi, K.; Potts, J.; Chiu, C. ; Hamilton, R. & Sanatani, S. (2009). Are implantable loop recorders useful in detecting arrhythmias in children with unexplained syncope ? *PACE*, Vol 32, No., (November 2009), pp1422-1427.

Armstrong, L.; Lawson, .J; Kamper, A.; Newton, J. & Kenny, RA. (2003).The use of implantable loop recorder in the investigation of unexplained syncope in older people. *Age and Ageing*, Vol.32, No.2, (March 2003), pp. 185-188.

Assar, M.; Krahn, A.; Klein, G.; Yee, R. & Skanes, A. (2003). Optimal duration of monitoring in patients with unexplained syncope. *American Journal of Cardiology*, Vol.92, (2003), pp.1231-123.

Babikar, A.; Hynes, B.; Ward, N.; Oslizok, P.; Walsh, K. & Keane, D. (2008). A retrospective study of the clinical experience of the implantable loop recorder in a pediatric setting. *International Journal of Clinical Practice*, Vol.62, No.10, (October 2008), pp.1520-1525.

Babuty, D.; Petitjean, F.; Fauchier, L. & Cosnay, P. (2001). Amazing sinus cardiac arrest. *Journal of Cardiovascular Electrophysiology*, Vol.12, No. 12, (December 2001), pp.1431.

Brignole, M.; Menozzi, C.; Moya, A.; Garcia-Civera, R.; Mont, L.; Alvarez, M.; Errazquin, F.; Beinas, J.; Bottoni, N. & Donateo, P. (2001). Mechanism of syncope in patients with bundle branch block and negative electrophysiological test. *Circulation*, Vol.104, No.17, (October 2001), pp. 2045-2050.

Brignole, M. ; Menozzi, C. ; Maggi, R. ; Solano, A. ; Donateo, P. ; Bottoni, N. ; Lolli, G.; Quarteri, F.; Croci, F. ; Oddone, D. & Puggioni, L. (2005a). The usage and diagnosis yield of the implantable loop-recorder in detection of the mechanism of syncope and in guiding effective antiarrhythmic therapy in older people. *Europace*, Vol.7, No.3, (May 2005), pp.273-279.

Brignole, M.; Moya, A.; Menozzi, C.; Garcia-Civera, R. & Sutton, R. (2005b). Proposed electrocardiographic classification of spontaneous syncope documented by an implantable loop recorder. *Europace*, Vol.7, No.1, (January 2005), pp. 14-18.

Brignole, M.; Sutton, R.; Menozzi, C.; Garcia-Civera, R.; Moya, A.; Wieling, W.; Andresen, D.; Benditt, DG. & Vardas, P. (2006). Early application of implantable loop recorder allows effective specific therapy in patients with recurrent suspected neurally mediated syncope. *European Heart Journal*, Vol.27, No.9, (May 2006), pp. 1085-1092.

Brignole, M.; Sutton, R.; Wieling, W.; Lu, SN.; Erickson, MK.; Markowitz, T.; Grovale, N.; Ammirati, F. & Benditt, DG. (2007). Analysis of rhythm variation during spontaneous cardioinhibitory neurally-mediated syncope. Implications for RDR pacing optimization: an ISSUE 2 substudy. *Europace*, Vol.9, No.5, (May 2007), pp. 305-311, ISSN

Chettaoui, R.; Kouakam, C.; Klug, D.; Marquie, C. & Lacroix D. (2002). Value of an implantable ECG monitor for the etiological diagnosis of syncope and recurrent unexplained syncopal attacks. *Archives des Maladies du Coeur et des vaisseaux*, Vol.95, No.1, (January 2002), pp. 29-36, ISSN

Chen, LY.; Benditt, DG. & Shen WK. (2008). Management of syncope in adults: an update. *Mayo Clinic Proceeding*, Vol.83, No.11, (November 2008), pp. 1280-1293.

Entem, FR.; Enriquez, SG.; Cobo, M.; Expositi, V.; Liano, M.; Ruiz, M.; Ollala, J. & Otero-Fernadez, M. (2009). Utility of implantable loop recorders for diagnosing unexplained syncope in clinical practice. *Clinical Cardiolology*, Vol.32, No.1,(January 2009), pp. 28-31.

Dinan, A.; de Toffol, B.; Pallix, M.; Breard, G. & Babuty, D. (2008). Cardiac arrest: it's all in the head. *Lancet*, Vol.371, No. 9622, (April 2008), pp.1476.

Deharo, JC.; Jego, C.; Lanteaume, A. & Djiane P. (2006). An implantable loop recorder study of highly symptomatic vasovagal patients. *Journal of American College of Cardiology*, Vol.47, (2006), pp.587-593, ISSN

Dion, F.; Saudeau, D.; Bonnaud, I.; Friocourt, P.; Bonneau, A.; Poret, P.; Giraudeau, B.; Régina, S.; Fauchier, L. & Babuty D. (2010). Unexpected low prevalence of atrial fibrillation in cryptogenic ischemic stroke: a prospective study. *Journal of Interventional Cardiac Electrophysiology*, Vol.28, No.2, (August 2010), pp. 101-107, ISSN

Edvardsson, N.; Frykman, V.; van Mechelen, R.; Mitro, P.; Mohii-Oskarson, A.; Pasquié, JL.; Ramanna, H.; Schwertfeger, F.; Ventura, R.; Vulgaraki, D.; Garutti, C.; Stolt, P. & Linker, N. (2011). Use of an implantable loop recorder to increase the diagnosis yield in unexplained syncope: results from the PICTURE registry. *Europace*, Vol.13, No.3, (February 2011), pp. 262-269., ISSN

Epstein, AE. (2008). ACC/AHA/HRS 2008 guidelines for device-bases therapy of cardiac rhythm abnormalities. *Journal of American College of Cardiology*, Vol.51, No.21, (May 2008), pp. 1-62.

Ermis, C.; Zhu, AX.; Pham, S.; Li, JM.; Guerrero, M.; Vrudney, A. ; Hiltner, L. ; Lu, F.; Sakaguchi, KG. & Benditt, DG. Comparison of automatic and patient-activated arrhythmia recordings by implantable loop recorder in the evaluation of syncope. *American Journal of Cardiology*, Vol.92, No.7, (October 2003), pp. 815-819.

Farwell, DJ.; Freemantle, N. & Sulke, N. (2006). The clinical impact of implantable loop recorders in patients with syncope. *European Heart Journal*, Vol.27, No.3, (February 2006), pp. 351-356.

Garcia-Civera, R. ; Ruiz-Granell, R.; Morell-Cabedo, S. ; Sanjuan-Manez, R.; Perez-Alcala, F.; Plancha, E.; Navarro, A. ; Botella, S. & LLacer, A. (2003). Selective use of diagnostic tests in patients with syncope of unknown cause. *Journal of American College of Cardiology*, Vol.41, No.5, (March 2003), pp.787-790.

Hindricks, G.; Pokushalov, E.; Urban, L.; Taborsky, M.; Kuck, KH.; Lebedev, D.; Rieger, G. & Pürerfellner, H. (2010). Performance of a new leadless implantable cardiac monitor in detecting and quantifying atrial fibrillation. Results of the EXPECT trial. *Circulation Arrhythmia Electrophysiology*, Vol.3, No.2,(April 2010), pp. 141-147, DOI: 10.1161/CIRCEP.109.877852.

Jons, C.; Jacobsen, U.; Joergensen, R.; Olsen, N. ; Dixen, U. ; Johannessen, A. ; Huikuri, H. ; Messier, M. ; McNitt, S. & Thomsen, P. (2011). The incidence and prognostic significance of new-onset atrial fibrillation in patients with acute myocardial infarction and left systolic fysfunction: a CRISMA study. *Heart Rhythm*, Vol.8, No. 3, (March 2011), pp342-348.

Kanjwal, K.; Karabin, B.; Kanjwal,Y. & Grubb, B. (2009). Differentiation of convulsive syncope from epilepsy with an implantable loop recorder. *International Journal of Medical Sciences*, Vol.6, No.6, (September 2009), pp.296-300.

Kapoor, WN.; Karpf, M.; Wieand, S.; Peterson, JR. & Levey, GS. (1983). A prospective evaluation and follow-up of patients with syncope. *New England Journal of Medecine*, Vol.309, No.4, (July 1983), pp. 197-204.

Kenny, A.; Richardson, D.; Steen, N.; Bexton R.; Shaw, F & Bond, J. (2001). Carotid sinus syndrome: a modifiable risk factor for non accidental falls in older adults (SAFE PACE). *Journal of American College of Cardiology,* Vol.38, No.5, (November 2001), pp. 1491-1496, ISSN 0735-1097/01.

Krahn, AD.; Klein, GJ.; Yee, R.; Takle-Newhouse, T. & Norris, C. (1999a). Use of an extended monitoring strategy in patients with problematic syncope. *Circulation*, Vol.99, No.3, (January 1999), pp. 406-410.

Krahn, AD.; Klein, GJ.; Yee, R. & Manda, V. (1999b). The high cost of syncope: cost implications of a new insertable loop recorder in the investigation of recurrent syncope. *American Heart Journal,* Vol.137, No.5, (May 1999), pp. 870-877.

Krahn, AD.; Klein, GJ.; Yee, . & Skanes, AC. (2001a). Predictive value of presyncope in patients monitored for assessment of syncope. *American Heart Journal,* Vol.141, No., (2001), pp.817-821.

Krahn, AD.; Klein, G.; Yee, R. & Skanes, AC. (2001b). Randomized assessment of syncope Trial (RAST). *Circulation,* Vol.104, No.1, (July 2001), pp.46-51.

Krahn, AD.; Klein, GJ.; Yee, R. & Skanes, AC. (2004). Detection of asymptomatic arrhythmias in unexplained syncope. *American Heart Journal,* Vol.148, No.2, (August 2004), pp.326-332.

Lombardi, F. ; Calasso, E. ; Mascioli, G. ; Marangoni, E. ; Donato, A. ; Rossi, S. ;Pala, M.; Foti, F.& Lunati, M. (2005). Utility of implantable loop recorder (Reveal Plus) in the diagnosis of unexplained syncope. *Europace,* Vol.7, No.1, (January 2005), pp.19-24.

Mason, P.; Wood, MA.; Reese, DB.; Lobban, JH.; Mitchell, MA. & DiMarco, JP. (2003). Usefulness of implantable loop recorders in office-based practice for evaluation of syncope in patients with or without structural heart disease. *American Journal of Cardiology,* Vol.92, No.9, (November 2003), pp.1127-1129.

Menozzi, C.; Brignole, M.; Garcia-Civera, R.; Moya, A.; Botto, G.; Tercedor, L.; Migliorini, R. & Navarro, X. (2002). Mechanism of syncope in patients with heart disease and negative electrophysiological test. *Circulation,* Vol.105, No.23, (June 2002), pp.2741-2745.

Miracapillo, G.; Costoli, A.; Addonisio, L.; Gemignani, L.; Manfredini, E.; Corbucci, G.; Severi, S. & Barold S. (2010). Left axillary implantation of loop recorder. *PACE,* Vol.33, No.8, (August 2010), pp.999-1002, DOI: 10.1111/j.1540-8159.2010.02764.x

Moya, A. ; Brignole, M.; Menozzi, C. ; Garci-Civera, R. ; Tognarini, S. ; Mont, L. ; Botto, G.; Giada, F. & Cornacchia, D. (2001). Mechanism of syncope in patients with isolated syncope and in patients with tilt-positive syncope. *Circulation,* Vol.104, No.11, (September 2001), pp.1261-1267.

Moya, A.; Sutton, R. ; Ammirati, F. ; Blanc, JJ. ; Brignole, M. ; Dahm, JB. ; Deharo, JC. ; Gajek, J. ; Gjesdal, K. ; Krahn, A.; Massin, M.; Pepi, M.; Pezawas, T.; Granell, RR.; Sarasin,

F.; Ungar, A.; va Dijk, J, Walma, E. & Wieling, W. (2009). Guidelines for the diagnosis and management of syncope (Version 2009). European Heart Journal, Vol.30, No.21, (November 2009), pp.2631-2671, DOI: 10.1093/eurheartj/ehp298.

Nierop, PR.; Van Mechelen, R.; Van Elsächer, R.; Luitjen, RHM. & Elhendy, A. (2000). Heart rhythm during syncope and presyncope: results of implantable loop recorder. *PACE*, Vol.23, No.10, (October 2000), pp.1532-1538.

Paruchuri, V.; Adhaduk, M.; Garikipati, NV.; Steinberg, JS. & Mittal S. (2011). Clinical utility of a novel wireless implantable loop recorder in the evaluation of patients with unexplained syncope. *Heart Rhythm*, (February 2011) (Epub ahead of print)

Pierre, B.; Fauchier, L.; Breard, G.; Marie, O.; Poret, Ph. & Babuty, D. (2008). Implantable loop recorder for recurrent syncope : influence of cardiac conduction abnormalities showing up on resting electrocardiogram and of underlying cardiac disease on follow-up developments. *Europace*, Vol.10, No.4, (April 2008), pp. 477-481.

Pezawas,T.; Stix, G.; Kastner, J.; Schneider, B.; Wolzt, M. & Schmidinger, H. (2008). Implantable loop recorder in unexplained syncope: classification, mechanism, transient loss of consciousness and role of major depressive disorder in patients with and without structural heart disease. *Heart*, Vol.94, No.4, (April 2008), pp.1-7.

Pokushalov, E.; Romanov, A.; Corbucci, G.; Artyomenko, S.; Turov, A.; Shirokova, N. & Karaskov, A. (2011). Ablation of paroxysmal and persistent atrial fibrillation: 1-year follow up through continuous subcutaneous monitoring. *Journal of Cardiovascular Electrophysiology*, in press.

Rugg-Gunn, F.; Simister, R.; Squirell, M.; Holdright, D. & Duncan, J. (2004). Cardiac arrhythmias in focal epilepsy: a prospective long term study. *Lancet*, Vol.364, No.9452, (December 2004), pp.2212-2219.

Sacher, F.; Probst, V. ; Iesaka, Y. ; Jacon, P.; Laborderie, J.; Mizon-Gérard, F.; Mabo, P.; Reuter, S.; Lamaison, D.; Takahashi, Y.; O'Neill, M.; Garrigue, S.; Pierre, B.; Jaïs, P.; Pasquié, JL. ; Hocini, M.; Salvador-Mazenq, M.; Nogami, A.; Amiel, A.; Defaye, P.; Bordachar, P.; Boveda, S.; Maury, P.; Klug, D.; Babuty, D.; Haïssaguerre, M.; Mansourati, J.; Clémenty, J. & Le Marec, H. (2006). Outcome after implantation of a cardioverter-Defibrillator in patients with Brugada syndrome. A multicenter study. *Circulation*, Vol.114, No.22 (November 2006), pp.2317-2324, DIO: 10.1161/CIRCULATIONAHA.106.628537.

Siedl, K.; Rameken, M.; Breunung, S.; Senges, J.; Jung, W.; Andresen, D.; va Toor, A.; Krahn, A. & Klein, G. Diagnostic assessment of recurrent unexplained syncope with a new subcutaneously implantable recorder. *Europace*, Vol.2, No.3, (July 2000), pp.256-262.

Sinha, AM.; Diener, HC.. Morillo, C.; Sanna, T.; Berstein, R.; Di Lazzaro, V.; Passman, R.; Beckers, F. & Brachmann, J. (2010). Cryptogenic stroke and underlying atrial fibrillation (CRYSTAL AF): Design and rationale). *American Heart Journal*, Vol.160, No.1, (July 2010), pp. 36-41.

Sivakumaran, S.; Krahn, A.; Klein, GJ.; Finan, J.; Yee, R.; Renner, S. & Skanes, AC. (2003). A prospective randomized comparison of loop recorders versus Holter monitoring in patients with syncope and presyncope. *American Journal of Medecine,* Vol.115, No.1, (July 2003), pp.1-5.

Solano, A.; Menozzi, C.; Maggi, R.; Donateo, P.; Bottoni, N.; Lolli, G.; Tomasi, C.; Crosi, F.; Oddone, D.; Puggioni, F. & Brignole, M. (2004). Incidence, diagnostic yield and safety of the implantable loop-recorder to detect the mechanism of syncope in patients with or without structural heart disease. *European Heart Journal*, Vol.25, No.13, (July 2004), pp. 1116-1119.

Soteriades, E.; Evans, JC.; Larson, MG.; Chen, MH.; Chen, L.; Benjamin,EJ. & Levy, D. (2002). Incidence and prognosis of syncope. *New England Journal of Medecine*, Vol.347, No.12, (September 2002), pp.878-885.

Sreeram, N.; Gass, M.; Apitz, C.; Ziemer, G.; Hofbeck, M.; Emmel, M.; et al. (2008). The diagnostic yield from implantable loop recorders in children and young adults. *Clinical Research Cardioliology*, Vol.97, No.5, (May 2008), pp.327-333.

Strickberger A, Benson W, Biaggioni I, Callans D, Cohen M, Ellenbogen K, et al AHA/ACCF Scientific statement on the evaluation of syncope. *Circulation,* Vol.113, No.17, (January 2006), pp.316-327.

Task force Guidelines on Management (Diagnosis and treatment) of syncope-Update 2004. The task force on syncope, European society of cardiology. *European Heart Journal*, Vol. 25, No.25, (November 2004), pp. 2054-2072.

Tomson, T.; Nashef, L. & Ryvlin, P. (2008). Sudden unexpected death in epilepsy : current knowledge and future directions. *Lancet Neurology*, Vol.7, No.11, (November 2008), pp.1021-1031.

The steering Committee of the ISSUE 3 study. (2007). International study on syncope of uncertain etiology 3 (ISSUE 3): pacemaker therapy for patients with asystolic neurally-mediated syncope: rationale and study design. *Europace*, Vol.9, No.1 (January 2007), pp. 25-30.

Vitale, E.; Ungar, A. ; Maggi, R. ; Francese, M. ; Lunati, M. ; Colaceci, R. ; Del Rosso, A. ; Castro, A. ; Santini, M. ; Giuli, S .; Belgini, L.; Casagranda, I. & Brignole, M. (2010). Discrepancy between clinical practice and standardized indications for an implantable loop recorder in patients with unexplained syncope. *Europace,* Vol.12, No10.,(October 2010), pp.1475-1479. DIO:10.1093/europace/euq302.

Zaidi, A.; Clough, P.; Cooper, P.; Scheepers, B. & Fitzpatrick AP. (2000a). Misdiagnosis of epilepsy: many seizure-like attacks have a cardiovascular cause. *Journal of American College of Cardiology*, Vol.36, No.1, (July 2000), pp. 181-184, ISSN 075-1097/00.

Zaidi, AM. & Fitzpatrick, AP. (2000b). Investigation of syncope: increasing the yield and reducing the cost. *European Heart Journal,* Vol.21, No.11, (June 2000), pp. 877-880.

Zellerhoff, C.; Himmrich, E.; Nebeling, D.; Przibille, O.; Nowak, B. & Liebrich, A. (2000). How can we identify the best implantation site for an ECG event recorder? *PACE*, Vol.23, No.10, (October 2000), pp. 1545-1549.

Part 3

Complexities and Possible Complications

7

Pacemaker Following Adult Cardiac Surgery

Silvero Miriam, Browne Leonardo and Solari Gabriel
Hospital San Juan de Dios de La Plata
Argentina

1. Introduction

The postoperative cardiac surgery status often determines a systolic and diastolic dysfunction, thus inducing the dependence of atrial contribution to ventricle telediastolic filling and a physiological dynamic contraction and so as to avoid ventricular segmental dyssynergia. The heart rate also plays an important role in maintaining an adequate cardiac output. Postsurgical pacemaker stimulation is useful in conduction disturbances and also helps to optimize cardiac index frequency dependent.
Another use may be the reduction or prevention of postoperative atrial fibrillation.
Before closing the chest electrode is usually placed in the right ventricle for an eventual postoperative univentricular stimulation. (Figure 1)

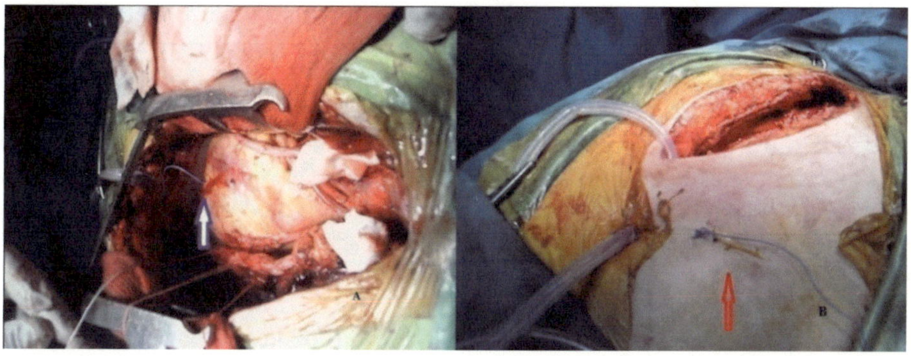

Fig. 1. A. Electrode suture wire in right ventricle. B. Wire comes out through the skin next to the incision.

In patients with left ventricular dysfunction and wide QRS complex, it may be advisable to implant another electrode in the left ventricle for biventricular pacing. (Figure 2)
In special circumstances atrial electrodes implantation would also be advantageous.
The requirement of temporary pacing (TPM) with further need of a permanent implantable pacemaker (PPM) after initial cardiac surgical procedures is usually less than 3%.
The need for TPM after cardiac surgery constitutes a rare complication but it is associated with increment morbidity and an increase of resource investment. It is also true that the requirement of a permanent pacemaker implant, if indicated on time, results in a survival similar to that of other patients who did not require a placement of a permanent pacemaker.

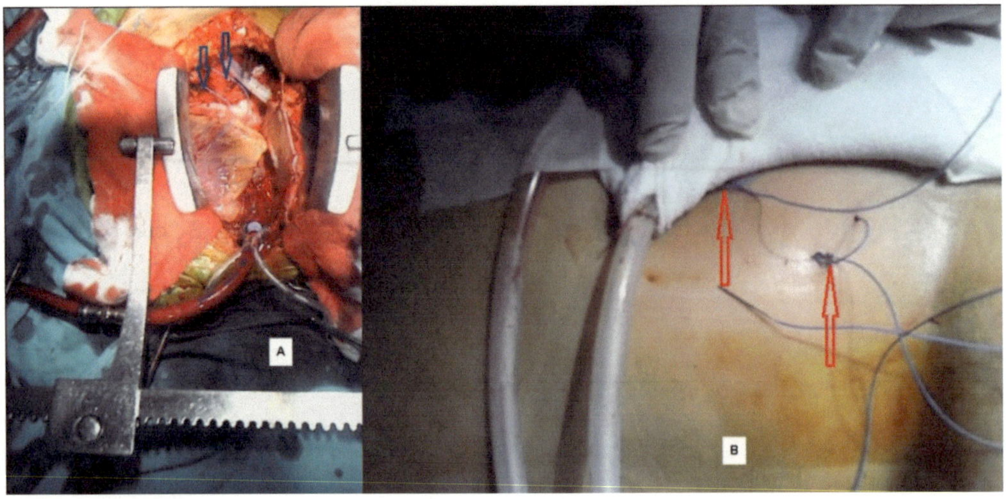

Fig. 2. A. Electrodes suture wires in right and left ventricles. B. Wires come out through the skin next to the incision.

The conduction defects associated with cardiac surgery are located at the sinus node, atrioventricular node or Purkinje His system and its branches.

The consequences depend on damage location and on whether it is an irreversible damage (such as direct traumatic injury of the conduction system during valve replacement) or temporary damage (such as ischemia observed in coronary artery bypass grafting (CABG)). First approach to the management of patients with conduction disturbances in the perioperative period during cardiovascular surgery to be taken into account are injury anatomical location and feasible aetiology. Therefore, it is indispensable to know the anatomical topography of conduction system, its relation with the rest of the cardiac structures and the irrigation type that receives from coronary arteries. For example, the appearance of complete atrioventricular (AV) block during aortic valve replacement surgery is an adverse prognostic marker, whereas the fascicular blocks are generally mild and transient. The latter occurs because in the first situation, direct injury by surgical manipulation would be involved as the atrioventricular bundle runs in the top of the wall of the septum next to the aortic annulus.

Identifying the mechanisms that cause injury to the conduction system, and recognizing risk factors may reduce its incidence, or at least prepare for this eventuality in order to make timely decisions.

In the informed consent, a percentage range of prevalence of PPM according to the patient's risk factors and type of surgery should be included. The importance of this information for the patient should not be underestimated.

2. Prevalence of pacing after cardiac surgery

Bradyarrhythmia after cardiac surgery may be due to injury of the conduction system during surgical manipulation in the area next to it or ischemia induced by aortic cross clamping (CXL), or a specific coronary disease. Thus, conduction disturbances are sometimes transient because the injury can be induced by reversible ischemic damage or posttraumatic edema. This would explain well the different incidences between those who require TPM and those eventually discharged with a PPM. Although permanent pacemaker indications are the same as those for non-surgical patients, it is controversial to determine cardiac surgery postoperatory timing of PPM implantation.

2.1 Temporary pacemaker

Temporary epicardial electrodes are routinely placed in patients after cardiac surgery, but position of ventricular leads and use of atrial leads are not uniform. There are recommendations, but no protocols.

The decision of to whom and where to place electrodes for subsequent pacing is formalized in some medical centers, in others is a discretionary decision between team intervening for each patient.

In CABG surgery has been compared sutured wires in right atrium, in left ventricular apex, in right ventricular apex, and right ventricular outflow tract before cardiopulmonary bypass entrance. In postoperative period, comparison of the groups showed that the addition of atrial activation during ventricular pacing resulted in higher cardiac indexes, higher systolic blood pressures, lower central venous pressures, and similar pulmonary arterial pressures. Right ventricular outflow tract pacing resulted in higher cardiac index than left ventricular apical pacing in patients with stenosis of the left anterior descending coronary artery (DCA) in 90% or more,while left ventricular apical pacing produced higher cardiac index in the absence of DCA lesion.

CABG intervention is described as a type of cardiac surgery less damaging to the conduction system and even so it may have an incidence of TPM of 45% at the end of surgery, but the number of patients who are discharged with PPM is significantly lower.

Must there be a different protocol for the placement or not of epicardial electrodes when the CABG is performed with cardiopulmonary bypass (ONCAB) or without it (OFCAB)?

The incidence of PPM is nearly the same in both cases: 5.5-6% for OPCAB and 6.8% for ONCAB. Where is the significant difference? Mean duration for TPM pacing is longer in ONCAB. Another point is that ONCAB has higher incidence of atrial fibrillation as pacing indication. The need for pacing before chest closure accurately identifies coronary patients who will require postoperative pacing after OPCAB or ONCAB.

Is routine use of temporary epicardial pacing wires unnecessary and must their use be limited?

It can also happen that a patient exits the surgery room without TPM and then needs to be paced in the recovery room. High level evidence conclusions are not yet found.

Patients undergoing CABG not including off-pump surgery, without a preoperative pacemaker, and no pacing wire placement present an incidence of 8.6 % of pacing during the postoperative period. Significant predictors for PPM on multivariate analysis are diabetes mellitus, preoperative arrhythmia, and pacing utilized to separate from cardiopulmonary bypass (CPB).

Valve surgeries, ascending aorta or intracavitary congenital interventions have higher incidence of TPM than CABG, and the gap finally requiring PPM between them is narrower.

2.2 Permanent pacemaker (Table 1)

Each year approximately 5% of 100,000 patients, who are undergoing cardiac valve surgery in the United States, will require postoperative PPM implantation before hospital discharge. Several studies with long list of patients, show concern about this issue.

Prevalence differs according to the type of surgery. In a retrospective review of 5,942 patients who underwent open-heart surgery to resolve acquired heart disease, it was observed that 2.1% of patients required PPM postoperatively; 4.6% of them underwent predominantly valve surgery, and 0.6% CABG surgery (Goldman, 1984). In a study of 10,421 patients a PPM prevalence of 0.4% to 1.1% after CABG, and 3.0 to 6.0% after valve operation was found. (Gordon, 1998)

Compared to the past, the incidence of post operatory PPM implantation decreases year after year due to improvements in surgical techniques, technological innovations and understanding of the mechanisms of injury that generates the arrhythmia. Paradoxically, the total number of PPM implanted is higher. As an explanation, we can say that severe ischemic heart disease (*NYHA* Class *III-IV)* in younger and older patients with longer life expectancy is increasing. In undeveloped countries there is also an increase in the population and in the incidence of rheumatic fever with valves affectation.

Reoperation, multivalvular, combined, complex surgeries (as Bentall-De Bono procedure), and myxomas ablation, among others have higher rates of PPM. On the other hand, it also appears that using valve repair techniques instead of replacement decreases its prevalence. In heart transplantation, the incidence is between 0 and 5%, but with the expansion of the inclusion criteria of donors, the percentage could attain more than 20% (older age donors). If tricuspid valve replacement or repair is included with another cardiac surgery, high incidences of PPM up to 28% can be reached. In the last two decades, more isolated tricuspid replacements have been performed (Infective endocarditis in intravenous drug users).

Author	%	**Surgery**
Gordon,1998	0,4-1,1	CABG
Gordon,1998	3-6	VS
Erdogan,2006	4,1	AVR
Imren,2008	2	CABG
Goldman,1984	0,6	CABG
Goldman,1984	4,6	VS
Emlein,1993	0,8	CABG
Del Rizzo,1996	1,3	ALL
Ben Ameur,2006	4	VS
Schurr,2010	4	AVR
Nardi,2010	3	AVR
Merin,2009	1,4	ALL
Limongelli,2003	3,2	AVR
Berdajs,2008	4,2	MV
Meimoun,2002	2,6	MV
Ashida,2000	6.7	VS

ALL= all type of cardiac surgery; AVR = aortic valve replacement; CABG = coronary artery bypass grafting; MV=mitral valve surgery; VS = valve surgery.

Table 1. Postoperative permanent pacemaker. Prevalence.

The reversibility of conduction defect continues recovering not just in the immediate postoperative period but also in the short, medium and long term. Thirty per cent in those with a narrow escape QRS, and 18% in others with wide QRS, no longer need the pacemaker during follow-up. Up to one third of patients recover at late follow-up.

3. Damage mechanisms in the conduction system during cardiac surgery

The main physiopathological mechanisms involved in the genesis of AV conduction disorders are myocardial ischemia, direct surgical injury,inadequate cardiac protection during surgery, and cardiac depressant medication (beta blockers, calcium blockers, etc.).
Mechanical trauma to the conduction system, arising secondary to valve operation, myomectomy for hypertrophic obstructive cardiomyopathy, or repair of ventricular septal defect, appears to be the most frequent cause.
Alternatively, ischemic injury of the sinoatrial node or conduction system might occur during any cardiac procedure as a result of inadequate myocardial protection during surgery time. Then, there are three postulates:

1. Operative procedures performed in close physical proximity to the sinoatrial or atrioventricular nodes or the His branch bundle.
2. Extensive coronary artery disease which compromises myocardial protection during intraoperative procedure, specially related to cardiopulmonary bypass and aortic cross-clamp duration.
3. Poor myocardial protection even without coronary disease.

(1) Risk of physical damage is increased in conduction system in patients who have repeated valve operations, in patients who underwent multiple valve replacement, and during debridement or reconstructive operation for active endocarditis. Similarly, debridement of a calcified aortic annulus after excision of the aortic valve might be the source of significant trauma to the conduction system. The surgical procedures added to CABG or aortic valve replacement (AVR); such as mitral valve replacement (MVR), sub aortic stenosis (SAS) resection, and ventricular septal defect (VSD) closure, are postulated as predict factors for the occurrence of postoperative AV conduction disturbances. This is not surprising: association between surgical manipulations at the fibrous skeleton of valves or septal wall, the immediate anatomical vicinity of the AV node, and the proximal conduction bundle entail a great possibility for the need of a PPM. These procedures have long development times and add to the manipulation risk, the factor mentioned in the second item (2), the risk of inadequate myocardial protection.
It has been suggested that patients with aortic valve disease have histological abnormalities of the conduction system because of elevated intraventricular pressures thus generating ischemia and degenerative disease of the conducting system. These tissues are more vulnerable to manipulation.
(2) In ischemic heart disease with involvement of the coronary artery supplying the conduction system, until it is revascularizated, there is a latent possibility of bradyarrhythmia or blockage. During surgery, the so-called "reperfusion arrhythmias" with the re-establishing of the flow in territories that had prior deficit can occur. If there is right dominance and the right coronary artery is obstructed, thus compromising blood septal flow with conduction abnormalities, which promote high incidence of need PPM, both in CABG as AVR regularly occur.
(3) When not performing an adequate myocardial protection adverse events are developed such as severe arrhythmias, ventricular failure requiring high doses of inotropic drugs or circulatory support, prolonged weaning from CPB, metabolic disorder, etc.

One must realize the mistake: temperature, cardioplegia type, long CXL time periods, appropriate surgical indication, and optimization of the patient status or several of these causes. Each patient deserves deep investigation.

4. Preoperative risk predictors of permanent pacemaker insertion

The preoperative identification of a high-risk subset of cardiac surgery patients who may require permanent pacing has an important implication to decide the number and location of temporary epicardial pacing wires to implant at the time of surgery. Their postoperative removal can cause bleeding, cardiac tamponade (cavity rupture), bypass graft injury, infection and other complications, but in many patients the absence of epicardial electrodes also carries a risk associated with delayed treatment of the bradyarrhythmia. It is important to know the factors to do the best in each case.

In relation to demographic and clinical features of patients, descriptive studies agree that the preoperative risk factors are: absence of preoperative sinus rhythm, female gender, advanced age (≥ 65 years), dense calcium in the aortic annulus, endocarditis, unstable angina, compromised septal blood flow, ventricular dilatation, renal failure, hypertension, some kind of drug medication and end-systolic left ventricle diameter.

Infective endocarditis is a particular condition that usually involves a sepsis state or incipient multiorganic failure involving heart and its structure, suffering hypoperfusion as a consequence of inability to keep adequate consumption-availability balance tissue oxygen. The conduction tissue is no exception to this rule: no perfusion, no proper function.

Regarding the preoperative rhythm, patients with first degree atrioventricular block (AVB) or fascicular block have higher incidence of permanent post operatory AVB. In valve surgery, the biggest risk is present in patients with right bundle branch block (RBBB). The incidence of left bundle branch block after aortic and mitral valve surgery is high, and having the previous RBBB, a trifascicular block develops more easily. However in coronary surgery, left bundle branch block (LBBB) is a more potent predictor of postoperative pacemaker need, than RBBB. (Table 2)

CABG	VALVE SURGERY
LBBB	**RBBB**
AF	**AF**
RBBB	BIFASICULAR BLOCK
BIFASICULAR BLOCK	LBBB
AVB	

AVB = atrioventricular block; AF = atrial fibrillation; CABG = coronary artery bypass grafting; LBBB = left bundle branch block; RBBB = right bundle branch block.

Table 2. Preoperative arrhythmias needed more pacing in the postoperative period according to the type of surgery.

In controversy, some authors found no additional relationship with age, gender, kind of valve disease, anemia, and use of digitalis or angiotensin converting enzyme inhibitor, preoperatory conduction disturbances, myocardial infarction (MI) or coronary arteries affected.

More meta-analysis studies should be made regarding these issues. The analysis can be adjusted by age group, type of surgery, previous systemic diseases, preoperative cardiac diseases, etc., if significant results cannot be obtained, a risk score must be built for each medical center.

There are attempts to validate risk scores as Koplan B,1993 validated with 4694 patients who underwent valve surgery :prediction Group n = 3,116 and a validation Group n =1,578. The exclusion criteria were patients who had an indication for PPM or an implanted cardioverter defibrillator (ICD) preoperatively, or who died within six days after surgery. Postoperative ICD implantation were considered to have a PPM only if they also had an indication for permanent pacing independent of their need for an ICD; otherwise they were classified in the no pacemaker group. The decision to implant a permanent pacemaker after surgery was at the physician's discretion in agreement with the current American College of Cardiology/ American Heart Association guidelines for permanent pacing. This study utilized demographic data, electrocardiogram (ECG), and surgical characteristics to predict the need for permanent pacing after cardiac valve surgery. (Table 3 and 4)

ECG Points	**Points**
Right bundle branch block	2
Left bundle branch block	1
PR interval >200	1
Multivalve surgery	
Tricuspid valve include	2
Tricuspid valve not include	1
Others	
Age ≥ 70	1
Prior valve surgery	1

ECG = electrocardiogram.

Table 3. Risk score to predict PPM after valve surgery. (Koplan B, 1993)

Score Points	**% PPM**
6	50
5	36
4	21
3	12
2	8,7
1	5,2
0	1,9

Table 4. Percent of patients in the validation group who required PPM. (Koplan B, 1993)

The risk score allows patients to know preoperatively the likelihood of a PPM and this should therefore be notified.

5. Intraoperative risk factors

It is crucial to know all perioperative risk factors, so that the patient knows and is aware of it in the preoperative informed consent. Counseling about the risk is part of medical ethics.

Gordon R. (1998) analyzed one hundred and thirty-four variables in a data base of 10,721 patients and identified those who had cardiac operations. All those variables are considered to be potential risk factors to date. (Figure 3)

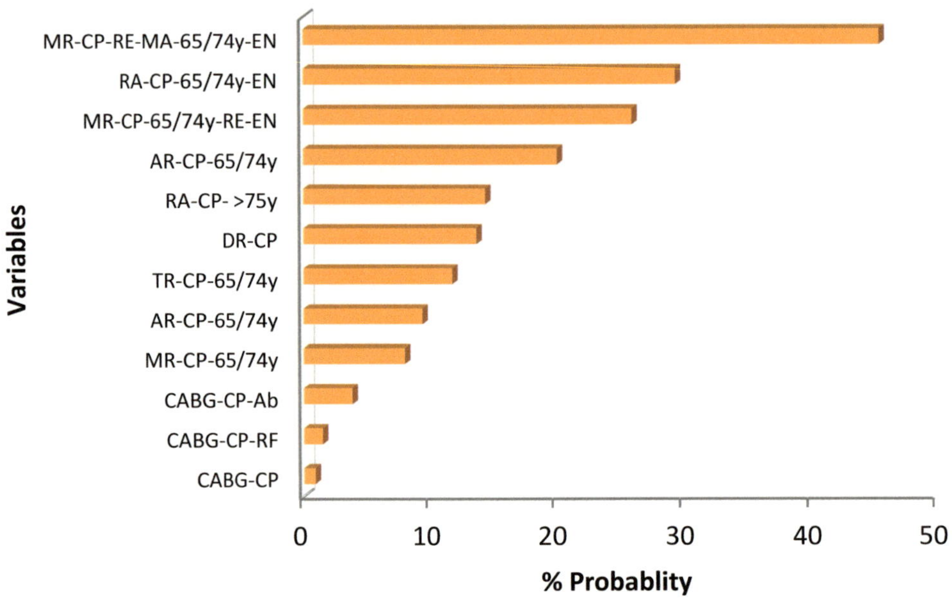

Ab = ablation; CABG = coronary artery bypass grafting; CP = cold cardioplegia; DR = Double valve repair or replacement; EN = active endocarditis; MA = mitral valve annulus reconstruction; MR = mitral valve repair or replacement; AR = aortic valve repair or replacement; RE = reoperation, RF = preoperative renal failure; TR = triple valve repair or replacement; Y = years.

Fig. 3. Predicted probabilities of permanent pacemaker requirement based on common operative variables. (Gordon R, 1998)

We can see in Figure 3 that trauma is the most frequent damage mechanism. Reoperation is repairing tissue which was manipulated and suture previously. Endocarditis is an inflammation status; it presents friable places, especially right and left fibrous trigones (Figure 4) whose boundary structures (valves themselves, coronary arteries and conduction system) are extremely close; the surgeon must work there. Older people have less tissue reconstructive capacity. In this score validation, the variable included as myocardial protection damage mechanism is cold cardioplegia, in this last item, the debate is still now open.

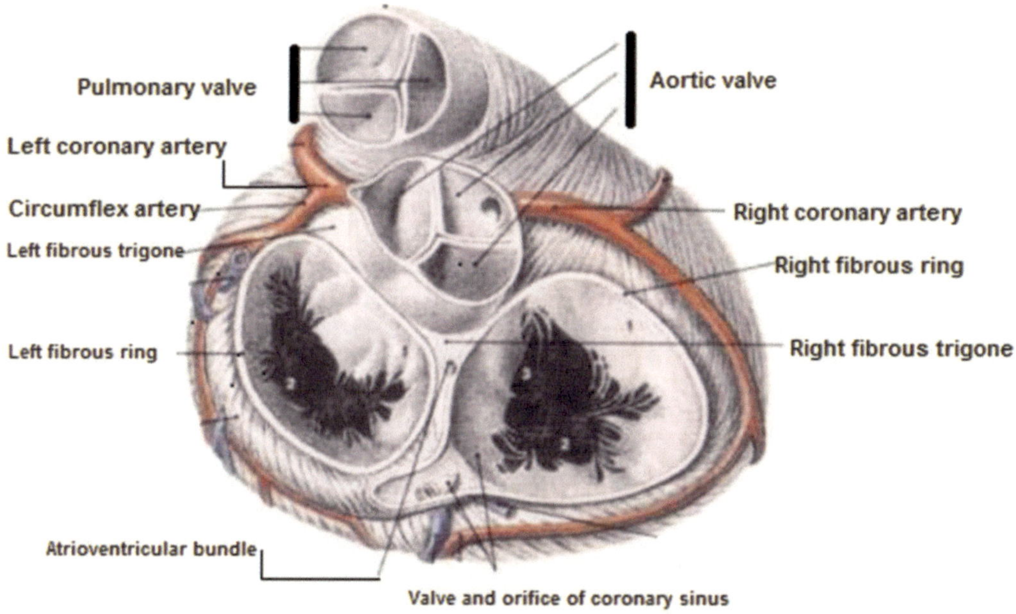

Fig. 4. Fibrous cardiac trigones

5.1 Valve surgery

So far, no studies determining in high value evidence what predictive risk factors are the strongest at the time of valve replacement might have forecasted postoperative PPM implantation. Each patient, each type of disease, intraoperatory and postoperatory events as well as decisions; are especially different and determine multiple variations.

5.1.1 AVR

Conduction abnormalities are commonly associated with aortic valve disease. During the 1960s, the incidence of complete heart block after AVR approached 13%. Recent reports indicate that the incidence has decreased to approximately 6%.

Preoperatory AVR risk factors are: female gender, age $\geq$ 65 years, systemic hypertension, myocardial infarction, conduction disturbances, greater preoperative left ventricle end-systolic diameter, poor left ventricle ejection fraction (< 35%), left atrial enlargement, left ventricular septum hypertrophy, calcified aortic root bicuspid aorta, annular calcification and aortic regurgitation.

Intraoperative factors are: additionally surgical procedure as CABG, redo surgery, CPB time, cross clamp time, stentless bioprosthetic and valve size.

The inserted wrong valve size chosen not only predisposes to PPM, but it also could need to be removed because the aortic disease becomes worse than before surgery.

Postoperative factors: electrolyte imbalance, myocardial infarction, cardiac arrest. All these situations that affect the consumption/availability of tissue oxygen, if not resolved, degenerates in an inability of physiological function on organs and systems. Cells cannot get oxygen, nor membranes achieve exchange.

Adding conduction system hypoperfusion and malfunction it is clear how conduction failure.

Persons aged ≥ 75 years in the coexisting aortic valve surgery with CABG, determine the double risk of PPM.
However, discussion exists as to whether surgery intended to this subset reflects a cost-effective approach to attaining life quality since it has high mortality (more than 5%).
Significant preoperative risk factors for early mortality (first week) include poor left ventricular function and preoperative pacemaker insertion. Predictors of late mortality (first month) include chronic obstructive pulmonary disease and urgency surgery.
Feature and valve configuration, might predispose to mechanical trauma of the conduction system during AVR: alteration of length of the membranous septum, calcification in the region of the atrioventricular bundle and its branches, and bicuspid valve; the latter can be congenital or fused by disease. (bicuspidization).
A pathologic study of the cardiac conduction system was performed in specimens that had undergone AVR, searching the impact of postoperative compression exerted by the valve, the suture and calcium ring.
Evidence found about higher incidence of traumatic recent lesions was: septum length less than 5 mm, mechanical injury to the conduction tissue attributed to residual deposits of calcium (its manipulation during surgery), and congenital bicuspid valve.
Especially in aortic regurgitation, the endocardium marked fibrous thickening in the left ventricular septum can cause degeneration of the driving system which run through it.
This thickening is caused by regurgitated blood flow that strikes the septum.
The intimate relationship between conducting tissue and prosthesic valve suggests that direct trauma at time of surgery might be involved: suture injury, pressure from residual calcic material, and impingement prosthesic valve against conduction system.
(Elahi M., 2006) introduces us to a new question: type and size of prosthesis influence in the incidence of implantation of PPM in AVR? In his research of 510 AVR isolates, smaller aortic prosthesis size (<21mm) was identified as a significant predictor of hospital mortality ($P < 0.05$) demonstrating that stentless valves required longer bypass and cross clamp times. This suggests that prevalence of PPM seems to be dependent on the size and type of prosthesis. PPM incidence is twice in a group with stentless valve (18% vs. 9.1%; $P = 0.01$).
In Providence Hospital in Michigan analyzed predictors in a study of 214 AVR with 6.3% incidence of PPM .There was no relationship with the type of valve. (Mechanical vs. Bioprosthetic) nor with its subtypes (stentless vs. stented).
(Totaro P., 2000) demonstrated that continuous rather than interrupted sutures were more often associated with postoperative AV conduction defects and PPM implantation (17.5% vs. 2.2%), but the two groups were not homogenous for age and cross clamp time.
¿Required time of valve placement, or its constituent material, or degree of degeneration of the aortic annulus, or the size of valve that has been decided to implant? ¿Wich is the variable? Further clinical trials, multicenter studies and meta-analysis are needed.

5.1.1.1 Trans-catheter self-expanding aortic bioprosthetic implantation (TAVI)

This last decade has innovated AVR technique with trans-catheter self-expanding aortic bioprosthetic implantation. It is performed while the heart is still beating without the need for a bypass or sternotomy. The procedure may be retrograde, performed via the transfemoral or subclavian or through a transapical approach. (Figure 5)
Often used in patients over 75 years with credibility as a valuable alternative to non surgical option. However, these patients are often affected by severe iliac-femoral arteriopathy too, rendering the transfemoral approach unemployable. This new technique does not escape PPM risk. The incidence is nearly 33%.It is extremely lofty. To address this high rate of complication it is necessary to carry out a careful evaluation of the aortic replacement with

this technique. Pre-existing right bundle branch block is an independent predictor of complete AV block after TAVI.

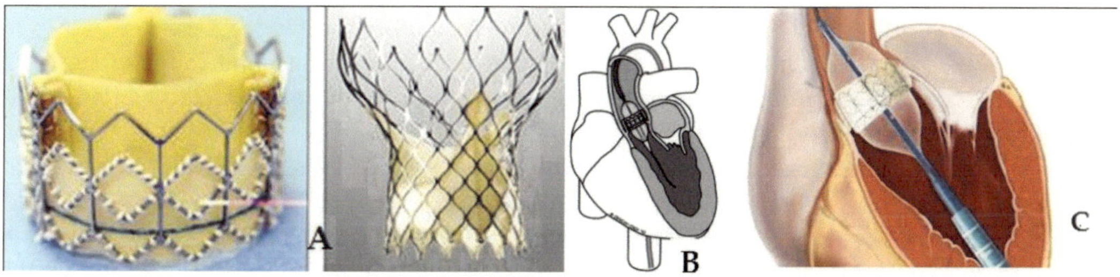

Fig. 5. **A** TAVI valves. **B** Transarterial approach. **C** Transapical approach.

In a European multicenter study including 16 centers, four hundred and forty four patients with a mean age of 82 years, only hold a post-intervention PPM incidence of 11,8%. The interesting point about this research is the inclusion of two different types of prosthesis and also different approaches. The bias of this analysis may arise from the variety of independent variables. However, the final outcome the post-intervention PPM implantationis lower, improving the results of those studies that use a single brand of valve or only one implantation approach.

Choice of prosthesis, approach election, indication time, patient's clinical status? What items improve incidence? We must find more specific evidence.

Another question to be answered: which is the appropriate technical surgery in elderly patients or must medical treatment be taken into account?

Older high-risk patients (Euro SCORE 19.9±18.8) with aortic stenosis are increasingly referred to TAVI but a subgroup of these cases is unsuitable for this and so conventional AVR is undertaken. The incidence of PPM is 7% (lower than TAVI). But re-operation for bleeding, renal failure, tracheotomy and sternal wound infection are frequent.

5.1.2 MVR

There are specific factors related to PPM in MV surgery. (Table 5)

Factors
Preoperatory
Pulmonar hypertension
Antiarrhythmic drugs
Sotalol
Digoxin
Mitral valve stenosis
Mitral annular calcification
Intraoperatory
Cross clamp time
Mitral valve replacement
Combined surgery(AVR-CABG)
Sternotomy approach
Reoperation

Table 5. Specific factors related to PPM in MV surgery.

The mitral valve apparatus is anatomically close to the atrioventricular conduction system, particularly the posterior-medial commissure of the anterior mitral leaflet, which lies close to the atrioventricular node (Figure 4).

Right now, it is important to refer to the different irrigation received by the AV node; in more than 70% of individuals it comes from the right coronary artery and for the rest, from the left. The coexisting coronary artery disease should not be underestimated. This should be expected in a well differentiated manner against the possibility of ischemia of conduction system during the MV surgery. Considering the topography of fibrous mitral and tricuspid rings the variants are:

1. The artery passes along the left lateral margin of the superior process and after reaching the proximal part of the annulus fibrosus of the posterior leaflet of the mitral valve the artery passes just lateral to the postero-medial commissure.
2. The artery runs in the middle of the space between the mitral and tricuspid valve.
3. The artery passes just adjacent but not in contact to the annulus of the septal leaflet of the tricuspid valve.

Trauma caused by manipulating the valve apparatus could result in ischemia because adjacent coronary artery flow is restricted by suture tug. The same manipulation is done around AV node. Tight suture can damage it. Face situation adding factors that become a vicious circle. The circumflex artery is the most affected by subocclusion. There is a relationship between iatrogenic circumflex lesions and coronary dominance, but no difference exists between replacement/repair.

Mechanisms underlying postoperative AVB following mitral valve replacement or annuloplasty are very interesting to research. In dry dissected human hearts, the AV node artery was discovered to run close to the annulus of the mitral valve in 23% of patients.

Reconstruction has recently become the technique of choice in the treatment of patients with mitral regurgitation of degenerative origin. This surgical technique is more complex and sometimes results in longer ischemic times. The longer intraoperative ischemia has been postulated as being responsible for the postoperative incidence of the AV node block in this type of intervention.

The extended transseptal approach provided a better exposure of the mitral valve compared to conventional approach. The operative times and the incidence of mortality and complications were similar to conventional technique. About 4.8% of patients required PPM.

Predictors of PPM in mitral valve repair using Carpentier's techniques: 23% perform AVB but is transient, and partially or completely resolves before the seventh postoperative day. No mitral type procedures including anterior versus posterior leaflet repair is related to AVB. Systemic hypothermia during surgery is the only independent predictor. Only 2.6% require PPM.

Surgery involving the aortic and mitral valves can increase the trend to receive PPM over three times, as an example 13.3% vs. 5.8%.

In the same manner as the AVR surgeries goal is to reduce the complications in elderly patients using TAVI, for mitral valve surgery also investigates the same goal: a minimally Invasive (right lateral minithoracotomy) versus sternotomy. The minimally invasive approach led to longer duration of surgery, cardiopulmonary bypass, and cross-clamp time. By sternotomy the number of postoperative arrhythmias and pacemaker implants was higher. In this surgical technique, long surgery times as cause of inadequate tissue perfusion, which is an important factor for severe postoperative arrhythmia, are discarded.

In this occasion, the traumatic would be the only damage mechanism. Validation of this statement could only be done on absolutely homogeneous group (Euro SCORE, disease severity, surgeon, perfusionist, anesthesiologist, etc).
The results on the incidence and risk factors for PPM according to the region where you get the results must be carefully analyzed. The bias is found for example between Latin America and North America. In the former, the main underlying valve disease for surgical indication is rheumatic fever while in the latter is fibroelastic mucopolysaccharide deficiency.

5.2 Redo surgery

The incidence to permanent pacemaker need after repeated cardiac surgery has approximately a fourfold increase. Factors commonly found are surgeries that involve two valves, preoperative endocarditis, increasing number of reoperations, the degree of hypothermia during cardiopulmonary bypass and advanced age. Additional univariable predictors included are CPB, aortic cross clamp increased time, and aortic valve replacement. (Lewis J, 1998) studied 558 consecutive patients undergoing at least one repeated cardiac operation: in this group, 54 patients (9.7%) required a permanent pacemaker. The need for a permanent pacemaker after reoperations did not result in significant long-term impairment of functional status or longevity compared with those who did not require a permanent pacemaker.

5.3 Myxomas

Atrial myxomas are the most frequent primitive cardiac tumors (50%). They appear between 30 and 60 years old, predominantly in women, and the most common location is the left atrium (75%) followed by the right atrium (15-20%) Only 4% are located in the ventricles. In 90% of cases there are solitary tumors but may be part of familiar syndromes (Carney).
In this case, there are at least two myxomas and the right atrium is the most affected cavity. Its symptoms are usually due to cavity obstruction. By their anatomical location, they may affect the conduction system and this can also be a symptomatic manifestation.
Not many publications deal with the need for PPM after the resection of these tumors. If the myxoma is located in the atrial septum, it is directly related to the need for PPM.
There are approximately 2.6 up to 18.8% of incidence of PPM.

5.4 Congenital heart disease surgery

The most common cardiac diseases that reach adulthood with surgical indication are atrial and ventricle septal defect, coarctation of aorta, persistent ductus arteriosus, bicuspid aortic stenosis, subaortic stenosis and ectasia of the aortic annulus in Marfan syndrome. The aortic and sub aortic stenosis was previously exposed in 5.1.1.
Not all congenital diseases that reach adulthood and are resolved after surgery can have endocardial PPM implantation. Epicardial pacing systems appear to have a higher incidence of lead failure predominantly in ventricle lead and are significantly less durable. This is a problem to be solved in each particular situation of the patient's evolution (Ebstein disease).
After congenital surgery, the recovery pacemaker's dependence occurs in 10% of patients with AVB after mid-term follow-up (40 days average).
Post-operative result in congenital heart diseases with septal defect is often impaired by the occurrence of disorders in atrio-ventricular conduction.

5.4.1 Septal defects

Interventricular communication (IVC) in adults is rare, most cases close spontaneously (before 10 years) or are surgically corrected during childhood. Its evolution depends on its location and size. There are 4 types: perimembranous, infundibular, anterior and trabecular core. The perimembranous and trabecular are the most frequent representing 90% of cases. The perimembranous persists for a longer term and constitutes 10% of adult congenital heart disease. The defect is located in the membranous septum with possible extension to the muscular region. Among the electrical abnormalities secondary to surgery 2% of complete atrioventricular block occur in immediate postoperative period, but it may appear after discharge as paroxysmal atrioventricular block. Incidence of PPM is nearly 2.5%. The defect near the conduction system and also the one with a larger diameter (≥ 1cm) are more likely to lock AVB followed by PPM. It should be kept in mind that larger defects require patch closure and sutures cover extensive zone of tissue. Inter-auricular communication (IAC) is the most common congenital heart disease predominant in adult (40%), with a female predominance and can manifest at any age. There are four types of IAC ostium secundum (most common defect at the atrial septum, i.e. foramen ovale type) sinus venosus (upper and lower), coronary sinus type and ostium primum type. The symptoms are: breath, atrial arrhythmia, cardiomegaly, right branch block bundle, paradoxical embolism or pulmonary vascular disease

The chronic course (diagnosed and untreated or non-diagnosed) is associated with left atrium increasing diameter, myocardial loss, and generalized conduction abnormalities, which favors the installation of sustained atrial fibrillation. Treatment in patients over 40 years is often cause for discussion.

Closure performed by surgery or percutaneous approach with Amplatzer ™ septal occluder (ASO) can be indicated at any age with the exception of pulmonary hypertension. Percutaneous closure can be the method of choice in isolated ostium secundum with appropriate edges, but it is an expensive procedure. Surgery is relegated to ostium secundum with defective edges or multi fenestrated. Surgical treatment gives better results than percutaneous technique and medical treatment. Septal occluder implant treatment shows superior results to surgery respect to some complications, but they were not significant in adults under 40 years.

There is certainly nothing wrong with continuing to do surgery in countries where the resources are limited. After surgical closure, atrial arrhythmias occur between 12% and 14% of patients (70% atrial fibrillation). PPM following AVB is related to age (>50 years),reoperation, cross clamp and CPB time. IAC complex types, simultaneous mitral insufficiency repair or other congenital procedure imply long surgery times.

5.5 Ascending aorta surgery. Marfan syndrome. Bentall- De Bono intervention

The intervention on the ascending aorta is always a challenge. The pathologies of surgical indications are: dilation (> 5cm), aneurysm, primary or secondary dissection of the artery (dilatation or aneurysm). These diseases may include in its pathophysiology aortic valve insufficiency. Combined intervention with artery and valve repair has a high index of AV block. The origin of the aneurysm may be degenerative (cystic, ecstatic, atherosclerotic), traumatic (blunt, penetrating, surgical and diagnostic), inflammatory, infectious, mechanical, dissecting and congenital. The most common congenital cause is Marfan syndrome which usually has annular aortic ectasia. The fundamental cause is a cystic media necrosis with high incidence of dissection and rupture.

Annulo-aortic ectasia is a dilation of the aortic root with the involvement of the Valsalva sinuses. In 1968, Bentall and De Bono proposed to replace aortic valve, Valsalva sinuses and the ascending aorta with a composite tube graft with aortic valve prosthesis. Also aortic root homografts are a valid alternative, specially in infection status; the main advantage of this therapy is that permanent anticoagulation is not needed. (Figure 6) Consequently, coronary ostiums have to be reimplanted on the prosthetic tube. This surgery is an adult cardiac surgery more technically complex and has a high incidence of complications such as bleeding, complete AVB, hemiparesis and high mortality. The causes of AVB are the extreme proximity to the conduction system, extreme hypothermia while the CPB is performed and/or circulatory arrest. The danger of inadequate perfusion and ischemia is aggravated because CPB is usually very prolonged (≥120 minutes). The incidence of PPM is about 5 to 14%.

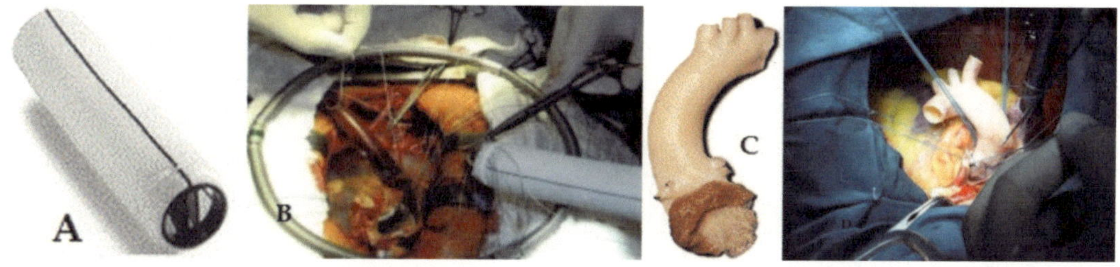

Fig. 6. **A**.Tube graft with aortic valve prosthesis, **B**. Bentall De Bono surgery. **C**. Aortic Homograft , **D**. Bentall De Bono surgery with homograft

5.6 CABG- myocardial protection

With longer CBP times, there is a lower myocardial protection quality. Duration bypass > 120 minutes is a significant predictor of long-term pacemaker dependency. More number of vessels bypassed in CBGA derives in longer CXL and CPB times, resulting in higher risk for PPM.

If myocardial protection is inadequate and uneven, it leads to perioperative myocardial infarction and low output syndrome, exacerbating postoperative conduction disturbances.

Although some evidence exists to suggest that the type (Crystalloid-Blood), the way (Antegrade-Retrograde), the temperature (Warm-Tepid-Cold) and the time delivery (Continuous-Discontinuous) of cardioplegia increase the risk of PPM insertion, reports are contradictory.

Normothermic cardioplegia is associated with a marked decrease in new and permanent conduction disturbances and CK-MB postoperative release. This suggests that a significant factor in the pathogenesis of conduction blocks is cold-related injury.

Cold blood cardioplegia represents a risk factor for PPM and this finding might be related to differences in delivery and not to cardioplegia composition.

It seems that continuous delivery provides improved myocardial protection and reduces the incidence of postoperative conduction disturbances.

Retrograde cardioplegia provides better results in venous sinus oxygen saturation.

Is it a panacea to use retrograde warm cardioplegia? The retrograde cardioplegia protects only the left coronary artery supply systems, in case of right origin of the atrio-ventricular bundle artery; this is not protected adequately during the surgical procedure, and thus may also be an origin of postoperative conduction disturbance.

Remote ischemic preconditioning (RIPC) induced by brief ischemia and reperfusion reduces myocardial injury in CABG surgery patients and improves ventricle function, proved by postoperative isquemic myocardial enzyme markers (Troponin I, Troponin T, pro-BNP) and hemodynamic measures. Volatile anesthetic agents can mimic ischemic preconditioning: delivery of >15 minutes of Sevoflurane or Desflurane for myocardium protection have the same or additive effect as RIPC.

Glucose-insulin-potassium (GIK) is a potentially useful adjunct to myocardial protection. Also high-dose insulin therapy protects by enhancing early metabolic recovery of the arrested heart during revascularization.

Non-diluted blood cardioplegia solution supplemented with L-arginine is associated with a significant decrease of myocardial lactate release after CXL and reperfusion during CABG surgery.

It is significant that reducing myocardial injury by using certain types of cardioplegia, adding protective substances, decreases the chance of arrhythmias and therefore pacing need.

The research for intraoperative PPM risk factors is important to improve outcomes. (Table 6)

Author	Surgery	n	Risk factors
Lewis,1998	REDO	54	VS. Number of reoperations and degree of hypothermia during CPB.
Erdogan, 2006	AVR	465	Total CPB and CXL time
Goldman, 1984	ALL	5,942	VS especially, tricuspid. Poor myocardial protection.
Del Rizzo,1996	ALL	3493	Redo surgery. VS: aortic and tricuspid. Cold blood cardioplegia. Postoperative IM
Schurr, 2010	AVR	3534	Postoperatory RBBB. Associated procedures: CABG. Aortic annulus size. CPB time .Redo.
Merin, 2009.	ALL	4,999	AVR.
Meimoun,2002	MVR	115	A lesser systemic hypothermia during surgery.
Huynh, 2009.	VAR	207	Cardiac arrest and dual valve surgery
Elahi, 2005	VAR	782	CPB > 100 minutes.CXL > 70 minutes.
Totaro, 2000	VAR	124	Continuous suture technique
Baerman, 1987	CABG	93	Number of bypassed arteries -CPB and CXL time.
Gundry, 1987.	CABG	468	Blood cardioplegia
Elahi, 1987.	VS	2,392	Reoperations .Longer cumulative CXL times, multiple-VS.

ALL = All heart surgery; AVR =aortic valve replacement; CABG = coronary artery bypass grafting; CPB = cardiopulmonary bypass; IM= myocardial infarction; MVR = mitral valve repair o replacement; REDO= reoperation; VS = valve surgery; CXL= aortic cross clamping.

Table 6. Intraoperative risk factors.

6. What to do to minimize the risk of PPM

It is necessary to minimize the risks of PPM, after a thorough analysis and validation of results trying to:

Solve preoperative non-sinus rhythm as possible.
Improve metabolic status as possible.
Minimally invasive approach (MVR).
Do valve repair instead of replacement where possible.
Do an optimal myocardial protection during CPB.
Minimize hypothermia times when it is not necessary.
Reduce CPB and aortic CXL times.
Continuous normothermic blood cardioplegia.
Improve adequate reperfusion.
Interrupted sutures in valve replacement.

7. Indications and estimated time for PPM implantation

Several variables are considered to place a PPM as well as the appropriate time to do so. (Table 7)

Variables considered to place PPM after cardiac surgery
Conduction disturbance
Start TPM time
Persistence arrhythmia in time
Surgery type
Patient's hemodynamic and clinical status
Complications's longer stay

Table 7. Variables considered to place PPM after cardiac surgery

High degree atrioventricular block, sick sinus syndrome, symptomatic bradycardia, slow atrial fibrillation and bifasicular block are the most frequent causes for implantation.
Postoperative complete atrioventricular block is the most important predictor of pacemaker dependency, enabling early decision on permanent pacemaker implantation.
The cardiac surgery allows direct access to the heart and therefore the possibility of implanting in atrials and/or ventricles temporary epicardial electrodes.
Although the common problems of poor sensing or capture, dislodgement or retention exist. There is no best appropriate status criteria for wires removal. Decision for optimal time for PPM implantation after cardiac surgery is a controversial item and should be individualized for each patient. The mean postoperative day of pacemaker implantation varies from 5 up to 7 days. Nevertheless, we can find averages between 3 and 31 days. (Table 8) An early PPM placement enables early mobilization and facilitates hospital discharge.
Each individual patient is affected by several risk factors including surgery type, preoperative rhythm, postoperative conduction abnormalities, different QRS complex morphology, and onset TPM time of postoperative course.
To Glikson, the maximum waiting time is no later than the sixth and the ninth postoperative days for wide-complex and narrow-complex escape, respectively. (Glikson, 1997)
Because of the extreme variability in the evolution of these arrhythmias Heart Association leaves to the physician's choice to decide when is the best time for PPM implantation, although they recommend waiting for at least 7 days in cases of second grade and third grade AVB in adolescents or patients undergoing congenital disease surgery.

Author	Surgery	Time (days)
Schurr, 2010	AVR	4.4 ± 3.8
Merin, 2009	ALL	5
Berdajs, 2008	MV	4
Glikson, 1997	ALL	6-9
Koplan, 2003	VS	8.4 ± 5.8
Huynh, 2009	AVR	6.1 ± 2.3
Dawkins, 2008	AVR	5

ALL = All heart surgery; AVR =aortic valve replacement; CABG = coronary artery bypass grafting; MV = mitral valve surgery; VS = valve surgery.

Table 8. Time elapsed between TPM and PPM placement, after cardiac surgery.

Prolonged immobilization from temporary pacing impedes patient recuperation and may increase the risk of pneumonia, deep venous thrombosis, and pulmonary embolism. Early pacemaker implantation may reduce morbidity and postoperative hospital stay.

7.1 Valve surgery

Waiting times to place a PPM in heart valve surgery are similar to other cardiac surgeries, unless combined with CABG and mitral valve repair; circumstances when it is prudent to wait for three or four more days for the spontaneous sinusal rhythm recovery (if it previously existed)

Hancock, 1988, advised permanent pacemaker implantation as soon as the third day in those patients with AVB after aortic valve surgery. For patients undergoing valve surgery, who develop complete AVB before the first postoperative 24 h and hold it for 48 hours, it is suggested to implement PPM before the first week.

Nevertheless, Zakhia Doueihi have observed that waiting for 10 days after surgery between 15 and 20% of valve patients with advanced AVB degree, spontaneously recover and do not require a permanent device. (Zakhia Doueihi, 1992)

The high percentage of cases with irreversible complete AVB in tricuspid valve replacement, along with difficulty of endocavitary pacemaker implantation after surgery has caused to take the usual attitude of implanting an electrode in the same surgery.

How much time should patients be monitored to expect appearance of arrhythmias after AVR? In the long-term monitoring (102 months) in survivors of AVR with a normal ECG, a 13.7% conduction disorders was reported, but only 1% PPM was required. Another research analyses PPM requirement after artificial aortic valve replacement is because of AV complete block and atrial fibrillation with slow ventricular response. Since the 9th up to 196th month, all these patients remained in good general NYHA state with permanent stimulation, and in complete AV block disappeared 24 months after AVR.

7.2 CABG surgery

Pathological lesions in the left anterior descending coronary artery compromising flow in the first perforator that do not provide an adequate circulation produce localized damage and conduction disturbances after coronary artery bypass grafting. This can be predicted from the preoperative angiographic anatomy.

After heart surgery, 35% of coronary patients with complete AVB and up to 70% of patients with sinus node disease are no longer dependent on the pacemaker over time.

In a short series of Baerman, 1987, the recovery of sinus rhythm in patients implanted with pacemakers for complete AVB was 54%.He also found that the third degree AVB appears in 4% of the patients and nearly all of them finally needed PPM.

8. Epicardic pacemakers complications

Intraoperatory epicardial electrodes are usually implanted on the anterior right ventricular muscle in areas without epicardial fat. It is an easily accessible area and it provides good pacing and sensing.

8.1 Failure of ventricular sensing and capture

Classic studies show that univentricular stimulation generates depolarization through multiple aberrant pathways in the unstimulated ventricle. Isolated right ventricular pacing reproduces the pattern of ventricular activation of left bundle branch block, so it has multiple deleterious effects. It may develop inter- and intraventricular left dyssynchrony, narrowing the left ventricular diastole, and an increasing relationship between diastolic times of both ventricles. All that has been said above precipitates a worse left ventricular filling, prolonged ventricular isovolumetric contraction-relaxation, lateral wall is contracted during diastole causing interventricular septal paradoxical movement. All these deleterious effects on left ventricular contractility and filling can be very harmful in the immediate postoperative period, especially in patients with systolic and/or diastolic ventricular dysfunction, with inotropic or intraaortic balloon pump dependency.

All these effects are pointing out that in certain patient groups postoperative epicardial biventricular pacing to improve cardiac output and postoperative course can be effective.

8.2 Others complications

These are bleeding from right ventricular laceration with tamponade, avulsion of a side branch from a saphenous vein coronary bypass graft, and perforation of the superior epigastric artery, gastric penetration, etc. They are emergency situations that put patient's life in danger, leading to urgent reoperation surgery, more days of mechanical ventilation and hospital stay, increasing mortality.

Removal of wires should be done under echocardiography control and in an operating room prepared for emergency reoperation.

9. Other pacemaker uses for heart surgery

9.1 Atrial fibrillation

Between the second and fourth postoperative day, postoperative atrial fibrillation has a variable incidence, about 30% for CABG surgery, 40% for valve surgery and 50% for combined surgery. It is an arrhythmia that is associated with hemodynamic instability, congestive heart failure, renal insufficiency, infection, neurologic injury and thromboembolism.

It is also associated with adverse outcomes and increased costs. Accordingly, therapy should be provided to prevent it. The assessment therapies do so is an area of active research with recent significant advances.

Multiple strategies are described to reduce incidence, most of them through drug treatment, primarily with beta blockers, amiodarone, magnesium, or combinations thereof. Except for magnesium in conventional doses, the others are not free of complications.

Premature atrial extrasystole produces dispersion of atrial refractoriness and induces a heterogeneous anisotropic conduction, especially in regions near the coronary sinus and the triangle of Koch. (Figure 7) These regional differences between refractory periods and the prolongation resulting in atrial activation, are precisely the best substrate for the creation of re-entry that supports the initiation and perpetuation of atrial fibrillation. Atrial pacing may prevent the occurrence of arrhythmia.

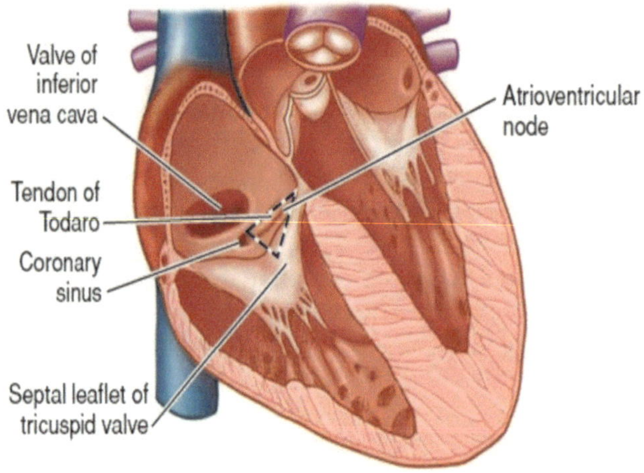

Fig. 7. Triangle of Koch, where the atrioventricular node lies.

During the 70's atrial pacing was not seen as a help for improving the cardiac output. Medical science is constantly changing day after day.
Two meta-analyses evaluated the atrial pacing prevention effect for postoperative atrial fibrillation. The findings analyses are quite similar. The biatrial and right atrial stimulation, at varying frequencies can reduce the incidence of postoperative atrial fibrillation from 2.6 to 1.8 times, respectively, while fixed frequencies only has proven effective in biatrial stimulation.Some studies agree that this therapeutic is safe and well tolerated, although to be effective should be combined with drugs. Biatrial mode pacing opens a promising new treatment opportunity.

9.2 Others uses

The problem with OPCAB is hemodynamic instability when heart is tilted for posterior's coronary arteries access. Decrease mean and systolic arterial pressure and increase left atrial pressure.
Several attempts have been proposed to improve this: Trendelenburg maneuver, right-side rotation (cardiac volume improve) of patient, β blockers, etc.; but all these methods have their own complications. Even one-lung ventilation (left lung excluded) was proposed. Without ventilation oscillation, the surgeon would find a quiet field to do bypass grafts faster. It was a failure because the heart shifts to the bottom thoracic cavity.
Mechanical stabilization with a restraining device and a suction device for immobilization are ways to resolve this situation.

In OPCAB, the effect of atrial epicardial pacing improves ventricular function. It increases cardiac output and mean and systolic pressures, and decreases central venous pressures, resulting in better tolerance at the exposure maneuver.

10. Conclusion

During cardiac surgery the placement of temporary pacemaker is usually necessary, especially for weaning from CPB. Epicardial electrode wires come out through the skin next to the incision. There are complications such as sensing and capture failures. Also during wire extraction trauma may occur. Predisposing factors for arrhythmia are pre- intra- and postoperative conduction disturbances, age ≥ 65 years; valve surgery and those surgeries where there is manipulation around to the conduction system, and inadequate myocardial protection.When arrhythmia persists more than 7 days, the placement of a permanent pacemaker is advisable.

It is important to make the decision to implant a permanent pacemaker. This implies to take into account arrhythmia damage mechanisms, times, and probable reversibility.

All these points must be informed to patients.

11. References

[1] Ashida Y Ohgi S, Kuroda H, Ishiguro S, and col. Permanent cardiac pacing following surgery for acquired valvular disease. Ann Thorac Cardiovasc Surg. 2000 Jun;6(3):161-6.

[2] Baerman JM, Kirsh MM, De Buitleir M and col. Natural history and determinants of conduction defects following coronary artery bypass surgery. Ann Thorac Surg. 1987; 44: 150- 3.

[3] Bateman TM, Gray RJ, Raymond MJ, Chaux A, and col. Arrhythmias and conduction disturbances following cardiac operation for the removal of left atrial myxomas. J Thorac Cardiovasc Surg. 1983 Oct; 86(4):601-7.

[4] Batra AS, Wells WJ, Hinoki KW, and col. Late recovery of atrioventricular conduction after Pacemaker implantation for complete heart block associated with surgery for congenital heart disease. J Thorac Cardiovasc Surg.2003; 125: 1291- 3.

[5] Ben Ameur Y, Baraket F, Longo S, Annabi N and col. Conductive disorders following open- heart valvular surgery. Concerning 230 operated patient. Ann Cardiol Angeiol (Paris). 2006 Jun; 55(3):140-3.

[6] Berdajs D, Schurr UP, Wagner A, Seifert B and col. Incidence and pathophysiology of atrioventricular block following mitral valve replacement and ring annuloplasty. European Journal of Cardio-Thoracic Surgery Volume 34, Issue 1, July 2008, Pages 55-61.

[7] Bethea BT, Salazar JD, Grega MA, Doty JR and col. Determining the utility of temporary pacing wires after coronary artery bypass surgery. Ann 2005 Jan; 79(1):104-7.

[8] Bolcal C, Emrecan B, Bingol H and col. Does combination of antegrade and retrograde cardioplegia reduce coronary artery bypass grafting-related conduction defects? Heart Surg Forum. 2006; 9:E866-70.

[9] Borracci R, Rubio M, Milani A and col. Abordaje transeptal para el reemplazo valvular mitral. Revista Argentina de Cardiología, VOL 78, N° 5 / SEPTIEMBRE-OCTUBRE 2010, pp 400-404

[10] Brazão A, Eugénio L, de Oliveira F, Antunes M. Surgery for acute type-An aortic dissection. Rev Port Cardiol. 1997 Jun; 16(6):525-32, 507.
[11] Bruschi G, De Marco F, Fratto P, Oreglia J and col. Alternative approaches for trans-catheter self-expanding aortic bioprosthetic valves implantation: single-center experience. Eur J Cardiothorac Surg. 2011 Jun;39(6):e151-8.
[12] Coma Samartín R., Carbonell de Blas R.; Castaño Ruiz M. Estimulación cardiaca temporal. Estimulación tras cirugía cardiaca. Rev Esp. Cardiol. 2007; 7 (Supl G):54-68.
[13] Cook DJ, Bailon JM, Douglas T and col. Changing incidence, type, and natural history of conduction defects after coronary artery bypass grafting. Ann Thorac Surg. 2005; 80: 1732-7.
[14] Cooper JP, Jayawickreme SR, Swanton RH. Permanent pacing in patients with tricuspid valve replacements. Br Heart J. 1995; 73: 169-72.
[15] Crystal E, Connolly SJ, Sleik K and col. Interventions on prevention of postoperative atrial fibrillation in patients undergoing heart surgery: a meta-analysis. Circulation. 2002; 106: 75 - 80.
[16] Daoud EG, Snow R, Hummel JD and col. Temporary atrial epicardial pacing as prophylaxis against atrial fibrillation after heart surgery: a meta-analysis. J Cardiovasc Electrophysiol. 2003; 14: 127 - 32.
[17] Dawkins S, Hobson AR, Kalra PR, Tang AT and col. Permanent pacemaker implantation after isolated aortic valve replacement: incidence, indications, and predictors. Ann Thorac Surg. 2008 Jan; 85(1):108-12.
[18] Del Nido P, Goldman B. Temporary epicardial pacing after open heart surgery: complications and prevention. J Cardiac Surg 1989; 4: 99 – 103.
[19] Del Rizzo DF, Nishimura S, Lau C, Sever J, Goldman BS. Cardiac pacing following surgery for acquired heart disease. J Card Surg. 1996 Sep-Oct; 11(5):332-40.
[20] Dias RR, Mejia OA, Fiorelli AI, Pomerantzeff PM.Analysis of aortic root surgery with composite mechanical aortic valve conduit and valve-sparing reconstruction. Rev Bras Cir Cardiovasc. 2010 Oct-Dec; 25(4):491-9.
[21] Dimarakis I, Rehman SM, Grant SW, Saravanan DM, and col. Conventional aortic valve replacement for high-risk aortic stenosis patients not suitable for trans- catheter aortic valve implantation: feasibility and outcome. Eur J Cardiothorac Surg. 2011 Feb 21. Epub ahead of print.
[22] Do QB, Pellerin M, Carrier M, and col. Clinical outcome after isolated tricuspid valve replacement: 20-year experience. Can J Cardiol. 2000; 16: 489-93.
[23] Edwin F, Aniteye E, Tettey M, Sereboe L and col. Permanent complete heart block following surgical correction of congenital heart disease. Ghana Med J. 2010 Sep; 44(3):109-14.
[24] Elahi M, Usmaan K. The bioprosthesis type and size influence the postoperative incidence of permanent pacemaker implantation in patients undergoing aortic valve surgery. J Interv Card Electrophysiol 2006; 15:113–118.
[25] Elahi M, Lee D, Dhannapuneni RR. Predictors of permanent pacemaker implantation during the early postoperative period after valve surgery. Tex Heart Inst J. 2006; 33(4):455-7.

[26] Eltchaninoff H, Prat A, Gilard M, Leguerrier A and col.Transcatheter aortic valve implantation: early results of the FRANCE (French Aortic National Core Valve and Edwards) registry. Eur Heart J. 2011 Jan; 32(2):191-7.
[27] Emlein G, Huang SK, Pires LA, and col. Prolonged bradyarrhythmias after isolated coronary artery bypass graft surgery. Am Heart J. 1993 Nov; 126(5):1084-90.
[28] Erdogan HB, Kayalar N, Ardal H, and col.Risk factors for requirement of permanent pacemaker implantation after aortic valve replacement. J Card Surg. 2006; 21: 211-5.
[29] Fan K, Lee KL, Chiu CS, and col. Effects of biatrial pacing in prevention of postoperative atrial fibrillation after coronary artery bypass surgery. Circulation 2000; 102: 755-60.
[30] Feldman S, Glikson M, Kaplinsky E. Pacemaker dependency after coronary artery bypass. Pacing Clin Electrophysiol. 1992; 15: 2037-40.
[31] Fernández P., Garro H., Pastori J., Chiale P. Indicaciones de implante de marcapasos definitivo en cirugía cardíaca. Revista del Conarec, Noviembre- Diciembre 2008 - Año 24 - Nº97:415-417.
[32] Flack JE 3rd, Hafer J, Engelman RM, Rousou JA and col. Effect of normothermic blood cardioplegia on postoperative conduction abnormalities and supraventricular arrhythmias. Circulation 1992; 86(5 Suppl): II-385–92.
[33] Forlani S, Moscarelli M, Scafuri A and col. Combination therapy for prevention of atrial fibrillation after coronary artery bypass surgery: a randomized trial of sotalol and magnesium. Card Electrophysiol Rev. 2003; 7: 168-71.
[34] Fukuda T, Hawley R L and Edwards J E. Lesions of conduction tissue complicating aortic valvular replacement. Chest 1976; 69; 605-614.
[35] Gerstenfeld EP, Hill MR, French SN, Mehra R and col. Evaluation of right atrial and biatrial temporary pacing for the prevention of atrial fibrillation after coronary artery bypass surgery. J Am Coll Cardiol. 1999 Jun; 33(7):1981-8.
[36] Glikson M, Dearani JA, Hyberger LK and col. Indications, effectiveness, and long-term dependency in permanent pacing after cardiac surgery. Am J Cardiol. 1997; 80:1309-1.
[37] Goldman BS, Hill TJ, Weisel RD, and col.Permanent cardiac pacing after open-heart surgery: acquired heart disease. Pacing Clin Electrophysiol. 1984 May; 7 (3 Pt 1):367-71
[38] Gordon RS, Ivanov J, Cohen G, and col. Permanent cardiac pacing after a cardiac operation: predicting the use of permanent pacemakers. Ann Thorac Surg. 1998 Nov; 66(5):1698-704.
[39] Grande AM, Fiore A, Massetti M, Viganò M. Iatrogenic circumflex coronary lesion in mitral valve surgery: case report and review of the literature. Tex Heart Inst J. 2008; 35(2):179-83.
[40] Gregoratos G, Abrams J, Epstein AE, and col. Guideline Update for Implantation of Cardiac Pacemakers and Antiarrhythmia Devices -summary article: a report of the American College of Cardiology/American Heart Association Task Force on Practice Guidelines (ACC/AHA/NASPE Committee to Update the 1998 Pacemaker Guidelines). J Am Coll Cardiol. 2002; 40: 1703 -19.
[41] Gulielmos V, Kappert U, Eller M, Sahre H and col.Improving hemodynamics by atrial pacing during off-pump bypass surgery. Heart Surg Forum. 2003; 6(6):E179-82.

[42] Gundry SR, Sequeira A, Coughlin TR, McLaughlin JS. Postoperative conduction disturbances: a comparison of blood and crystalloid cardioplegia. Ann Thorac Surg. 1989 Mar; 47(3):384-90.
[43] Habicht J, Scherr P, Zerkowski H, Hoffmann A. Late conduction defects following aortic valve replacement. J Heart Valve Dis 2000; 9:629 –32.
[44] Hancock EW. AV block after aortic valve replacement. Hosp Pract (Off Ed). 1988; 23: 41-48.
[45] Haworth P, Behan M, Khawaja M, Hutchinson N and col. Predictors for permanent pacing after transcatheter aortic valve implantation. Catheter Cardiovasc Interv. 2010 Nov 1; 76(5):751-6.
[46] Holzhey DM, Shi W, Borger MA, Seeburger J, and col.Minimally invasive versus sternotomy approach for mitral valve surgery in patients greater than 70 years old: a propensity-matched comparison. Ann Thorac Surg. 2011 Feb; 91(2):401-5.
[47] Huynh H, Dalloul G, Ghanbari H, Burke P, and col. Permanent pacemaker implantation following aortic valve replacement: current prevalence and clinical predictors. Pacing Clin Electrophysiol. 2009 Dec; 32(12):1520-5.
[48] Imren Y, Benson AA, Oktar GL, Cheema FH and col.Is use of temporary pacing wires following coronary bypass surgery really necessary? (Torino). 2008 Apr; 49(2):261-7.
[49] Jahangiri M, Laborde JC, Roy D and col. Outcome of patients with aortic stenosis referred to a multidisciplinary meeting for transcatheter valve. Ann Thorac Surg. 2011 Feb; 91(2):411-5.
[50] Jilaihawi H, Chin D, Vasa-Nicotera M, Jeilan M, and col. Predictors for permanent pacemaker requirement after transcatheter aortic valve implantation with the Core Valve bioprosthesis. Am Heart J. 2009 May; 157(5):860-6.
[51] Kikura M, Sato S. The efficacy of preemptive Milrinone or Amrinone therapy in patients undergoing coronary artery bypass grafting. Anesth Analg. 2002; 94: 22-30.
[52] Kim MH, Deeb GM, Eagle KA, and col. Complete atrioventricular block after valvular heart surgery and the timing of pacemaker implantation. Am J Cardiol. 2001; 87: 649 - 51.
[53] Koplan BA, Stevenson WG, Epstein LM and col. Development and validation of a simple risk score to predict the need for permanent pacing after cardiac valve surgery. J M Coll Cardiol. 2003 Mar 5; 41(5):795-801.
[54] Lazzara RR, Park SB, Magovern GJ. Cardiac myxomas: results of surgical treatment. J Cardiovasc Surg (Torino). 1991 Nov-Dec; 32(6):824-7.
[55] Lewis JW Jr, Webb CR, Pickard SD, and col. The increased need for a permanent pacemaker after reoperative cardiac surgery. Thorac Cardiovasc Surg. 1998 Jul; 116(1):74- 81.
[56] Li L, Luo W, Huang L, Zhang W, and col. Remote preconditioning reduces myocardial injury in adult valve replacement: a randomized controlled trial. 2010 Nov; 164(1):e21-6.
[57] Limongelli G, Ducceschi V, D'Andrea A, Renzulli A and col. Risk factors for pacemaker implantation following aortic valve replacement: a single centre experience. Heart 2003 Aug; 89(8):901-4.
[58] Maisel WH, Rawn JD, Stevenson WG. Atrial fibrillation after cardiac surgery. Ann Intern Med. 2001; 135: 1061- 73.

[59] Matthews IG, Fazal IA, Bates MG, Turley AJ In patients undergoing aortic valve replacement, what factors predict the requirement for permanent pacemaker implantation. Interact Cardiovasc Thorac Surg. 2011 Mar; 12(3):475-9.
[60] McLeod CJ, Attenhofer Jost CH, Warnes CA, Hodge D 2nd and col. Epicardial versus endocardial permanent pacing in adults with congenital heart disease. 2010 Sep; 28(3):235-43.
[61] Meimoun P, Zeghdi R, D'Attelis N, Berrebi A and col. Frequency, predictors, and consequences of atrioventricular block after mitral valve repair. 2002 May 1; 89(9):1062-6.
[62] Merin O, Ilan M, Oren A, Fink D and col. Permanent pacemaker implantation following cardiac surgery: indications and long-term follow-up. Pacing Clin Electrophysiol. 2009 Jan; 32(1):7-12.
[63] Mitchell LB, Crystal E, Heilbron B, Page P. Atrial fibrillation following cardiac surgery. Can J Cardiol. 2005; 21: B45-50.
[64] Mitchell LB. Prophylactic therapy to prevent atrial arrhythmia after cardiac surgery. Curr Opin Cardiol. 2007; 22: 18- 24.
[65] Molnár T, Farkas K, Palkó A, Eszlári E and col. Gastric penetration of epicardial pacemaker leads 8 years after cardiac surgery. Endoscopy. 2010; 42 Suppl 2:E273-4.
[66] Mosseri M, Meir G, Lotan C, et al. Coronary pathology predicts conduction disturbances after coronary artery bypass grafting. Ann Thorac Surg 1991; 51: 248–52.
[67] Moya Mur J.; Oliva De Anquin E. Centella Hernández T. y col. Selección del mejor lugar de estimulación tras cirugía cardiaca evaluando la asincronía con strain tras diferentes estimulaciones. Rev Esp Cardiol.2010; 63:1162-70.
[68] Nardi P, Pellegrino A, Scafuri A, Bellos K, and col.Permanent pacemaker implantation after isolated aortic valve replacement: incidence, risk factors and surgical technical aspects. J Cardiovasc Med (Hagerstown). 2010 Jan; 11(1):14-9.
[69] Oter Rodríguez R, Montiel J, Roldán Pascual T, and col. Guías de práctica clínica de la Sociedad Española de Cardiología en marcapasos. Rev Esp. Cardiol. 2000; 53: 947 - 66. 10.
[70] Puskas JD, Sharoni E, Williams WH, Petersen R, and col. Is routine use of temporary epicardic pacing wires necessary after either OPCAB or conventional CABG/CPB? Heart Surg Forum. 2003; 6(6):E103-6.
[71] Raichlen JS, Campbell FW, Edie RN, Josephson ME and col. The effect of the site of placement of temporary epicardial pacemakers on ventricular function in patients undergoing cardiac surgery. Circulation.1984 Sep; 70(3 Pt 2):I118-23.
[72] Raza SS, Li JM, John R, Chen LY, and col. Long-Term Mortality and Pacing Outcomes of Patients with Permanent Pacemaker Implantation after Cardiac Surgery. Pacing Clin Electrophysiol. 2011 Jan 5. doi: 10.1111/j.1540-8159.2010.02972. Nov; 11(5):556-60.
[73] Roten L, Wenaweser P, Delacrétaz E, Hellige G and col. Incidence and predictors of atrioventricular conduction impairment after transcatheter aortic valve implantation. Am J Cardiol. 2010 Nov 15; 106(10):1473-80.
[74] Scafuri A, Nardi P, Forlani S, Bassano C and col. Bentall-DeBono intervention: 8 years of clinical experience. Ital Heart J Suppl. 2000 Jun; 1(6):783-9.

[75] Schurr UP, Berli J, Berdajs D, Häusler A and col. Incidence and risk factors for pacemaker implantation following aortic valve replacement. Interact Cardiovasc Thorac Surg. 2010 Nov; 11(5):556-60.

[76] Scrofani R, Carro C, Villa L, Botta M and col. Cardiac myxoma: surgical results and 15-year clinical follow-up. Ital Heart J Suppl. 2002 Jul; 3(7):753-8.

[77] Scully HE, Armstrong CS. Tricuspid valve replacement. Fifteen years of experience with mechanical prostheses and bioprostheses. J Thorac Cardiovasc Surg. 1995; 109:1035 - 41.

[78] Silvero M. Boullosa J. Implicaciones Anestesiológicas en el Síndrome de Carney.Revista Anestesia en México; Vol. 21 Nro 1 (Enero-Abril 2009) ,68-72.

[79] Sniezek-Maciejewska M, Małecka B, Bednarek J, Machejek J and col. Patients history following artificial aortic valve and pacemaker implantation. Przegl Lek. 2004; 61(6):718-21.

[80] Totaro P, Calamai G, Montesi G, Barzaghi C, Vaccari M. Continuous suture technique and impairment of the atrioventricular conduction after aortic valve replacement. J Card Surg 2000; 15:418–422.

[81] Tseng EE, Lee CA, Cameron DE, Stuart RS and col.Aortic valve replacement in the elderly. Risk factors and long-term results. Ann Surg. 1997 Jun; 225(6):793-80.

[82] Wisheart JD, Wright J E C, Rosenfeldt F. L, Ross J. K. Atrial and ventricular pacing after open heart surgery. Thorax 1973; 28:9-14.

[83] Yao YT, Li LH. Sevoflurane versus propofol for myocardial protection in patients undergoing coronary artery bypass grafting surgery: a meta-analysis of randomized controlled trial. Chin Med Sci J. 2009 Sep;24(3):133-41.

[84] Zakhia Doueihi R, Leloux MF, De Roy L, Kremer R. Permanent cardiac pacing for prolonged second and third degree atrioventricular block complicating cardiac valve replacement. Acta Cardiol. 1992; 47: 157 - 66.

[85] Zieroth S, Ross H, Rao V and col. Permanent pacing after cardiac transplantation in the era of extended donors. J Heart Lung Transplant. 2006; 25: 1142-7.

8

Early Complications after Pacemaker Implantations

Kabayadondo Maidei Gugu and de Meester Antoine
Jolimont Hospital
Belgium

1. Introduction

The clinical benefit of cardiac pacemakers has been long proven through numerous studies. Millions of pacemakers have been implanted worldwide and, as a result the quality of life for these patients has been drastically improved, not forgetting the reduced morbidity and mortality. The first stimulations through transthoracic electrodes were pioneered by Zoll in the early fifties (Zoll, 1952)), then came percutaneous endocardial pacing in 1959 (Furman & Schwedel. (1959).. A "permanent" pacemaker using epicardial electrodes was first described in 1960 (Chardack, 1960). Pacemakers and implantation techniques have progressed rapidly since the then; Generators are more reliable, more compact, filled with micro-electronic components, can be controlled automatically and remotely and thus providing more options for programmation and monitoring and a longer pacemaker life span (Kusomoto & Goldschlager, 1996; Trohman, et al, 2004). Leads are thinner and more resistant to damage and thus equally longer-lasting.
The latest European guidelines published in 2007 confirmed the classic indications; symptomatic bradyarrhythmias including sinus node dysfunction and atrioventricular or intraventricular conduction disturbances (Vardas et al., 2007). The guidelines also recommended cardiac pacing for specific conditions (vasovagal syncope, hypertrophic cardiomyopathy, heart failure with prolonged QRS duration, etc). Since over 10 years, left ventricular resynchronisation therapy has proved to be beneficial to patients presenting heart failure with complete left bundle block in association with optimal medical treatment; the European guidelines were updated for this indication in 2010 (Dickstein,2010)
The correct implantation of a pacemaker is capital for optimal function. A recent trend shows pacemaker implantation can be performed as successfully in the electrophysiology study environment as in the operating room (Garcia-Bolao & Alegria, 1999). This requires a centre with a qualified team of cardiologists as well as experienced nursing and technical staff. Continued education for the team and follow-up of complications is essential. The cardiologists' or surgeons' experience, and the volume of pacemakers implanted in the centre, plays a role in reducing post-implantation complications; thus, guidelines discourage this procedure in centres with a low volume of implantation.
Despite these precautions, some early complications, occurring within the first 6 weeks after implantation, may be observed. Their incidence is probably underestimated (approximately 7%), as is their severity (Kiviniemi et al., 1999; Klug et al., 2003). Less than 5% have to incur reintervention. Per-procedure mortality is extremely rare; only one case was observed in the cohort of 650 patients implanted at Columbia-Presbyterian Medical Centre. The dutch

database FLOOWPACE PM has indexed/listed six variables associated with at least one complication prior to hospital discharge; a low body mass index, history of heart failure (one of the principal indications for implantation), a subclavian venous access, an active fixation auricular pacing lead, and double lead implantation. These patients should be considered at risk for complications (van Eck et al., 2007).

2. Clinical cases

Early complications of pacemaker implantation are not uncommon, even in an experienced team of cardiologists or surgeons. Before discharge, careful evaluation of the pacing system is required. Diagnosis of malfunction is not always evident. Most of the patients needed an invasive procedure or medical intervention to prevent further morbidity.
Through practical clinical examples, we aim to elaborate the principal complications of electronic implanted cardiac devices, as well as discuss situations in which the presence of such a device needs to be kept in mind for the work-up of disorders that may or may not seem pacemaker-related.

2.1 Case 1 - Latrogenic pneumothorax resulting from subclavian puncture

A 61 year old man presents to his general practitioner with right thoracic pain and dyspnoea, progressively worsening since three days. He was discharged from cardiology a week before, for implantation of a double chamber pacemaker for sick sinus syndrome with symptomatic atrial fibrillation and bradycardia. Clinical examination revealed good cicatrisation of the implantation site, normal cardiac sounds with no murmur, but abolished respiratory sounds in the right lung. Twelve-lead electrocardiogram (EKG) showed a sinus rhythm with paced ventricular response (typical left bundle block pattern). Chest X-ray confirmed the presence of a complete right pneumothorax (Figure 1). The patient was therefore treated with a chest tube and his recovery was uneventful. The additional hospital stay was three days.

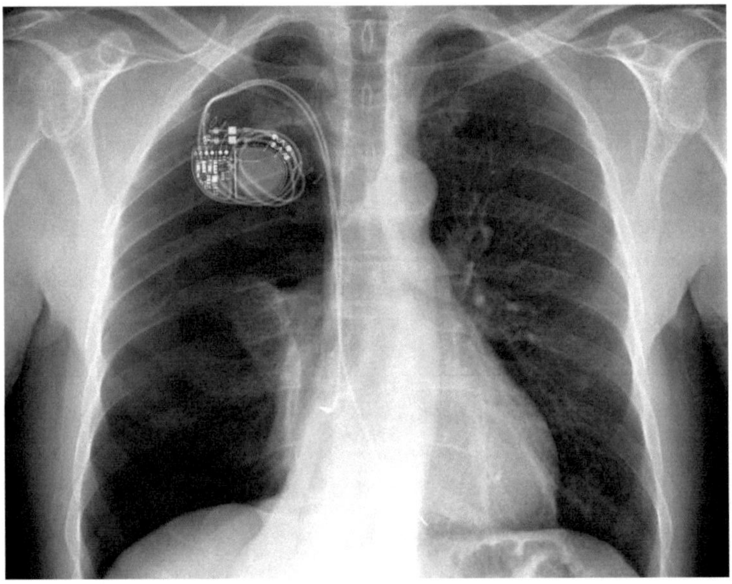

Fig. 1. Chest X-ray showing complete right pneumothorax, which was treated with a chest tube.

Comments: Iatrogenic pneumothorax after subclavian venous access is a rare complication whose incidence varies from 1-5% depending on the series, on the realisation of routine post-procedural chest X-ray and on the exact definition of this complication (consideration of both complete and partial pneumothorax, the need for chest tube insertion, hemothorax or gas embolism) (Res et al., 2004). It is usually an immediate complication and is rarely witnessed after discharge. To avoid this complication, access through a central cephalic vein is possible. However, this technique is subject to failure in approximately 20%. The operator's anatomical knowledge and experience reduce this risk. Pneumothorax is usually asymptomatic and resolves spontaneously in most cases. It is to be suspected in all patients presenting with dyspnoea, unexplainably low blood pressure and variable or elevated stimulation thresholds. Chest tube placement with aspiration is necessary if pneumothorax exceeds 10% of lung volume, if tension pneumothorax or hemothorax are diagnosed.

2.2 Case 2 - Skin necrosis, suture line failure, and lead erosion due to a large pocket hematoma

An 80 year old male needed pacing for complete atrioventricular block is re-admitted three months after implantation. Despite daily wound care by a home-based nurse, the suture line at the site of implantation would not cicatrize. Patient history included myocardial infarction for which percutaneous cardiac intervention (PCI) with a bare metal stent was performed, as well as receiving classical medical treatment that included clopidogrel and aspirin on a daily basis. After implantation, a large hematoma formed in the generator pocket. A conservative treatment was initially proposed. On re-admission, the hematoma had almost completely disappeared, but severe skin necrosis was impeding site closure to the extent that the leads were visible with the naked eye. The absence of infection, as proved by numerous negative swab cultures, allowed for the pacemaker generator to be re-implanted under the pectoralis muscle.

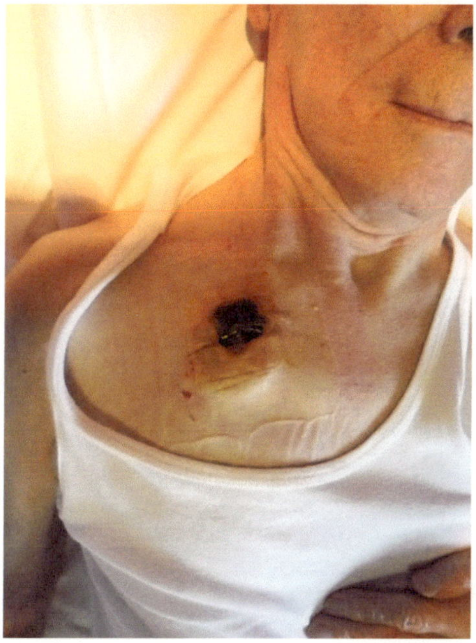

Fig. 2. Hematoma. Lack of suture line healing, pacemaker leads visible.

Comments: Pocket hematoma is the most frequent complication (5% of cases) and can lead to prolonged hospital stay and in the latter case, re-implantation (1-2%) (Kiviniemi et al., 1999 ; Wiegand et al., 2004). Risk factors include use of high doses of low molecular weight heparin, of the association aspirin-clopidogrel, and inexperienced operator. Aspirin alone or an oral anticoagulant like warfarin, to take international normalized ratio (INR) of < 2.0, does not increase the risk of hematoma. Electrocautery or a second look to the pocket is useful to minimize bleeding and the risk of large hematoma. Selective use of topical thrombin is reserved for high risk patients; in Reynolds's series, the incidence of significant hematoma dropped from 20.8% to 8%. Sometimes drain placement may be necessary and sufficient. Evacuation of hematoma is realised in less than 0.5% with a major risk of infection; potential reasons include persistent bleeding, pain refractory to analgesics, failed healing and skin necrosis.

2.3 Case 3 - Recurrent syncope due to lead displacement

A 60 year old female patient with no medical history and under no current treatment was admitted for complete atrioventricular block causing shortness of breath and dizziness. Implantation of a double chamber pacemaker was performed with ease. P/R sensings were measured at 3.1 mV and 7.8 mV respectively, and both thresholds for stimulation are 0.5 volt/0.4 msec. The next day, the patient represented with dizziness and faints. Lead displacement was suspected. EKG no longer showed physiological stimulation and chest X-ray confirmed lead displacement (Figure 3). Lead repositioning and active fixation was performed successfully.

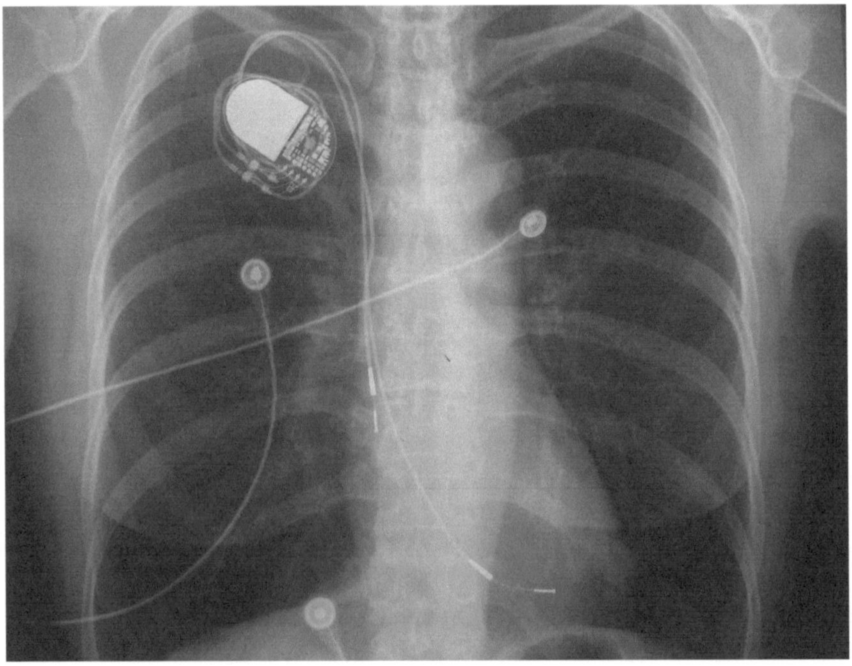

Fig. 3. Chest X-ray showing migration of both atrial and ventricular leads.

- Failure to OUTPUT: no pacemaker activity. NO SPIKE
  - battery failure or EOL (end of life), battery trauma
  - lead problems : lead fracture, lead dislodgement, fractured lead insulation, poor lead connection
  - oversensing causes (myopotentials, electromagnetic interference, cross-talk phenomenon)
  - "cross-talk" phenomenon
  - extreme electromagnetic interference
  - pseudo-malfonction : hystérésis, normal algorithmes (AV conduction)

- Failure to CAPTURE: no depolarisation of the cavity. SPIKE without P/QRS complexes
  - normal situation : Functional non-capture—output delivered during refractory period
  - inappropriate programming of the pacemaker (too low safe margin)
  - lead problems : lead fracture, lead dislodgement, fractured lead insulation, poor lead connection
  - myocardial perforation
  - elevated pacing threshold :
    - myocardial infarction (necrosis) at the lead tip
    - drugs (eg, flecainide)
    - dyskaliemia
    - metabolic abnormalities (eg, acidosis, alkalosis)

- Oversensing (Oversensing occurs when a pacemaker incorrectly senses cardiac/noncardiac electrical activity and is inhibited from pacing):
  - Myopotentials or muscular activity (particularly the diaphragm or pectoralis muscles)
  - cross-talk phenomenon
  - electromagnetic interference (eg, Magnetic Resonance Imaging (MRI)
  - lead fracture and fractured lead insulation

- Undersensing (Undersensing occurs when a pacemaker incorrectly misses intrinsic depolarization and paces despite intrinsic activity)
  - Normal device function—misinterpretation : triggered mode, fusion and pseudo-fusion beats, functional undersensing (long refractory periods, blanking period, safety pacing, oversensing)
  - poor lead positioning (poor intrinsic signal amplitude), lead dislodgment, lead fibrosis or thrombosis
  - magnet application
  - battery depletion
  - drugs (eg, flecainide, amiodarone)
  - metabolic abnormalities (eg, acidosis, alkalosis)
  - dyskaliemia (eg, hyperkaliemia)
  - hypothyroidism
  - ischemia and myocardial infarction
  - or electrical shock (transient)

Table I. Pacemaker Troubleshooting and early complications of pacemaker insertions

Comments: Lead displacement can be found in 2-10% of cases depending on the series (Kiviniemi et al., 1999 ; van Eck et al., 2007). Atrial leads migrate more often than ventricular leads. Active fixation reduces the risk, especially in patients having undergone cardiac surgery. Manifestations include undersensing, failure to capture and increase in pacing thresholds. Repositioning of leads is primordial. Causes of undersensing include lead displacement, fibrosis at the site of fixation of the lead, myocardial ischemia and necrosis, some antiarrhythmic agents (flecainide), dyskaliemia, or transient undersensing following an electric shock (Table I) (de Meester, 2008). When lead displacement is induced by the patient, following a repetitive rotational movement (twisting of the box) and leading to winding of the leads around the generator, we talk of Twiddler's syndrome; this is observed in certain psychiatric cases, or when the pocket is too big for the pacemaker generator.

2.4 Case 4 - Minor right ventricular perforation

A 77 year-old patient had a physiological pacemaker implanted for symptomatic sinus bradycardia, with sinus arrest. A few days after the intervention, she presented with continuous chest pain. Upon clinical examination, blood pressure was 130/80 mmHg, heart sounds were regular but a pericardial friction rub was audible. EKG showed a sinus rhythm with ventricular capture. Chest X-ray revealed a ventricular lead projecting further than the apex (Figure 4). Cardiac ultrasounds confirmed myocardial perforation by the lead and a minimal pericardial effusion. We decided to abstain from removing the lead, which would have been to some extent invasive in this elderly patient. Treatment by anti-inflammatory drug was installed and was sufficient for pain relief.

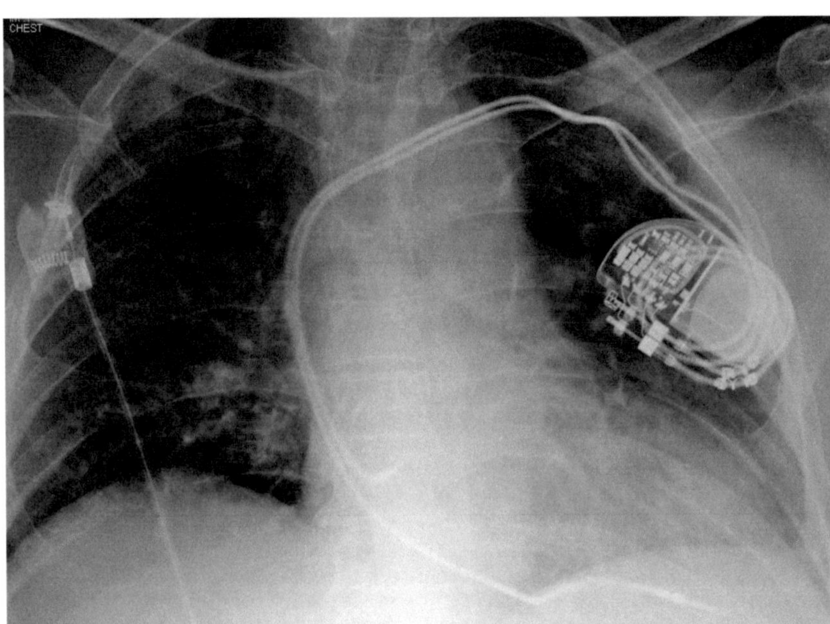

Fig. 4. Chest X-ray showing atrial and ventricular leads, with the ventricular lead clearly beyond the cardiac shadow

Comments: Cardiac perforation is a serious complication, with risk of tamponnade and death. It occurs in less than 2% of cases (Ellenbogen et al., 2002). Clinical symptoms are variable, including chest pain, shortness of breath and more rarely hypotension and shock. Advanced age, use of active fixation leads and operator inexperience are contributing factors (Mahapatra et al., 2005). Furthermore, atrial leads seem to perforate more frequently (Hirschl et al., 2007). The new Magnetic Resonance Imaging (MRI)-compatible leads are more rigid, but increased frequency of perforation does not seem to be induced by the use of these leads. Treatment is not standardised, but removal (and replacement) of these leads is crucial in the case of tamponnade and shock. Pericarditis without perforation has been observed in 5% of cases and must lead to close follow-up. Figure 5 illustrates a case of tamponnade. The patient remained stable after drainage.

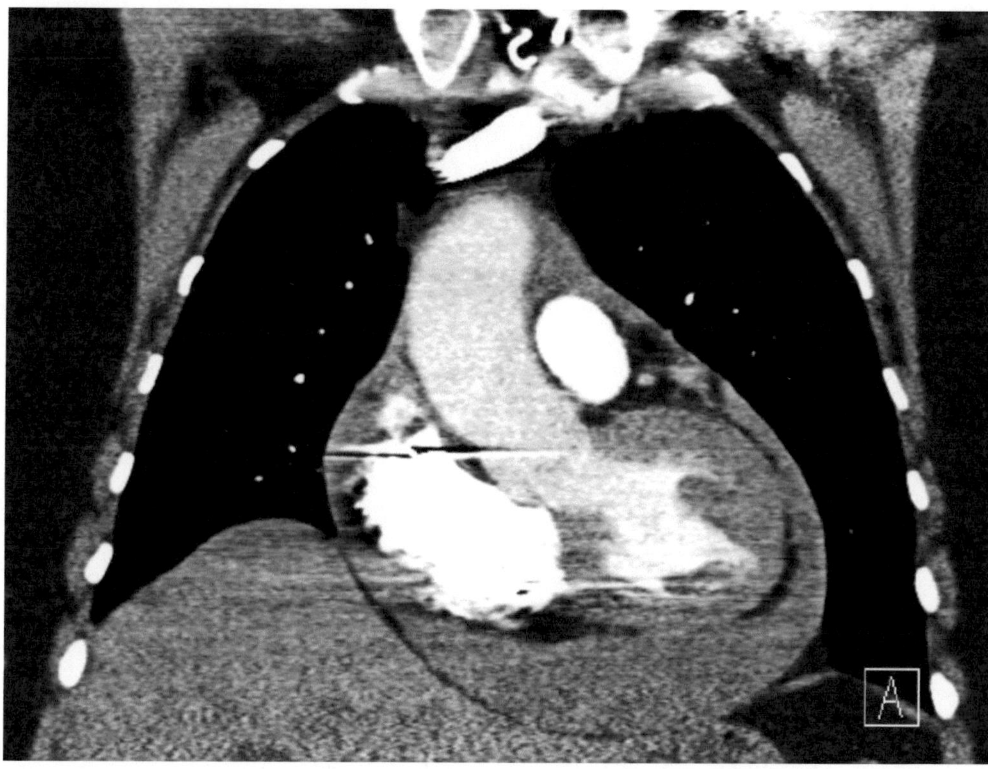

Fig. 5. Chest scan showing significant pericardial effusion, responsible for pre-tamponnade and shock.

2.5 Case 5 - Skin erosion and exterisation of the generator

An 85 year old female patient is admitted for malaise and confusion. Medical history is positive for asthma treated regularly by corticoids and B2 mimetic aerosols. EKG shows a complete atrioventricular block and, after excluding all reversible causes, a physiological pacemaker is implanted. No complications are noted during her hospital stay. Having regained her autonomy and the confusional episode resolved, the patient returns to her old age home with instructions for routine care for the following weeks. A follow-up is programmed at six weeks and the cardiologist is confronted with a case of skin erosion and exteriorisation of the pacemaker generator (Figure 6). Due to the high risk of infection in this case, the device is removed and a new device is implanted on the contra-lateral side after six weeks of antibiotherapy and with negative hemocultures.

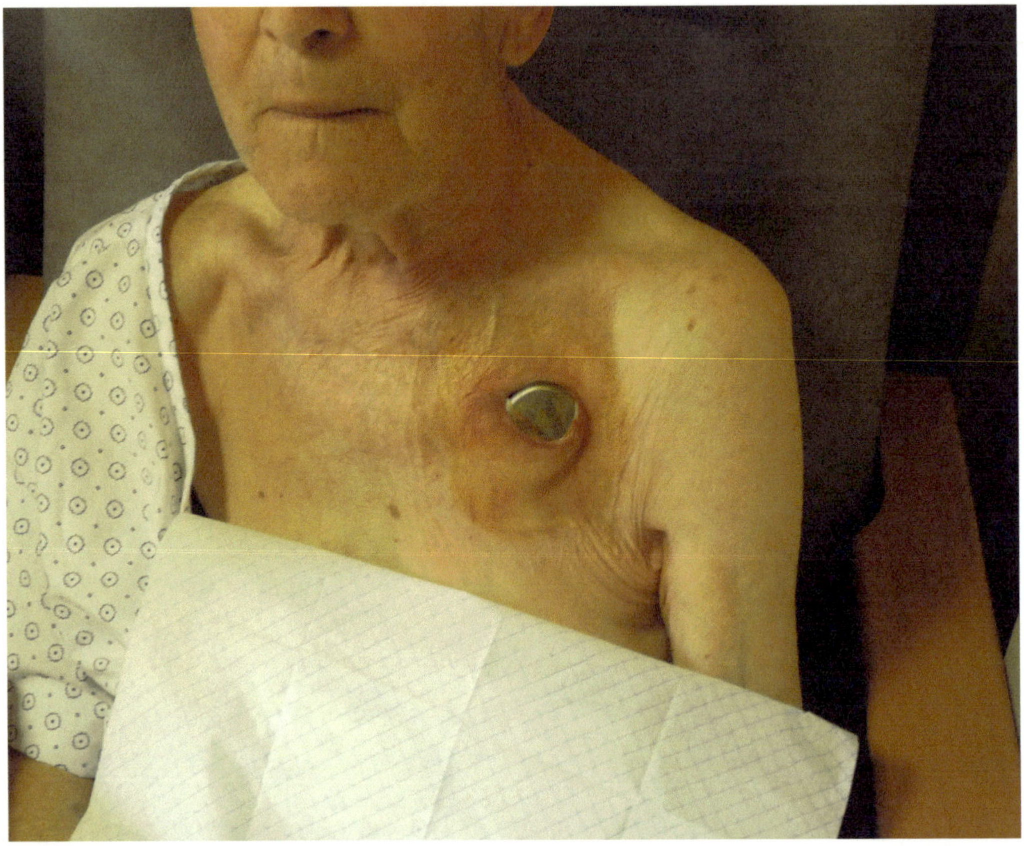

Fig. 6. Erosion and exteriorisation of pacemaker generator in our elderly patient.

Comments: Skin erosion is caused by the pacemaker generator, and is usually a result of pocket infection. Other precipitating factors can be present, for example, the extremely fragile skin of elderly patients, a pocket that is too small, precarious subcutaneous fat, chronic use of corticoids, and use of abrasive disinfectants (Kiviniemi et al., 1999). Exteriorisation of a generator, and/or a lead, is always associated with bacterial contamination, making removal of the material an obligation, accompanied by antibiotherapy and eventually re-implantation on the contra-lateral side. Skin erosion is hence to be sort for and detected before exteriorisation. This is rarely an early complication, and incidence is estimated to be 1%.

2.6 Case 6 - Ventricular lead malposition and right bundle branch block morphology on EKG

A 55 year old patient with history of hypertension, obesity, diabetes, anterior myocardial infarction and severe left ventricular dysfunction has a defibrillator implanted in primary prevention of sudden death. The follow-up is satisfactory with acceptable sensing, impedance and threshold stimulation values on the device programmer. EKG shoes a sinus rhythm with evident old anterior infarction. Chest X-ray, performed in a recumbent position and under non-optimal condition seems satisfactory and the patient is discharged. Upon follow-up one month later, the parameters of the defibrillator are still satisfactory, but the ventricular stimulation shows atypical right bundle block. Chest X-ray confirms the suspected left ventricular stimulation, via a permeable foramen ovale (Figure 7). Lead replacement is indicated seeing the high risk of thrombo-embolic complications in this young patient.

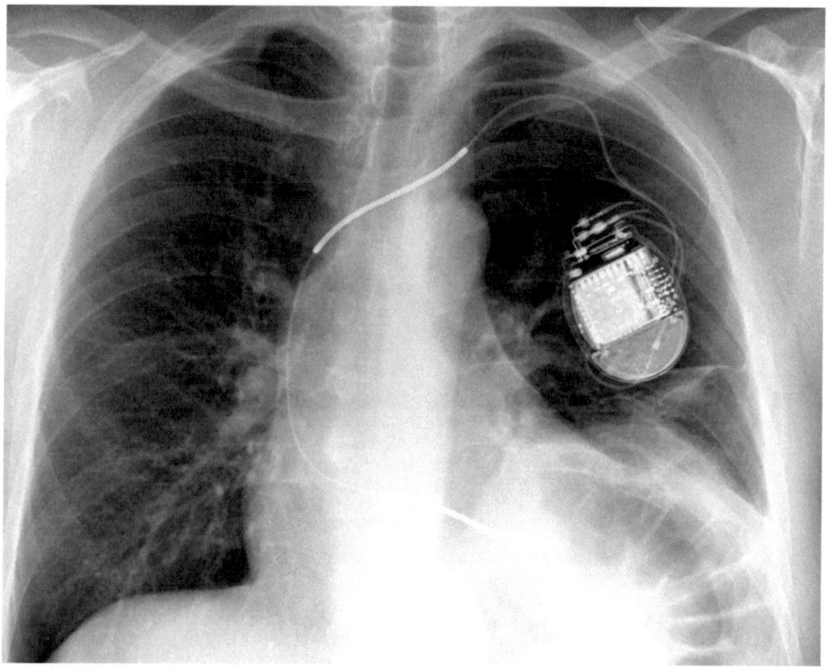

Fig. 7. Chest X-ray showing a ventricular lead that is located higher than usual; this lead is in the left ventricle, having gone through a patent foramen ovale.

Comments: an erroneous lead placement is extremely rare. It remains possible in patients with a patent foramen ovale or an atrial septal defect. Less than twenty cases are reported in the literature (Allie et al, 2000; Blommaert et al., 2000 ; Van Gelder al, 2000; Le Dolley et al, 2009). An EKG during stimulation and chest X-ray in an upright position (antero-posterior and lateral takes) are recommended. The risk of thrombo-embolism, including stroke, of mitral insufficiency should be evaluated. Repositioning of the lead or long term anticoagulation should be considered. When right bundle branch block pacing morphology appears in a patient with a permanent or temporary transvenous right ventricular pacemaker, myocardial perforation or malposition of the pacing lead must be ruled out, even though the patient may be asymptomatic. The overall causes of right bundle branch block morphology include:

- erroneous left ventricular lead placement in patient with an atrial septal defect
- biventricular stimulation or cardiac resynchronisation therapy (CRT) (Figure 8)
- epicardial lead placement.
- some cases of "normal" right ventricular apical stimulation

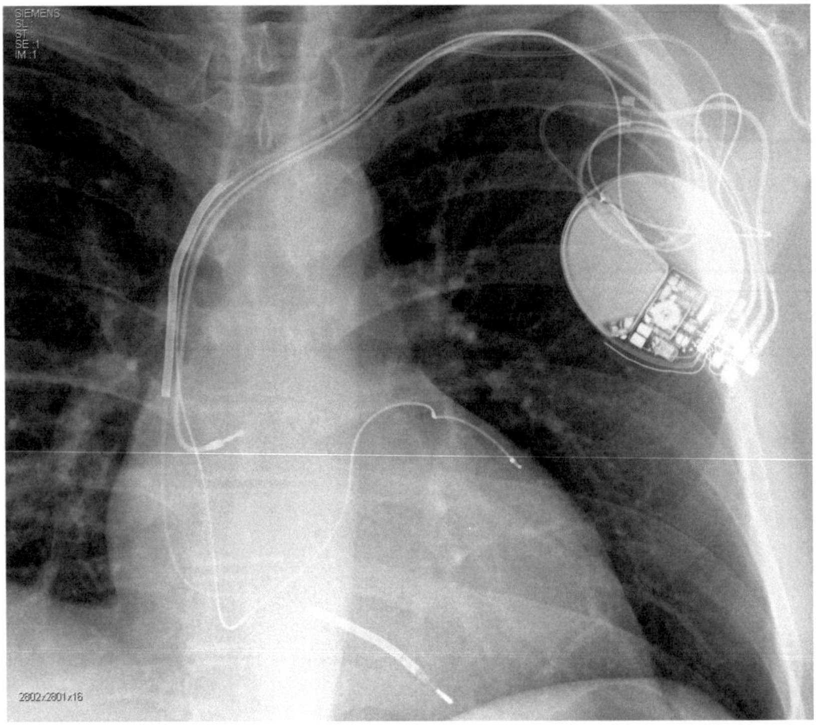

Fig. 8. Chest X-ray showing implantation of 3 leads including a left ventricular lead placed in a branch of the coronary sinus (cardiac resynchronisation therapy).

2.7 Case 7 - Twiddler syndrome in a psychiatric patient

A 68 year old patient, with a history of chronic obstructive pulmonary disease and psychosis, underwent pacemaker implantation for repeated loss of consciousness due to sinus hypersensitivity. Carotid sinus massage resulted in 10 second pauses. The pacemaker was set in double chamber mode and after satisfactory programmation control (P-R sensing 2.5 mV and 12.5 mV, impedance at 564 ohms and 496 ohms respectively, stimulation thresholds at 0.5 volts/0.4 msec), the patient was discharged to his psychiatric institution. At one month follow-up, the patient has no complaints, though anamnesis is laborious. Check-up of the stimulator shows absence of detection of both P and R waves, and absence of atrioventricular capture despite maximal stimulation. Displaced leads are suspected and confirmed by chest x-ray (Figure 9). The patient later admits to having manipulated the pace generator by repeatedly twisting it around. Correct repositioning and fixation of the leads were conducted.

Comments: Twiddler's syndrome is describes as the migration of cardiac stimulator leads due to repetitive rotatory movements of the generator in its pocket, secondary to manipulation by the patient himself, which may be intentional or non-intentional (for example, sportsmen). In certain cases, the stimulation of displaced leads can cause pectoral muscle contraction, or life-threatening symptoms in the case of pacemaker dependency (Nicholson et al, 2003; Castillo & Cavusoglu, 2006; Essoh et al., 2010) (Figure 10).

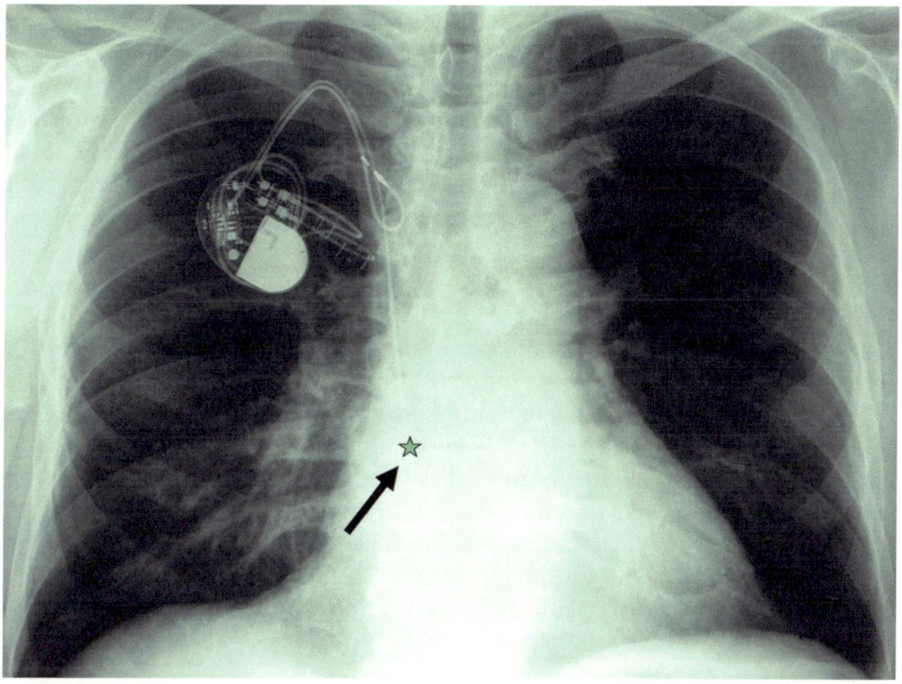

Fig. 9. Chest X-ray showing displaced lead (ventricular lead tip indicated by the star).

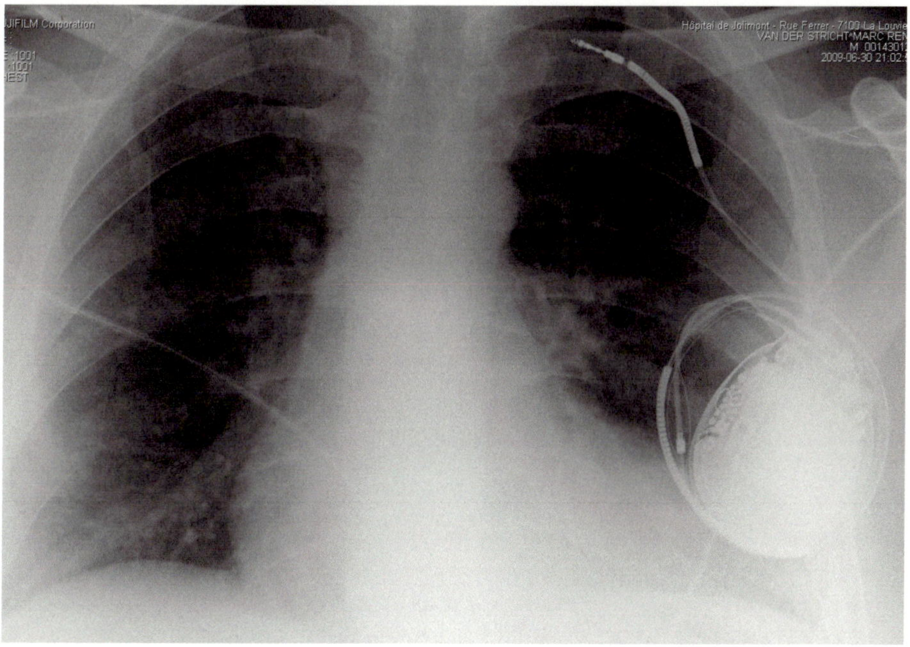

Fig. 10. Chest X-ray showing dual-coil ventricular lead displacement, causing pectoral permanent stimulation, in a case previously reported by our team (Essoh et al, 2010). Repositioning the lead was required and successfully reported.

Risk factors include obesity (adipose tissue being less firm in these patients), female sex, elderly patients, patients known as having stigmata for character disorders (obsessive compulsive tendencies, dementia). Treatment consists of repositioning the leads, and changing them in the event of fracture. Several surgical techniques have been proposed to avoid recurrence; implanting the pacemaker generator under the aponevrosis, active lead fixation (almost always the case with implantable cardioverter-defibrillators), Parsonet's dacron pouches. Patient education, and psychiatric treatment if indicated, should be proposed.

2.8 Case 8 - Early venous thrombosis after defibrillator with resynchronisation (CRT-D) placement

A 73 year old male has a defibrillator with resynchronisation implanted for ischemic cardiomyopathy after an anterior infarction left him with a left ventricular ejection fraction of 25%. He had presented an episode of ventricular tachycardia with syncope. Implantation of the device was by the subclavian route. There were no immediate post-operative complications and good parameters were recorded for all three leads. Three weeks later, the patient complains of discomfort in the left arm, followed by oedema of the whole arm, forearm and hand (Figure 11); ultrasound and vascular tomodensitometry confirmed complete thrombosis of the left subclavian vein, of the axillary vein, leading up until the convergence of the jugular vein. Anticoagulation therapy was commenced and evolution was slow but favourable in the following weeks.

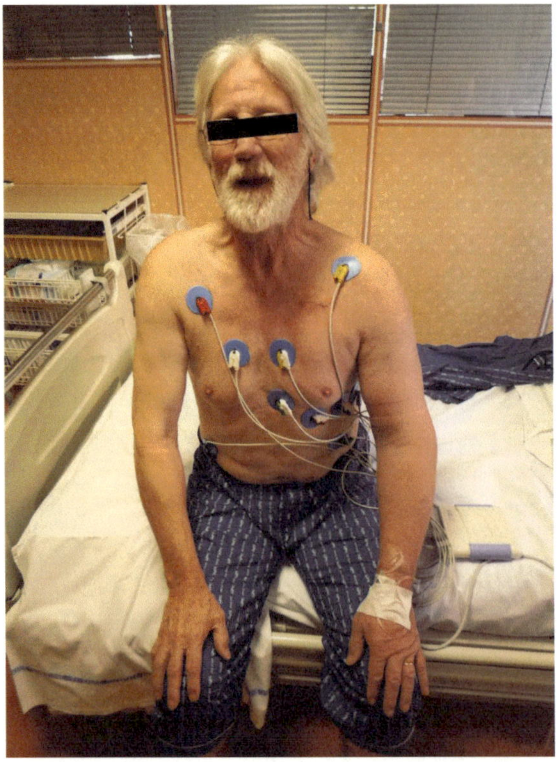

Fig. 11. Oedema of the left arm, forearm and hand caused by massive thrombosis of the subclavian vein after defibrillator with Cardiac Resynchronisation Therapy (CRT-D).

Comments: Subclavian vein thrombosis is not uncommon. It can occur in about 30% of cases, but usually remains asymptomatic due to the rapid development of collateral circulation (Oginosawa et al., 2002). Less than 5% of patients are symptomatic, presenting mainly with pain or oedema of the arm closest to the implantation site. Risk is higher in cases where three leads are implanted (Cardiac Resynchronisation Therapy (CRT), when the patient is under hormonal therapy, when personal history of thrombo-embolic event is present, with temporary ipsilatérale transvenous lead, during upgrade of a simple pacemaker to a pacemaker with resynchronisation, dual coil leads, and when the ejection fraction is less than or equal to 40% (Da Costa et al., 2003 ; Rozmus et al., 2005). The risk of thrombosis does not differ for pacemakers and implantable cardioverter-defibrillators. Preventive measures may be necessary (platelet aggregation inhibiting drugs or anticoagulation therapy).

2.9 Case 9 - Unusual tachycardia after implantation of a double-chamber pacemaker

A 75 year old male is admitted for repeated fainting caused by major sinus dysfunction as shown by a 24 hour Holter monitor which revealed pauses of up to 8 seconds and paroxystic atrial fibrillation. Medical history was negative and patient was on no current treatment. EKG at rest showed a sinus rhythm with a frequency of 68 bpm and normal repolarisation. A physiological pacemaker is implanted in the operating room. After the intervention, the patient feels palpitations and an EKG recording shows probable pacemaker-mediated tachycardia (Figure 12). Programmation control shows a P-R sensing of 15.8 mV and 1.2 mV respectively, and threshold values for stimulation both inferior to 0.5 volts for 0.4 msec; a connection error is confirmed during threshold verification. Programming in AAI mode would result in VVI pacing, and programming in VVI mode would result in AAI pacing. Re-intervention allowed the correction of this connection error.

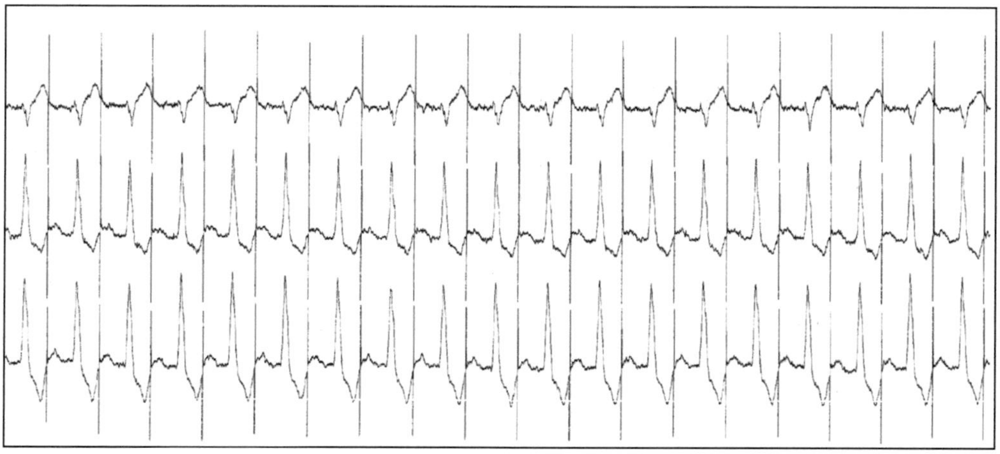

Fig. 12. Tachycardia due to an error in the connection of the atrial and ventricular leads. We note the same QRS configuration as with VVI pacing from the apex.

Comments: Atrial and ventricular lead connection errors are rare at implantation, but have already been documented (Barold et al, 2010). Programmation verification allows rapid detection of the switch ("green wire on the green button and red wire on the red button"). A control of the programmation of a stimulator is mandatory before patient discharge. It allows detection and correction of such an error, as well as early detection of a lead displacement. Different types of tachycardia are to be excluded:

- Classical "endless loop" or pacemaker mediated tachycardia is rare with the double chamber generators of today.
    - it is usually initiated by an extra-systole with a retrograde p wave which is easily detected and sustains the circuit. Pacemaker mediated tachycardia can also be provoked by ventricular extra-systoles, by atrial over-detection (myopotentials, interferences) or underdetection and failure to capture
    - long post-ventricular atrial refractory period (PVARP), excluding retrograde P wave and retrograde conduction, may prevent pacemaker mediated tachycardia
- Runaway Pacemaker is due to a malfunction of the pacemaker generator resulting in life-threatening rapid tachycardia (up to 200 bpm).
    - the generator may malfunction for various causes, including battery failure or external damage.
    - the use of a magnet can reduce the rate of the rhythm induced by the defiant pacemaker. Generator replacement is necessary.
- Atrioventricular nodal reentrant tachycardia. In this case, the stimulator does not intervene in the circuit.
    - figure 13 shows the initiation of the common type (slow-fast) of atrioventricular nodal reentrant tachycardia ; this is a typical example where the arrhythmia is triggered by an atrial extrasystole which blocks the rapid pathway of the atrioventricular node and allows flow through the slow pathway and thus initiation of the supraventricular tachycardia circuit
    - radiofrequency ablation is the treatment of choice.
- Other reentrant tachycardia includes
    - atrial flutter
    - orthodromic circus movement tachycardia using an accessory pathway in the retrograde direction and the AV node in the anterograde direction (concealed or not, in the Wolff-Parkinson-White syndrome)
    - atrial tachycardia (paroxysmal and nonparoxysmal)

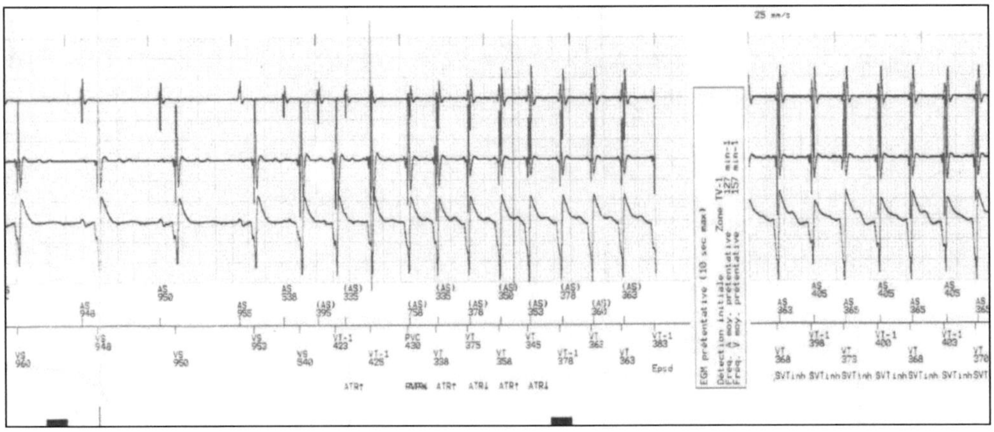

Fig. 13. Baseline rhythm strip showing atrial, ventricular and shock intracardiac electrogram leads, and marker atrial and ventricular channels. This is an example of initiation of common atrioventricular node reentrant tachycardia; see text.

2.10 Case 10 - Recurrent malaise after pacemaker implantation

A man aged 65 with history positive for high blood pressure, diabetes and renal failure actually undergoing haemodialysis receives a pacemaker for complete atrioventricular block with syncope. His treatment includes ramipril, aspirin and insulin. No immediate post-operative complications occur. Just before a haemodialysis session a few days later, the patient complains of feeling faint. An EKG shows evident signs of hyperkaliemia (very wide QRS complexes with tall peaked T waves and obliteration of the ST segment, as well as a long PR interval) and of double chamber stimulation without atrial or ventricular captures (Figure 14). Blood work-up confirms severe hyperkaliemia (potassium 7.8 mEq/L). The atrioventricular underdetection and the absence of capture are caused by the high level of potassium and corrected as soon as kaliemia is normalised by haemodialysis.

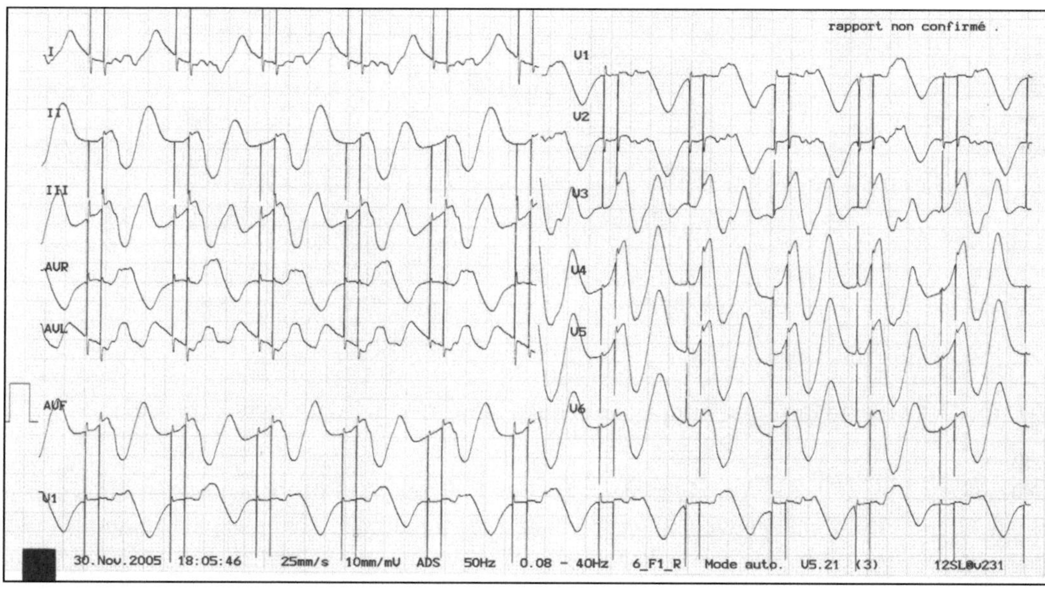

Fig. 14. Twelve-lead EKG showing signs of hyperkaliemia and defiant AV detection and stimulation.

Comments: Causes of atrioventricular underdetection and failure to capture are shown in table I. Hypokaliemia is another cause of life-threatening undersensing (de Meester et al, 1996). Correction of the cause is essential for adequate pacemaker function. The risk of triggering ventricular fibrillation, due to a ventricular stimulation during the vulnerable T wave period (R-on-T phenomenon), is present, as is present in asynchronous VOO stimulation or the use of a magnet (Oupadia et al., 1998).

2.11 Case 11 - Important dyspnoea and malaise at follow-up

A 68 year old patient was admitted for class III dyspnoea according to the New York Heart Association (NYHA) score and repeated episodes of malaise since implantation of a single chamber pacemaker in another centre. Her personal history is positive for hypertension and sick sinus syndrome with atrial fibrillation associated with a slow ventricular rhythm and pauses of more than 8 seconds, hence the indication for cardiac pacing. Her treatment is comprised of ramipril, amlodipin and an oral anticoagulant, (acenocoumarol). Clinical examination is unremarkable. Blood pressure was 130/80 mmHg. Twelve-lead EKG shows regular ventricular stimulation at 70 beats per minute, and a basal sinus rhythm. Dissociated P waves are seen (Figure 15). Pacemaker syndrome is suspected, and confirmed. The pacemaker was reprogrammed to VVI 30 bpm to avoid deleterious ventricular stimulation in this patient.

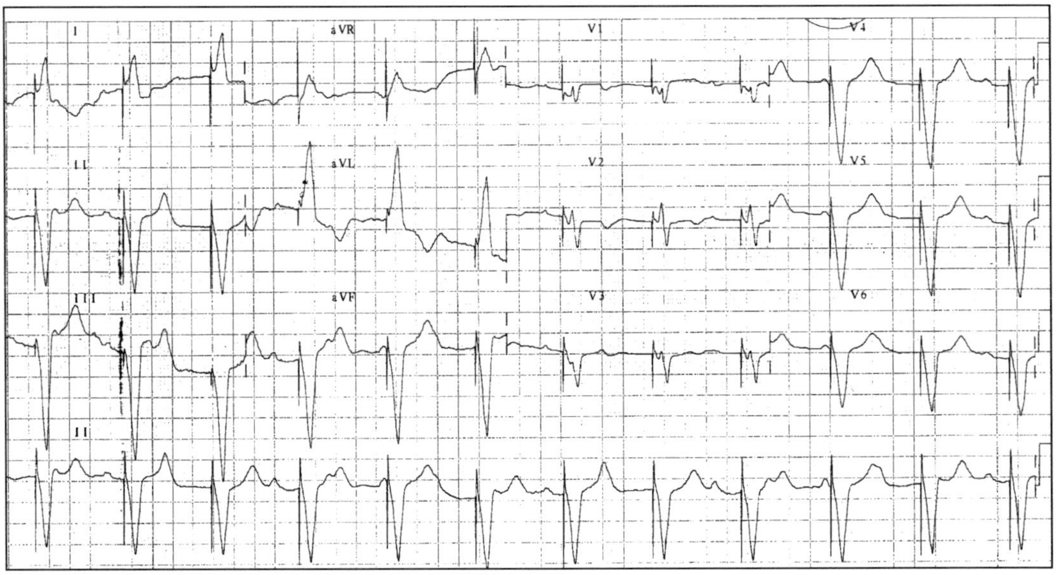

Fig. 15. Twelve-lead EKG showing a dissociated sinus rhythm with right ventricular stimulation.

Comments: This is not a veritable implantation complication but the erroneous choice of a single chamber pacemaker whereas a physiological (or double chamber) stimulator would have avoided the problem. Pacemaker syndrome is described as a combination of symptoms evoking cardiac failure and hypotension in a patient with a cardiac stimulator (Chalvidan et al., 2000). It is caused by the loss of atrioventricular synchronism leading to a drop in cardiac output, elevated atrial pressure and hypotension. The Mode Selection Trial (MOST) investigators defined pacemaker syndrome as occurring if either one of two different criteria occurred (Link et al., 2004). The first criterion was new or worsened dyspnea, orthopnea, elevated jugular venous pressure, rales, and oedema with ventricular (VA) conduction during ventricular pacing. The second criterion was symptoms of dizziness, weakness, presyncope, or syncope, and a >20 mmHg reduction of systolic blood pressure when the patient had VVIR pacing compared with atrial pacing or sinus rhythm. Its incidence is 7-20% of stimulators in VVI mode with a sinus rhythm. Pacemaker syndrome can also be seen in AAIR mode and in double chamber modes (VDD, DDI, DDD) if the stimulator if programmation is sub-optimal or the stimulation mode is incorrectly selected. Dyspnoea should, besides pacemaker syndrome, evoke:

- chronotrope insufficiency, especially during exertion, requiring programmation in rate-responsive mode.
- Wenckeback functioning in DDD mode
- intermittent dysfunction (sensing and pacing)

2.12 Case 12 - Acute infection of the pocket and the cardiac device

A 45 year old female patient suffering from idiopathic congestive cardiomyopathy with a left ventricular ejection fraction of 35%, class III dyspnoea on the New York Heart Association (NYHA) scale, left bundle branch block morphology, with a QRS duration of 175 msec, on EKG and under optimal medical treatment for over three months receives a pacemaker with left ventricular resynchronisation. Implantation was complicated immediately by left ventricular lead displacement. A Starfix Attain OTW 4194 (Medtronic Inc., Minneapolis, MN, USA) was necessary for stability (The Attain Starfix's design includes three soft, polyurethane lobes near the lead tip that, when expanded, enable stable lead placement in the target location) (de Meester, 2010). After one month, the implantation site becomes suppurative (Figure 16). Local wound care and 10 day antibiotherapy did not help. Bacteriological studies revealed the presence of pseudomonas aeruginosa. Treatment required complete ablation of the material and prolonged antibiotherapy. Re-implantation on the counter-lateral side in this case was performed two months after the end of the antibiotic course.

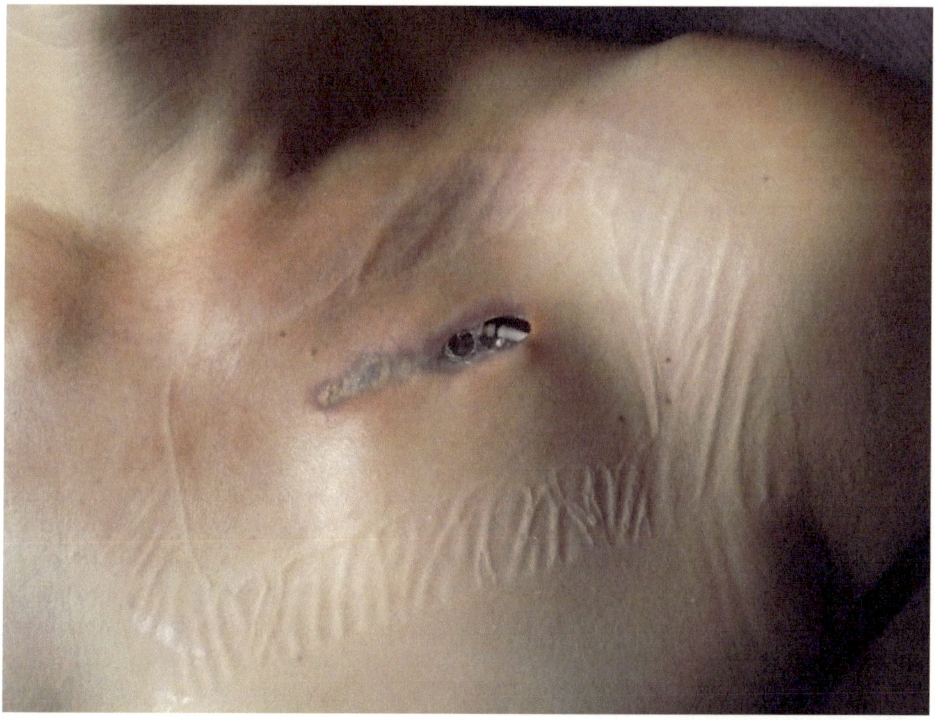

Fig. 16. Photograph showing suppurative wound with visible pacemaker leads. Ablation of all material was necessary.

Comments: Suture or pocket infection is not a rarity during the first month and incidence is estimated to be 1% (del Rio et al., 2003 ; Klug et al., 2007). Principal risk factors are re-intervention, diabetes, old age, corticoids, operator inexperience, and renal failure. Antibiotic prophylaxis prior to pacemaker implantation has a protective effect. In the case of very early infection, a per-operatory contamination by cutaneous flora (staphylococcus aureus) is the principal source of infection (Kearney et al., 1994 ; Da Costa et al., 1998).

Successful treatment of an infected device requires removal of the entire system and administration of antimicrobials. Infection after one month usually originates from the lead (and not the pocket). Sepsis is uncommon and diagnosis includes positive blood cultures (80% of cases) and transesophageal echography showing lead anomalies. Skin erosion at pocket site and other local signs of infection are common. Staphylococcus epidermidis or other gram negative bacteria are most commonly found.

3. Conclusions

Early complications after pacemaker and other cardiac device implantation are not uncommon. Hematoma, skin erosion and pocket infection, as well as lead displacement are the most common of these complications and should be looked for and recognised during routine follow-up, as well as during work-up of any patient presenting a new symptom in the first couple of weeks after implantation. Operator inexperience and implantation in a low-volume centre increases the risk of these complications. Adhesion to good practice and recommended guidelines is indispensable.

4. References

Allie, DE; Lirtzman, MD; Wyatt, CH; Vitrella, DA; Walker, CM. (2000); Septic paradoxal embolus through a patent ovale after pacemaker implantation. *Ann Thorac Surg,* 69: 946-8.

Barold, SS; Stroobandt, RX; Sinnaeve, AF. (2010). Cardiac Pacemakers and Resynchronization Step by Step: An Illustrated Guide, *Wiley-Blackwell editors.*

Blommaert D, Mucumbitsi J, De Roy L. Images in cardiology. Ventricular pacing and right bundle branch block morphology: diagnosis and management. Heart. 2000; 83: 666.

Castillo, R & Cavusoglu, E. (2006). Twiddler's syndrome: an interesting cause of pacemaker failure. *Cardiology,* 105: 119-21.

Chalvidan, T ; Deharo, JC ; Djiane P. (2000). Les syndromes du pacemaker. *Ann Cardiol Angeol,* 49 : 224-9

Chardack, WM; Gage, AA; Greatbatch, W. (1960) A transistorized self-contained, implantable pacemaker for the long-term correction of heart block. *Surgery,* 48: 643.

Da Costa, A; Lelièvre, H; Kirkorian, G et al. (1998). Role of the preaxillary flora in pacemaker infections: a prospective study. *Circulation,* 97: 1791-8.

Da Costa, SS; Scalabrini Neto, A; Costa, R; Caldas, JG; Martinelli Fihlo, M. (2002); Incidence and risk factors of upper extermity deep vein lseions after permanent transvenous pacemaker implant: a 6-month follow-up prospective study. *Pacing Clin Electrophysiol,* 25: 1301-6.

del Rio, A; Anguera, I; Miro, JM; Mont L, Fowler VG, Azqueta M, et al. (2003). Surgical treatment of pacemaker and defibrillator leads endocarditis. *Chest,* 121: 1451-9.

de Meester, A ; Jacques, JM ; Jopart, P ; Chaudron, JM. (1996). Syncope chez une patiente porteuse d'un stimulateur cardiaque. *Louvain Med,* 115: 465-71.

de Meester, A. (2008). Manuel pratique de cardiologie aiguë. 3ème édition. Antoine de Meester éditeur. European Graphics, Strépy-Bracquegnies.

de Meester, A; van Ruyssevelt, P; Blaimont, M; Prioux, D; Marcovitch; O. (2010). Déplacement de la sonde ventriculaire gauche: existe-t-il une possibilité de remédier à ce problème? *J Cardiol,* 22 : 295-9

Dickstein, K; Vardas, PE; Auricchio, A et al for the Task Force Members (2010). 2010 focused update of ESC guidelines on device therapy in heart failure. *Eur Heart J*, 31: 2677-87.

Ellenbogen, K.A.; Wood, M.A. & Shepard, R.K. (2002). Delayed complications following pacemaker implantation. *Pacing Clin Electrophysiol*, 25, 1155-8

Essoh, E ; Badot, D ; Marcovitch, O ; de Meester, A. (2010). Docteur, j'ai le hoquet à l'épaule! Une cause rare de dysfonctionnement d'un défibrillateur implantable. *Louvain Med*, 129 : 237-40.

Furman, S; Schwedel, JB. (1959). An intracardiac pacemaker for Stokes-Adams seizures. *N Engl J Med*,261: 948.

Garcia-Bolao, I; Alegria, E. (1999). Implantation of 500 consecutive cardiac pacemakers in the electrophysiology laboratory. *Acta Cardiol*, 54: 339

Hirschl, DA; Jain, VR; Spindola-Franco, H; Gross, JN; Haramati, LB. (2007). Prevalence and characterisation of asymptomatic pacemaker and ICD lead perforation on CT. *Pacing Clin Electrophysiol*, 30: 28-32.

Kearney, R; Eisen, HJ; Wolf, JE. (1994). Nonvalvular infection of the cardiovascular system. *Ann Intern Med*, 121: 219-30

Kiviniemi, MS; Pirnes, MA;, Eranen, HJ et al. (1999). Complications related to permanent pacemaker therapy. *Pacing Clin Electrophysiol*, 22: 711

Klug, D ; Marquie, C ; Lacroix, D ; Kacet, S. (2003). Complications de la stimulation cardiaque definitive. *Arch Mal Cœur*, 96 : 546-53.

Klug, D; Balde, M; Pavin, D, et al. (2007). Risk factors related to infections of implanted pacemakers and cardioverter-defibrillators: results of a large prospective study. *Circulation*, 116: 1349-56.

Kusomoto, FM; Goldschlager, N. (1996) Cardiac pacing. *N Engl J Med*, 334: 89-97

Le Dolley, Y; Thuny, F; Bastard, E; Riberi, A; Tafanelli, L; Renard S, et al. (2009). Pacemaker Lead Vegetation Trapped in Patent Foramen Ovale. *Circulation*, 119: e223-4

Link, MS; Hellkamp, AS; Estes, NAM, et al. (2004). High incidence of pacemaker syndrome in patients with sinus node dysfunction treated with ventricular-based pacing in the Mode Selection Trial (MOST). *J Am Coll Cardiol*, 43: 2066–71

Mahapatra, S.; Bybee, K.A.; Bunch, T.J.; Espinosa, R.E.; Sinak, L.J.; McGoon, M.D. & Hayes, D.L. (2005). Incidence and predictors of cardiac perforation after permanent pacemaker placement. *Heart Rhythm*, 2, 907-11

Nicholson, WJ ; Tuohy, KA ; Tilkemeier, P. (2003). Twiddler's syndrome. *N Eng J Med*, 34: 1726-7.

Oginosawa, Y; Abe, H; Nakashima, Y. (2002). The incidence and risk factors for venous obstruction after implantation of transvenous pacing leads. *Pacing Clin Electrophysiol*, 25: 1605-11.

Oupadia, P & Ramasswamy, K. (1998). "R-on-T phenomenon" Images in Cardiology. *N Engl J Med*, 338: 1812.

Res, JCJ; de Priester, JA; van Lier, AA; van Engelen, CLJM; Bronzwaer, PNA; Tan P-H; Visser, M. (2004); Pneumothorax resulting from subclavian puncture: a complication of permanent pacemaker lead implantation. *Neth Heart*, 12: 101-5.

Rozsmus, G; Daubert, JP; Huang, DT; Rosero, S; Hall, B; Françis, C. (2005). Venous thrombosis and stenosis after implantation of pacemakers and defibrillators. *Pacing Clin Electrophysiol*, 13: 9-19.

Sohail, MR; Uslan, DZ; Khan, AH et al. (2007). Management and outcome of permanent pacemaker and implantable cardioverter-defibrillator infections. *J Am Coll Cardiol,* 49:1851-9.

Trohman, RG; Kim, MH; Pinski, SL. (2004) Cardiac pacing: the state of the art. *Lancet,* 364: 1701-19.

van Eck, JWM; van Hemel, NM; Zuithof P, et al. (2007). Incidence and predictors of in-hospital events after first implantation of pacemakers. *Europace,* 9: 884-9.

Van Gelder, BM; Bracke, FA; Oto, A; Yildirir, A; Haas, PC; Seger, JJ, et al. (2000). Diagnosis and management of inadvertently placed pacing and ICD leads in the left ventricle: a multicenter experience and review of the literature. *Pacing Clin Electrophysiol,* 23: 877-83.

Vardas, PE; Auricchio, A; Blanc, JJ et al for the Task Force Members. Guidelines for cardiac pacing and cardiac resynchronisation therapy. (2007). *Europace,* 9: 959-98.

Wiegand, U.K.; LeJeune, D.; Boguschewski, F.; Bonnemeier, H.; Eberhardt, F.; Schunkert, H.; & Bode, F. (2004). Pocket hematoma after pacemaker or implantable cardioverter defibrillator surgery: influence of patient morbidity, operation strategy, and perioperative antiplatelet/anticoagulation therapy. *Chest,* 126, 1177-86

Zoll, PM. (1952). Resuscitation of the heart in ventricular standstill by external electric stimulation. *N Engl J Med,* 247: 768.

9

Lead Extraction in Congenital Heart Disease Patients – Indications, Technique and Experience

Philip Chang, Miguel Salazar, Michael Cao and David Cesario
Keck School of Medicine at U.S.C
USA

1. Introduction

Implantation of pacemakers and implantable cardioverter defibrillators (ICDs) are common procedures associated with very low complication rates(1-3). Device therapy is frequently used in the management of adult congenital heart disease (ACHD) patients given the high prevalence of arrhythmic complications encountered in this population. The ACHD population continues to grow at a rapid pace. It is estimated that that there are currently more surviving adults with severe congenital heart disease (CHD) than children(4). The prevalence of arrhythmias and conduction disorders in adults with surgically treated CHD as well as those with specific congenital defects associated with conduction system abnormalities has led to an increasing need for implantable devices (both pacemakers and ICDs) in these patients (5). Unfortunately, as the indications for device implantation in patients with CHD have increased, so have the rate of device related infections and other complications leading to a growth in referrals for lead extraction in this expanding patient population(6-8). A thorough understanding of the role that lead extraction plays in this growing subgroup of patients is therefore critical for any implanting and extracting practitioner.

2. Specific challenges in the adult CHD population

At times patients with complex CHD in need of a permanent implantable device (pacemaker or ICD) require epicardial lead placement. This is due to complex anatomy or vascular limitations that prevent access to the venous circulation or due to the presence of intracardiac shunts that may increase the risk of embolic events with intracardiac leads. However, successful transvenous lead placement is often possible in patients with CHD, and these procedures are done with increasing frequency in the cardiac catheterization laboratory(9; 10). Transvenous lead systems are preferable to epicardial leads due to their generally lower capture thresholds and their greater durability and longevity(11). Procedural risk and peri-procedural morbidity is also significantly reduced with a transvenous approach. Yet, many patients with CHD are young and anatomic considerations often place additional stress on leads requiring multiple device pulse generator or lead replacements over time(12). Both lower age at implantation and a diagnosis of CHD have been associated with increased risks of lead failure over time(13).

3. Lead extraction indications

In adults with CHD, as well as in the general population of patients with implantable devices, the main indications for lead extraction include lead fracture, venous stenosis with associated superior vena cava (SVC) syndrome, infection and patient discomfort related to implanted materials. Lead malfunction rates in the published literature - ICD leads in particular - range from 16 to 20% at 10 years(14; 15). Although this rate may not hold true for all modern leads, it is of significance in patients with CHD since many receive implants at an early age and have a cumulative risk of developing device-related complications.

Over the past decade, due to expanded indications for ICDs and a resultant dramatic increase in the number of devices implanted, the incidence of device infections has been rising(16; 17). Infection of any of the components of the device system can lead to sepsis and death. Prompt extraction of the entire device system coupled with intravenous antibiotics is a viable and effective treatment option to prevent these complications.

4. General experience

For the reasons stated above, transvenous leads are now favored over epicardial leads in the pediatric and young adult CHD population. Published data on lead extraction in CHD patients is steadily growing but currently consists of single-center experiences with patient numbers far smaller than typical adult studies.(6; 18; 19) Due to the extreme heterogeneity of the ACHD population, interventions such as device extraction are often generalized to the entire CHD population, as the number of each individual defect type is often too small for meaningful comparison and reporting. We have summarized, in table format, the three largest published reports on lead extraction in ACHD patients published to date (Table 1)(10; 19; 20).

	Number of patients	Number of leads	Number of leads Removed	Technique	Mean duration of lead implantation	Indication	Minor complication	Major complications	Deaths
Cecchin et al.	144	203	162 (80%)	Laser and Torsion device.	7.6 +-4.3 years	Infection (8%);Lead failure (65%); Device upgrade (12.5%)	2.80%	2.80%	None
Khairy et al.	16	23	21(91%)	Laser	9.0 ± 5.2 years	Infection 44%; Lead failure 25%; Device upgrade 25%; pain 6%	N/A	1 (6.3%)	None
Cooper et al.	14	21	20 (95%)	Laser	42.0 ± 18.9 months	Lead failure (93%)	3 required transfusions	None	None

Table 1.

5. Planning the procedure

The ACHD population presents several unique challenges to physicians planning a device extraction. Before bringing these patients to the electrophysiology (EP) lab, the operator needs to become extremely familiar with the patient, their anatomy, the device and leads. A thorough understanding of the patient's anatomy and device history is paramount to all other aspects of the procedure. Understanding the anatomy in an adult with CHD includes knowing the original defect, previous surgeries and interventions performed on the patient, residual defects, chamber sizes, and vascular connections.

In addition to the standard history, physical exam and chest x-ray (posterior-anterior and lateral) to assess the number and relative locations of the lead(s), a detailed review of previous surgical reports, echocardiography reports, advanced imaging studies, and clinical progress notes should be done in preparation for lead extraction in CHD patients. Echocardiography remains a standard component in the anatomical evaluation of CHD patients and transthoracic and transesophageal modalities should be used to assess for residual intracardiac shunts, valve function, chamber sizes, and basic lead courses and locations. We routinely perform trans-esophageal echocardiograms (TEEs) prior to or during our device extractions. This is particularly important in ACHD patients for several reasons. Pre-procedural TEEs can confirm the diagnosis of device infection and define large vegetations on the leads that may contra-indicate percutaneous extraction, particularly in patients with intra-cardiac shunts. Given, the risk of cerebral emboli in such patients, these devices are often best removed through open surgical extraction. Cardiac computed tomography (CT) is quickly becoming an important tool in the care of ACHD patients by providing excellent images for anatomic and functional features of CHD. Additionally, venous anatomy and patency can also be assessed with cardiac CT. Finally, angiography can be performed at the time of the device procedure to further assess for venous patency, baffle obstruction or baffle leaks.

Not only will CHD patients with devices have a broad variety of defects but their device and lead implant history may be equally complicated. Some CHD patients carry a long history of device-related procedures dating back to early childhood years with epicardial systems, subcutaneous leads and arrays, pericardial leads, and transvenous implants together with their associated generator changes. For others who have undergone transvenous implantation, it is possible to encounter patients with multiple leads and venous obstruction. The operator also needs to be familiar with the lead itself including its fixation mechanism and type of insulation material. The manufacturer and their representatives can be valuable assets in obtaining this information. Interrogation of the device prior to the procedure will also reveal whether the patient is dependent on its pacing functions in order to determine if a temporary pacemaker will need to be placed during the procedure. At times, careful device interrogation may show apparent recovery of intrinsic atrio-ventricular conduction and that the patient has not been device dependent. Such patients may not require immediate re-implantation and can be closely monitored to assess their current pacing requirements. Any decision to delay or forego device re-implantation must be weighed against the possibility that conduction disease can progress over time in patients with CHD and that transient or permanent conduction block can recur over time. At the time of the procedure, interrogation of all the leads must be done. This is particularly important if a lead is to be re-used.

In ACHD patients with infected device systems, a pre-procedural consultation with an infectious disease specialist may be warranted to provide recommendations for proper intravenous antibiotic therapy and timing of device re-implantation if patients are device dependent.

The decision to perform complex lead extractions or to abandon leads is another important consideration in CHD device procedures. Venous access and patency remain great concerns in ACHD patients with devices and this may lead the electrophysiologist to undertake complex extractions on multiple leads in an effort to preserve the vascular space and previously implanted lead courses, knowing that these patients will likely return several additional times in the future for similar procedures. Laser and RF extraction sheaths should be present and easily available during CHD lead extractions.

Additionally, ACHD patients are at increased risk for extraction related complications. Surgical support should always be coordinated before CHD lead extractions and measures should be in place in the event that emergent surgical intervention is required. Interventional cardiology involvement should also be in place in the event of certain complications and to provide expertise in the event that leaks or stenoses require balloon dilation, stenting or percutaneous device closure. Patch and baffle leaks or tears can occur during extraction resulting in the acute mixing of blood pools to varying extents depending on the size of the tear. Certain leaks may be amenable to percutaneous device closure while others may require surgical intervention. Patients should be counseled on these possibilities and the potential involvement of surgeons or interventional cardiologists to address them. Combined procedures involving both the electrophysiologist and interventional cardiologist can be arranged to facilitate transvenous device procedures that otherwise would have been contraindicated given anatomic limitations in CHD patients(21).

6. Specific anatomic lesions

6.1 Transposition of the Great Arteries

Transposition of the great arteries (TGA) is a defect where the usual right ventricle (RV)-pulmonary artery (PA) and left ventricle (LV)-aorta relationships are reversed such that the RV is in continuity with the aorta while the LV is anatomically connected to the main PA (See Figure 1). In general, there are 2 types of transposition that include this reversed ventricle-to-great artery relationship. The first form, commonly referred to as "D-TGA", involves an otherwise structurally normal heart with isolated transposition of the great vessels off the ventricles. The second form, frequently called "L-TGA" or congenitally corrected transposition of the great arteries (CCTGA), involves transposed great arteries with additional atrial-to-ventricular transposition such that the right atrium empties into a morphologic LV while the left atrium empties into a morphologic RV.

Surgical repair of both forms of TGA can involve an atrial switch procedure, either of the Mustard or Senning variety (See Figure 2). In general, the atrial switch involves baffling blood from the superior and inferior vena cavae, within the atria, over to the left sided atrio-ventricular (AV) valve and ventricle. Pulmonary venous return is routed within the atria to empty into the right sided AV valve and ventricle(22). The current approach to the repair of D-TGA involves the arterial switch procedure where the aorta, coronary arteries and PA are removed from their respective ventricles and switched such that the aorta and coronaries are connected to the LV while the PA is anastomosed to the RV, thereby restoring normal ventricle-great artery continuity. Atrial switches are still incorporated in combination with an arterial switch procedure in the so-called "double switch" procedure for anatomical repair of CCTGA.

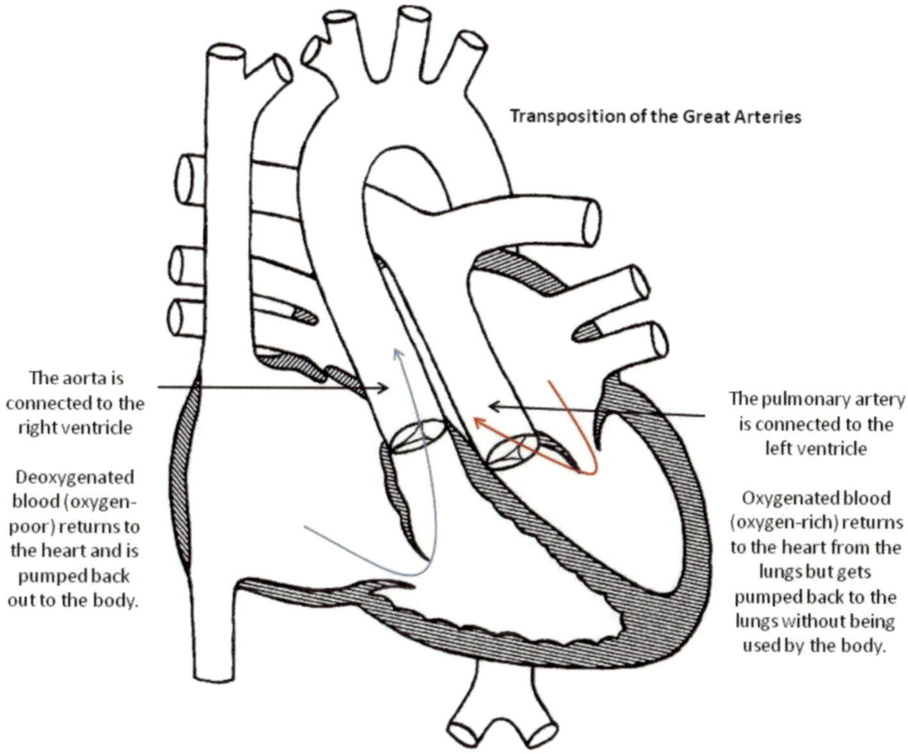

Fig. 1. Transposition of the Great Arteries.

Arrhythmias are frequently encountered in TGA patients who have undergone atrial switch procedures. Sinus node dysfunction and atrial arrhythmias are often encountered in atrial switch patients and can be addressed with device implantation and/or catheter ablation(23). Ventricular arrhythmias and risk of sudden death have been addressed with ICD implantation in palliated TGA patients and have been associated with compromised systemic RV function(8).

Atrial baffles present an element of complexity to lead implantation and extraction. The traditional approach of placing the atrial lead in the right atrial appendage or along the lateral right atrial wall is no longer possible. Leads are generally placed through the SVC and atrial baffle over to the left atrial wall. A location along the lateral atrial wall or in the left atrial appendage where reasonable sensing and pacing thresholds are achieved is selected for active lead fixation. In similar fashion, the ventricular lead also courses through the baffle to the left sided AV valve and is fixated in the left sided ventricle.

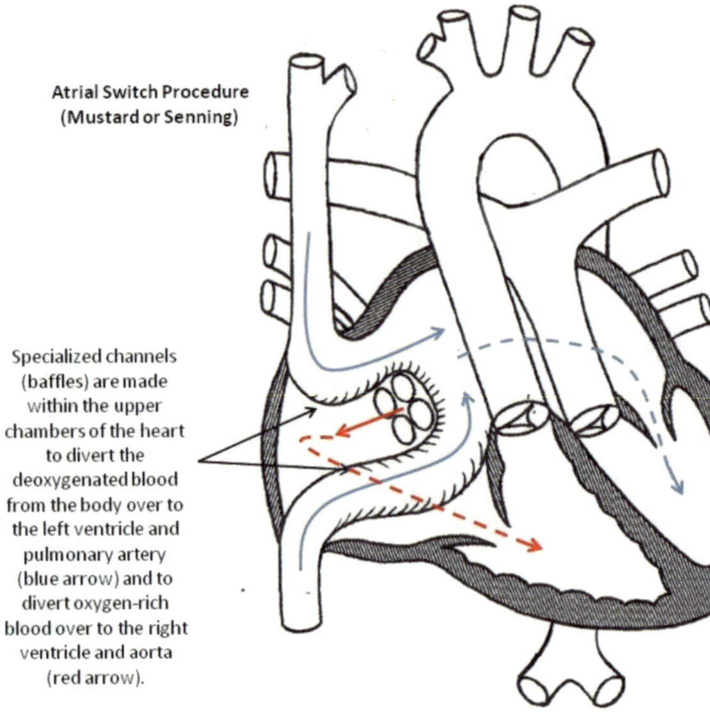

Fig. 2. Atrial Switch Procedure.

6.2 Tetralogy of Fallot

Tetralogy of Fallot (TOF) is among the most common forms of cyanotic CHD encountered in pediatric patients. In the current surgical era, complete repair is frequently undertaken in early infancy. The defect consists of a primary abnormality in ventricular septal formation where the conal or outflow region of the ventricular septum is mal-aligned relative to the rest of the ventricular septum and anteriorly deviated into the space normally occupied by the right ventricular outflow tract. This defect results in positioning of the aorta over the crest of the ventricular septum (overriding aorta) and the formation of a large ventricular septal defect (VSD) coupled with varying degrees of right ventricular outflow tract obstruction. The RV undergoes compensatory hypertrophy completing the fourth component of TOF.

Complete surgical repair consists of closure of the VSD with various materials along with a variety of interventions to augment the size of the right ventricular outflow tract. This often involves a right ventriculotomy incision, resection of obstructive muscle bundles in the sub-pulmonary region, and trans-annular incisions and patch placement to increase the effective size of the pulmonary valve and main pulmonary artery segment. While ventricular level shunting and outflow tract obstruction are generally eliminated, patients are left with varying degrees of pulmonary insufficiency and impaired right ventricular hemodynamics.

It is well recognized that repaired TOF patients are at risk for a variety of arrhythmic disturbances. Atrial arrhythmias and sinus and AV node dysfunction are not infrequent. Ventricular arrhythmias related to macroreentry around incisions and patches and poor ventricular hemodynamics have been well described(24; 25).

Lead extraction in repaired TOF patients can generally follow a similar approach to that in non-CHD patients. Special attention should be given to previous device and surgical histories. Many patients have undergone prior device implants with resultant vascular obstruction and others have undergone old approaches to device management with separate pacemaker and ICD systems implanted at the same time to address bradycardia and ventricular arrhythmias or sudden death risk. Therefore, assessing vascular access becomes an important part of pre-procedural planning and great care must be taken to preserve transvenous access for the placement of new leads.

6.3 Septal and AV Canal defects

Patients with atrial and ventricular septal defects are usually repaired in early childhood with excellent outcomes. Those with atrio-ventricular canal (AVC) defects comprise a spectrum of patients with variable long-term outcomes.

Atrial septal defects (ASDs) come in several varieties, the most common being the secundum ASD where a septal hole exists that is enclosed circumferentially by atrial septal tissue. This defect is easily repaired through patch closure or primary suture closure during surgery or through percutaneous means with a variety of deployable devices. Primum type and sinus venosus type defects are more complicated forms of ASDs. In sinus venous ASDs, the septal defect is located adjacent to the caval junctions with the atrium. Anomalous pulmonary venous return is frequently associated with sinus venosus ASDs and surgical repair is needed and often involves baffling of the anomalous pulmonary venous blood flow back to the left atrium. In primum type ASDs the defect is located inferiorly with the lower rim being bounded by the AV valve itself.

Ventricular septal defects (VSDs) can involve any part of the ventricular septum and may come in the form of isolated holes in the septum, mal-alignment types as in TOF, or deficiencies in the septum related to abnormal formation of the AVC and incorporation of embryologic endocardial cushion tissue into the ventricular septum. Defects in the membranous septum occur most frequently followed by muscular septal defects, both of which can usually be addressed through surgical patch closure. AVC type VSDs involve deficiencies of the inlet ventricular septum and the superior border of the defect involves the AV valve. Surgical closure is the dominant way of addressing VSDs however, percutaneous device-based methods can be employed to close certain types of muscular and membranous defects.

AVC defects represent a group of septal defects that are associated with varying degrees of AV valve anomalies (See Figure 3). Partial AVC defects consist of a primum type ASD with a cleft mitral valve. Transitional AVC defects involve a primum type ASD, small or occluded VSD component, and abnormal left and right AV valves. Complete AVC defects involve a large septal defect that spans both the atrial and ventricular septae and a single, common AV valve. Surgical repair of such defects requires an extremely experienced surgeon who will be able to separate and re-create the AV valves and their supporting valve architecture while also closing the atrial and ventricular septal defects.

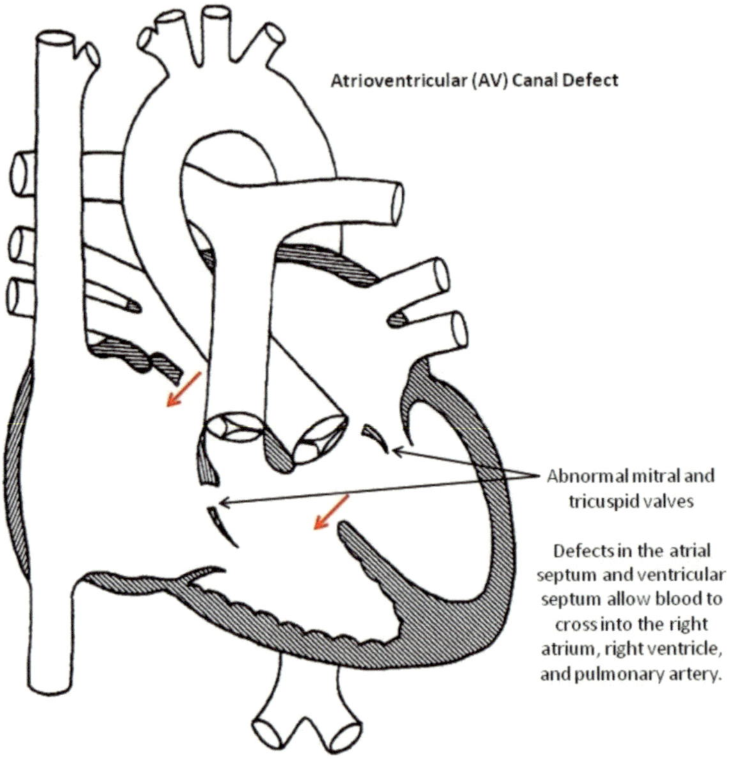

Fig. 3. AV Canal Defect.

Arrhythmias and conduction system disease can arise in septal defect patients. Prior cardiac surgery with an atriotomy incision and cannulation for cardiopulmonary bypass can result in sinus node dysfunction. AV node dysfunction occurred in the earlier surgical era of VSD repairs as the conduction system fibers ran close to the defects and were often injured by patches and/or suture material. Finally, in AVC type defects, the conduction system is inferiorly displaced, which also makes it prone to surgical trauma during repair attempts.
Lead extraction in patients with standard forms of atrial or ventricular septal defects can be undertaken in a manner similar to non-CHD patients. Repaired AVC defect patients can have unique anatomical features related to abnormal AV valve architecture and large ventricular septal patches. Finally, pre-procedural imaging is critical to determine the presence or absence of residual septal shunting after surgical repair.

6.4 Complex lesions (single ventricle hearts)

Patients with severe forms of CHD involving single ventricle anatomy and physiology often require device-based therapies to treat sinus or AV node dysfunction and to treat and prevent lethal arrhythmias. Single ventricle patients are palliated surgically with an eventual Fontan procedure where systemic venous blood is channeled directly to the pulmonary arterial tree (See Figure 4). The single ventricle is isolated and used to pump exclusively to the systemic circulation. Fontan circulation involves the passive flow of systemic venous blood back to the lungs and is dependent on low vascular resistance within the pulmonary vasculature to promote venous return. Multiple forms of the Fontan procedure have been devised with most patients in the current surgical era having either a lateral tunnel or extra-cardiac Fontan conduit placed to channel inferior vena caval blood flow to the lungs. Superior caval blood is channeled to the lungs through a bidirectional Glenn anastomosis where the SVC is removed from the right atrium and connected in an end-to-side fashion to the right pulmonary artery. Classic Fontan patients have a direct anastomosis of the right atrium to the pulmonary arteries. Lateral tunnel and classic Fontan variants maintain an anatomical connection of the right atrial tissue with the systemic venous pathway.

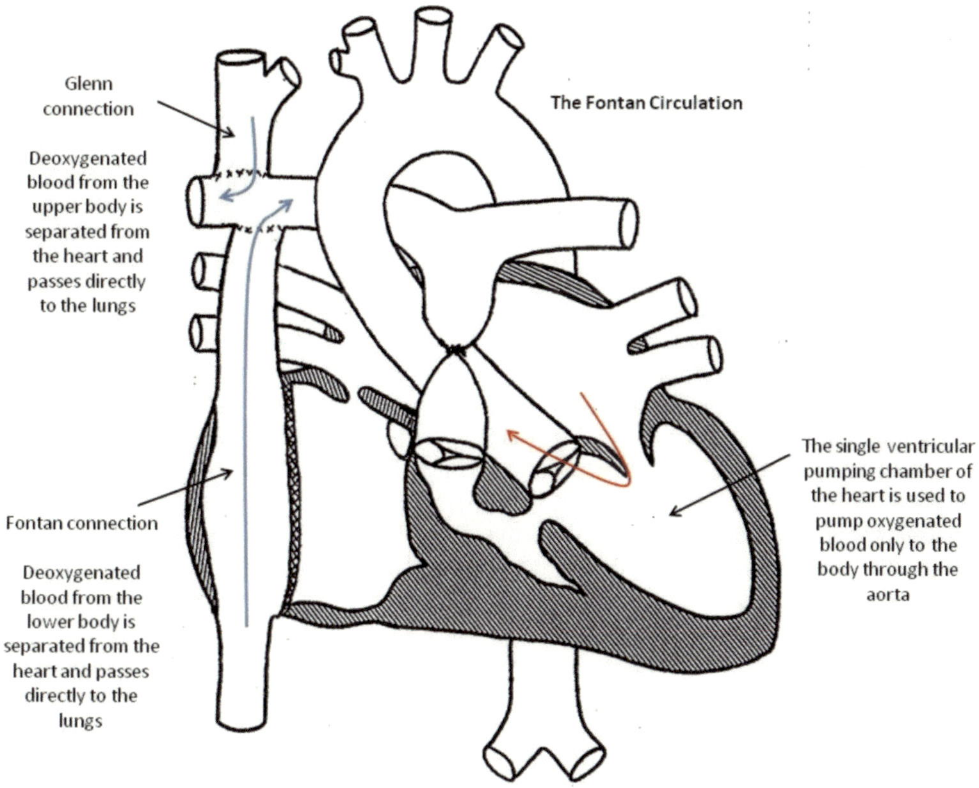

Fig. 4. The Fontan Circulation.

Pacemaker and ICD therapy in Fontan patients is frequently applied through epicardial routes with few patients having transvenous atrial leads(26; 27). Therefore, device procedures will predominantly involve sternotomies with direct visualization to sever old leads and place new leads in a different location on the myocardium. Transvenous atrial leads have occasionally been used in Fontan patients with isolated sinus node disease, particularly those with lateral tunnel or classic Fontan forms that permit venous to atrial access for lead placement. For patients with transvenous atrial leads, extraction can be performed but careful attention must be paid to risks of thromboembolic complications, risks of conduit tears, and bleeding. In addition, placement of a new transvenous atrial lead may be challenging given a lack of reasonable endomyocardial targets with good sensing and pacing thresholds.

7. General technique for lead extraction using the implant vein

If the patient is pacemaker dependent, a temporary wire can be inserted from the groin or from the contra-lateral internal jugular or subclavian veins. Our center has found that placement of a temporary screw-in lead attached to an externally placed pacemaker pulse generator similar to what is implanted under the skin (tempo-permanent device) can be a useful tool in device dependent patients requiring extraction secondary to infection. This approach allows patients to have stable back-up pacing while receiving intravenous antibiotics and remaining ambulatory on the floor, until they are cleared for permanent device re-implantation.

To begin the extraction procedure, a small incision is made at the site of the previous pulse generator. Careful dissection is then undertaken in an effort to free up the leads and the device from the pocket. Dissection is performed along the leads all the way down to the suture sleeves which are cut and removed.

The dissected leads are then disconnected and tested. Further dissection is then undertaken to the venous entry point. Straight stylets are then inserted down the central lumen of each lead and an unsecured figure of eight stitch is done around the lead bodies to aid in hemostasis. If the lead is an active fixation lead, an attempt at retracting the fixation screw should be made. We have frequently used a laser sheath for these complex extraction cases. In preparation for laser lead extraction, the dissected lead is cut with heavy scissors. A sizing tool is inserted into the lead's inner coil to help select the appropriate size of locking stylet. Next, the locking stylet is introduced and advanced to the distal part of the lead and expanded. This stylet will be used to provide counter traction from the proximal part of the lead. Additionally, we tie a suture around the insulation and lead body and pass this suture through the laser sheath to provide further tension on the distal end of the lead. The laser sheath alone, or in combination with its outer Teflon sheath, is then inserted over the lead. Under fluoroscopic guidance, the sheath is carefully guided to the vein-lead interface. Staying coaxial to the lead, the laser sheath is advanced while counter-traction is kept on the lead with the locking stylet and the suture. Serial laser pulses are delivered during laser sheath advancement to heat the tissue and aid in the lysis of adhesions. The outer sheath can also be advanced into the vein and carefully rotated to help disrupt adhesions. Additionally, significant scarring and calcifications can develop along the leads, especially as they course through baffles.(See Figure 5) Baffle stenosis can be present and involve existing pacemaker or defibrillator leads, thereby necessitating baffle stenting and increasing the difficulty of extraction and re-implantation(28; 29). Dense calcifications may limit the efficacy of laser applications and careful dissection through these regions may require blunt dissection with the laser sheath and/or outer sheath and necessitates that the operating physician exhibit great patience and care during this portion of the procedure. This advancement is continued until the lead body is free or the sheath is advanced all the way down to the myocardial tissue where the lead is fixated. The same procedure is repeated for each lead to be removed.

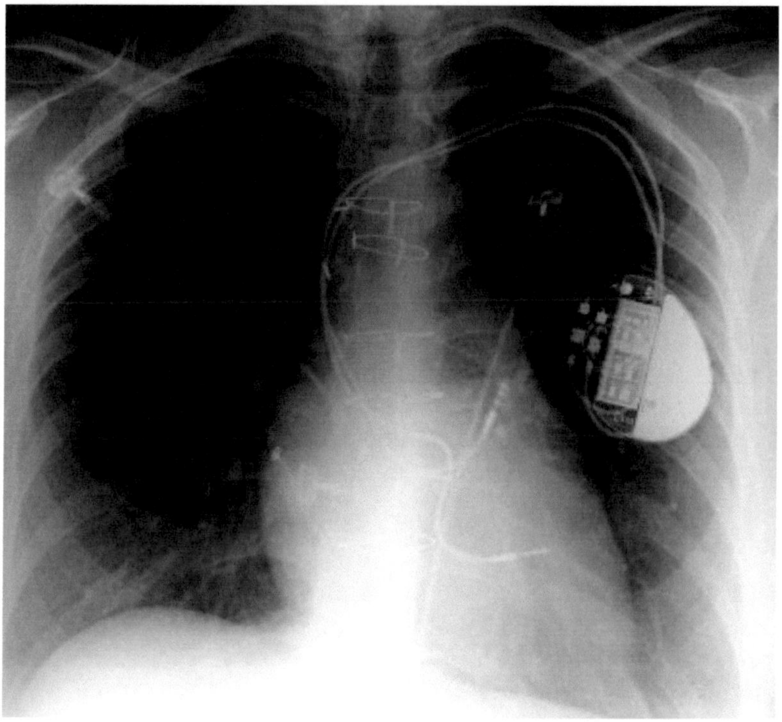

Fig. 5. A PA chest X-ray demonstrating a ventricular lead coursing through the systemic baffle in a patient with D-Transposition of the great arteries.

In the case of system infections, proper debridement of the pocket is also recommended, with complete removal of the capsule and debridement and removal of any scar tissue. The pocket should be thoroughly irrigated with antibiotic solution. In most patients the pocket can be loosely closed with interrupted sutures to allow drainage, unless there is gross pus present in the pocket. In such cases, a Jackson-Pratt drain is placed in the pocket and delivered through a healthy portion of tissue below the incision. The pocket is then sutured with interrupted and evenly spaced non-absorbable sutures. Alternatively, if there is great concern over abscess formation and re-accumulation of pus, the wound can be left open and packed with antibiotic soaked gauze and allowed to heal by secondary intention.

As many referrals for lead extraction are secondary to lead or device infection, the timeline for re-implantation in these patients becomes critical. As a general rule, the white blood cell count needs to be within normal limits or trending down and blood cultures need to be negative for at least 48 hours before considering re-implantation of a new system. These guidelines are not standard though and will vary from center to center. The duration of intravenous antibiotic treatment after re-implantation depends on the type of bacterium cultured, but generally lasts for 4-6 weeks. Input from an infectious disease consultant regarding duration of antibiotic therapy and optimal timing for re-implantation is essential.

8. Operator experience

Analysis of lead extraction outcomes suggests that the frequency of complete procedural success improves dramatically after the first 10 procedures have been performed. Lower complication rates are associated with a prior experience of 30 procedures. The complication rate tends to keep improving after the first 30 procedures as the operator gains further experience.

There is no specific data for the CHD population, but since the rate of complications appears to be similar, these general guidelines may also apply. In general it is probably best that extractions in patients with CHD be done at centers with the necessary expertise and experience in both complex lead extractions and the management of adults with CHD.

9. Complications

The overall published complication rate for CHD patients undergoing lead extraction is consistently low (10; 19; 20). The rate of major complications varies from 2.8 to 21% (10; 20). Major complications include induction of ventricular fibrillation and cardiac perforation with risk of tamponade. Minor complications include pocket hematoma, superficial infection and excessive bleeding requiring transfusion.

10. Conclusions

Adults with CHD and implanted devices present unique challenges to the practitioner performing lead extractions. While the general indications for lead extraction and the technical aspects of the procedure are similar in both CHD patients and those with structurally normal hearts, close attention needs to be paid to several features of CHD patients. First the electrophysiologist must be aware of the specific CHD defect in each patient and the associated ramifications of prior surgical- and catheter-based interventions, complex device histories, and the importance of preserving the vascular space. Overall, the use of laser sheaths to assist in lead extraction has greatly increased the safety and efficacy of this procedure in both the general population and adults with CHD(19; 30). There remains a relative paucity of published data on device extraction in ACHD patients. However, the published reports suggest that device extraction is a safe and efficacious procedure in this patient population.

Due to the highly variable anatomic substrates and additional complexities, all ACHD device extractions require meticulous pre-procedural planning. Comprehensive review of the clinical and surgical history, inclusion of appropriate advanced imaging studies, incorporation of available tools as well as involvement of surgical and interventional services should all be routinely practiced to ensure successful outcomes while minimizing morbidity in a patient population that has had substantial exposure to medical and surgical interventions in the past.

11. References

[1] Ellenbogen KA, et al. 2003. Complications arising after implantation of DDD pacemakers: the MOST experience. *Am J Cardiol.* 92, 740-741.

[2] Bailey SM, Wilkoff BL. 2006. Complications of pacemakers and defibrillators in the elderly. *Am J Geriatr Cardiol.* 15, 102-107.

[3] Poole JE, et al. Complication rates associated with pacemaker or implantable cardioverter-defibrillator generator replacements and upgrade procedures: results from the REPLACE registry. *Circulation.* 122, 1553-1561.

[4] Marelli AJ, et al. 2007. Congenital heart disease in the general population: changing prevalence and age distribution. *Circulation*. 115, 163-172.
[5] Ih S, et al. 1983. The location and course of the atrioventricular conduction system in common atrioventricular orifice and in its related anomalies with transposition of the great arteries--A histopathological study of six cases. *Jpn Circ J*. 47, 1262-1273.
[6] Cesario D, et al. 2009. Device extraction in adults with congenital heart disease. *Pacing Clin Electrophysiol*. 32, 340-345.
[7] Perloff JK, Warnes CA. 2001. Challenges posed by adults with repaired congenital heart disease. *Circulation*. 103, 2637-2643.
[8] Gatzoulis MA, et al. 1999. Outpatient clinics for adults with congenital heart disease: increasing workload and evolving patterns of referral. *Heart*. 81, 57-61.
[9] Gammage MD. 2000. Pacing approaches to the patient with a univentricular heart and the factors associated with choice of pacing site. *Pacing Clin Electrophysiol*. 23, 144.
[10] Khairy P, et al. 2007. Laser lead extraction in adult congenital heart disease. *J Cardiovasc Electrophysiol*. 18, 507-511.
[11] Radbill AE, et al. System survival of nontransvenous implantable cardioverter-defibrillators compared to transvenous implantable cardioverter-defibrillators in pediatric and congenital heart disease patients. *Heart Rhythm*. 7, 193-198.
[12] Shah A, et al. 2006. Stable atrial sensing on long-term follow up of VDD pacemakers. *Indian Pacing Electrophysiol J*. 6, 189-193.
[13] Fortescue EB, et al. 2004. Patient, procedural, and hardware factors associated with pacemaker lead failures in pediatrics and congenital heart disease. *Heart Rhythm*. 1, 150-159.
[14] Hardeland R. 2009. Neuroprotection by radical avoidance: search for suitable agents. *Molecules*. 14, 5054-5102.
[15] Hauser RG, et al. 2008. Safety and efficacy of transvenous high-voltage implantable cardioverter-defibrillator leads in high-risk hypertrophic cardiomyopathy patients. *Heart Rhythm*. 5, 1517-1522.
[16] Uslan DZ, Baddour LM. 2006. Cardiac device infections: getting to the heart of the matter. *Curr Opin Infect Dis*. 19, 345-348.
[17] Voigt A, et al. Continued rise in rates of cardiovascular implantable electronic device infections in the United States: temporal trends and causative insights. *Pacing Clin Electrophysiol*. 33, 414-419.
[18] Friedman RA, et al. 1996. Lead extraction in young patients with and without congenital heart disease using the subclavian approach. *Pacing Clin Electrophysiol*. 19, 778-783.
[19] Cooper JM, et al. 2003. Implantable cardioverter defibrillator lead complications and laser extraction in children and young adults with congenital heart disease: implications for implantation and management. *J Cardiovasc Electrophysiol*. 14, 344-349.
[20] Cecchin F, et al. Lead extraction in pediatric and congenital heart disease patients. *Circ Arrhythm Electrophysiol*. 3, 437-444.
[21] Daehnert I, et al. 2001. Echocardiographically guided closure of a patent foramen ovale during pregnancy after recurrent strokes. *J Interv Cardiol*. 14, 191-192.
[22] Konstantinov IE, et al. 2004. Atrial switch operation: past, present, and future. *Ann Thorac Surg*. 77, 2250-2258.

[23] Kanter RJ, Garson A, Jr. 1997. Atrial arrhythmias during chronic follow-up of surgery for complex congenital heart disease. *Pacing Clin Electrophysiol*. 20, 502-511.
[24] Khairy P, et al. Arrhythmia burden in adults with surgically repaired tetralogy of Fallot: a multi-institutional study. *Circulation*. 122, 868-875.
[25] Walsh EP, et al. 1988. Late results in patients with tetralogy of Fallot repaired during infancy. *Circulation*. 77, 1062-1067.
[26] Takahashi K, et al. 2009. Permanent atrial pacing lead implant route after Fontan operation. *Pacing Clin Electrophysiol*. 32, 779-785.
[27] Welisch E, et al. A single institution experience with pacemaker implantation in a pediatric population over 25 years. *Pacing Clin Electrophysiol*. 33, 1112-1118.
[28] Undavia M, et al. 2008. Laser lead extraction and baffle stenting to facilitate dual chamber implantable defibrillator upgrade in a patient with L-transposition of the great arteries status-post Senning/Rastelli repair: a case report and review of literature. *Pacing Clin Electrophysiol*. 31, 131-134.
[29] Chan AW, et al. 2002. Percutaneous treatment for pacemaker-associated superior vena cava syndrome. *Pacing Clin Electrophysiol*. 25, 1628-1633.
[30] Wilkoff BL, et al. 1999. Pacemaker lead extraction with the laser sheath: results of the pacing lead extraction with the excimer sheath (PLEXES) trial. *J Am Coll Cardiol*. 33, 1671-1676.